WAKE THE FIT UP

By

Paul Birch

Table of Contents

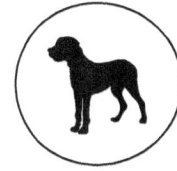

Dedication

Apparently, more than 350 million people on this planet suffer from depression. It's probably more than that but 50 million were no doubt curled up in bed ignoring the world, so didn't get round to completing the survey.

More women seem to be affected by this illness than men, but anybody at any time can experience this serious health condition regardless of gender, age or status. Many people aggravate their symptoms by over-eating, self-harming or drug abuse, leading to a spiral of self-destructive behaviour and their self-esteem at rock bottom. For some it becomes too much, they can't cope, so they kill themselves. However, the majority of sufferers conform to the maxim that anti-depressants are the answer and temporarily mask the melancholy by popping pills. Others find a different path to salvation. A long-term solution to their woes. A way out.
Which is exactly what I did.

This book is dedicated to anybody that is struggling with depression. I feel your pain because I've been there. But let me tell you now, life can get considerably better although it's up to you to make the changes.

Hi, my name is Paul, I'm 45 years old and I've suffered from depression for most of my adult life.
To most of my friends and family, that statement will come as a hell of a shock.
READER: *Why?*
I couldn't admit to them that I had a problem. I was too embarrassed, guilty and ashamed of my condition. I suppose I thought of depression as a weakness and as a man, it wasn't something I could talk about with friends.
READER: *Why not, that's ridiculous?*
I know, but I can tell you exactly what they'd have said, *'Mate, just man up and pull yourself together'*. That's just how most men communicate and there's such a social stigma towards depression, that us blokes can't converse maturely and rationally about the subject.
Anyway, I felt trapped, isolated, miserable and just... **bleeuurrgghh!!**
So I'd put on a front, a façade.
I've always been the *'funny'* one, the *'good craic to be around'* one, the *'strong, dependable'* one, not the *'Oh shit, he's bloody topped himself'* one.

This is really difficult to admit, to you, to anyone really but I've actually attempted to commit suicide three times...
READER: *Oh! How did you get on?*
Yeah it worked and I'm now typing these words from beyond the grave... **Duh!!**
Obviously I failed, like most things in my life.
However, after the third aborted attempt, I knew I had to make some radical changes to my life.
I had to alter my mindset, to think differently, lead a positive life instead of feeling sorry for myself.

Luckily, I managed to find the perfect antidote to my specific issues and over a decade later, I now lead a moderately happy life. And if I can do it, then you can too.

Which is why I've written this book, to help **you...** OK, one of the reasons.

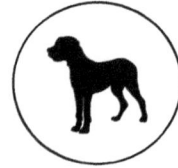

Introduction

She was called Amanda and when I initially started to advertise my services as a Personal Trainer, she was the first person to contact me. This is a copy of her original e-mail and her request for assistance:

Hi Paul,
I'm a 29 year old female looking to lose five stones. I know that sounds like a lot but in order for me to just fall into a 'healthy' weight bracket, I feel I need to reach ten stones, as my height is 5'3. I haven't actually weighed myself for a while but I can tell as my clothes feel very snug, that I will be touching fifteen stone, which is the heaviest I have ever been.

Normally, I am an average size 12 to 14 in clothes and 10 to 11 stone in weight, but these last couple of years, I have really piled on the weight and have reached a fitted size 18.
I have started to avoid social situations and don't wear, or even buy nice clothes anymore, just stick to baggy cardigans. I used to take a lot of pride in my appearance but now I have a wardrobe full of beautiful clothes which just don't fit.

I think I need an intense programme because the trouble with me is that I start but very quickly get impatient when I don't see dramatic results. I find it very hard to exercise for a long period of time because I get out of breath by just climbing stairs, and I certainly can't do jogging at the moment because it puts a lot of strain on my knees.
I do enjoy walking but I sweat profusely whenever I try and struggle a bit up hills.
I actually still have a gym membership but never go as I can't keep up with exercise classes, so just don't have the confidence or motivation to attend.
I find it's far easier to sit on the sofa eating junk food, watching the telly, rather than getting all puffed out, trying to undo the damage I have done to myself.

I am not usually this open and honest with someone I don't know and I'm quite embarrassed admitting all of this but I am hoping you can give me some advice or tips that might just make a difference.
Even as I write this, I am thinking I am so ashamed about what I have done to myself, putting all this weight on by comfort eating but I guess it is my way of dealing with emotions.

Time scale – in an ideal world, overnight! Back to the real world, I think about 12 months. I am going to be 30 years old next September and my goal is to be a size 10 by then.
I am going to a diet club meeting this week to try and gain some control back from my eating habits. Counting points and looking up food in books. Hmm! I have been there done that. I start with such positivity on these diets but the trouble with me, is if I don't see the weight coming off fast and clothes starting to feel less fitted, I just give up, lose motivation and get disheartened.

I really have no patience when it comes to losing weight. But I am trying to tell myself now, that it will take time for me to get back to my usual self.
I hate having photographs taken and try to avoid mirrors, as when I do catch my reflection, it's like the face is me but not this body.
My health is really, really suffering and I am constantly tired, red faced and sweating.
It is awful. In the process of feeding and numbing my emotions with chocolates and crisps, I haven't realised the damage I have done to myself over the years. I look and feel so old; I just don't feel like me anymore.

So that's me!!
Sorry for rambling on and on but I just wanted you to get a clear picture of where I am at.

Please can you help?!

WOW!!

As you can imagine, that was extremely tough for Amanda to write and no doubt it wasn't her first attempt. Like most people who've suffered excessive weight gain she was deeply unhappy, embarrassed about her size and unsurprisingly her health was starting to suffer. But Amanda accepted there was a problem, identified her goal, had a preferred time frame and wanted to sort it.

However, that was the easy bit; the hardest part was actually starting.

She wanted to lose about five stone and ideally within a year. That's thirty-two kilograms, which in old money is about seventy pounds. Or even better, approximately the same weight as thirty-two bags of sugar.
Think about that.
This woman wanted to lose five stone, which is the equivalent of losing thirty-two bags of sugar from her body.
THIRTY… FUCKIN'… TWO.
Holey moley, sweet baby Jesus.

That's approximately two and a half bags of sugar, a month.
For twelve months.

It was certainly achievable but extremely difficult nevertheless.

How the hell would she possibly start to accomplish this? Luckily it's not rocket science. It's very straightforward. In fact, we all know how to do it, there's no special secret.

EAT LESS SHIT, DO MORE SHIT

Although admittedly, that appears to be easier said than done.

I offered to help Amanda for free because she would've been my very first client, but for some reason she changed her mind and actually refused my assistance. I spent a few weeks e-mailing her, hoping she would reconsider but she just wouldn't meet me to discuss her weight loss goals. Therefore I had no other option than to forget about her, and continue to focus on other people who were more willing to take some action. I e-mailed her some basic tips on nutrition and low-level fitness, and then left her to it.

Over the years I occasionally wondered how she was getting on, and if she'd managed to finally chuck out those baggy cardigans and become a size ten again.

Then I found out.

It wasn't cancer, or a heart attack, or a car accident, nope, Amanda decided to take her own life. Depressed, overweight and alone, she obviously felt that she had no other choice. She was thirty-eight years old.

I could blather on about a wasted life and what a shame it was etc, etc but I didn't really know her, I didn't know how tough her life was, what emotions and problems she was dealing with, or why she felt the only option was suicide. Therefore who was I to judge?

But her death really affected me.

I was bloody gutted for her of course but it also reminded me of how perilously close I came to killing myself a decade before.

The first two times were pathetic cries for help and I didn't really put my full energy and commitment into either attempt, but I gave the third one a thoroughly decent bash.

ATTEMPT NUMBER ONE – I was being bullied at school because I wore catalogue clothes, was ignominiously dropped from the footy team and my lack of a pubic bush, somehow gave my teenage peers further ammunition to mock and ridicule me. In addition, I fuckin' hated my step-dad, what with his penchant for violence and scornful abuse. So I'd had enough. I placed a plastic bag over my head and began the liberation by asphyxiation.

But let me tell you, it was bloody dangerous I could hardly breathe, so I ripped it off within 2.4 seconds. Sod that for a game of soldiers, I'm sure life will be fine. I was beginning to see some sprinkling of hair in the ol' previously sparse, nether regions and I could've sworn I heard my mum mention something about divorce.

ATTEMPT NUMBER TWO – Girlfriend cheated on me. Woop-de-doo I hear you ask but it pissed me right off, so the obvious solution and a great way to *'show her'*, was to pop my clogs. The ultimate revenge. Ha! Ha! Ha! Didn't quite work out that way. Got ridiculously drunk, took several aspirins, puked up all over the bedspread, had a terrible hangover. Girlfriend took pity, stayed in loveless relationship for six more months and eventually it reached it's sad, inevitable conclusion. Life went on.

ATTEMPT NUMBER THREE – Single, hated my job and pretty skint, I wasn't living the life I wanted to live and just felt… so alone. To this day, I don't really know why I didn't go through with it. I even wrote a note. Woe is me and all that jazz. I'd drunk a few bottles of wine, taken loads of paracetamol but somehow I knew it wasn't the answer and something deep within me, made me stop. My family probably, I didn't want them to find me. It wasn't their fault, I was just being selfish but that's depression for you, logic goes out of the window because all you want is an end to the misery. One final act of control.

Anyway, I forced myself to be sick, had a bit of a cry and vowed to find another way out. I realised I had a serious problem and I needed to find a solution.

Which leads me neatly back to Amanda and the reason why you're currently reading these words.

Apparently, there's a book in all of us but I'll tell you something, it's damn difficult to find. I'd struggled for twenty years to actually find something interesting to write about. Something that people would actually want to read.

Well, I don't know who *'they'* are but *'they'* say that you should write about what you know.

What the hell do I know?

I know that sex sells but I don't think my technique on how to last eighteen, maybe thirty seconds at a push, is gonna set the pulses racing. I know that when you inform people that you're writing a book, they laugh in your face and smugly wish you *'all the best'* but I can't write about that. I also know that you can't lick your own elbow (reader tries, pulls a stupid face and realises nope, no you can't) but I'm not going to fill the pages of a book regarding that particular nugget of info.

What am I truly passionate about?

Obviously my family and my mates but not much else really, apart from music and erm, Liverpool Football Club (c'mon the Reds), yep that's me… sad but undeniably true.

Although, I suppose my real passion, in fact obsession and the only thing it seems that I'm really good at, is keeping fit and healthy. Fortunately for me, I managed to combat depression by finding salvation in fitness. I became fascinated by physiology and wanted, nay needed for my own wellbeing, to know everything about the subject, so I qualified as a Personal Trainer.

And as a sweat jockey this doesn't just mean that I am authorised to wear tight fitting vests, guzzle protein shakes, shave my chest and sport tribal tattoos. It also means that I have the fitness and nutritional knowledge to help the obese lose weight, the depressed feel happier, and the anxious more confident about themselves.

So that was it, sorted, I'd write something about fitness but it's such a saturated market, I needed an angle. And that angle was Amanda.

Sadly, it was too late to help her but it's not too late to help **you**.

One of the major causes of excessive weight gain is *'comfort eating'*. People get bored, so they eat. They're upset, so they eat. They hate their job, so they eat. They're lonely, so they eat. They're depressed, so they eat. They get even bigger, so they eat. It becomes a vicious, self-destructive cycle with sufferers not knowing how to break the pattern.

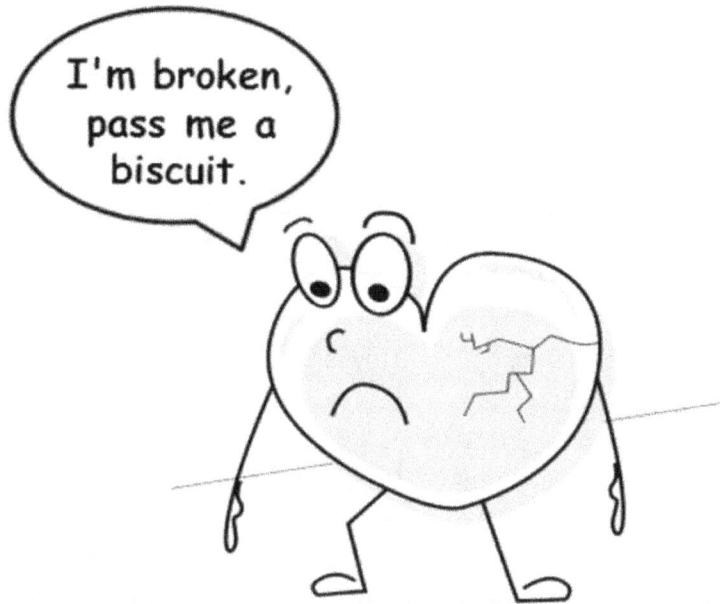

This is what some of my other clients said regarding this topic and no, I'm not referring to the nutty chocolate bar.

JOHN, 48 - *For as long as I can remember, I've associated food with comfort. I have vivid childhood memories of being upset and knowing I'd only be happier once I had my hands wrapped around a chocolate bar, or munching through a packet of crisps. Now when I get stressed or if I have a wobble and feeling down, I don't eat to bury my emotions, instead I talk to friends, go for a run, listen to music or just put a comedy on the box.*

ALEX, 30 - *I was ever so lonely and I yearned to be loved. I desired affection and when I didn't get either, I replaced those emotions with food and alcohol. And lots and lots of it. Life seems so much simpler when you're gorging on a cream bun or sinking a few bottles of wine.*

NATASHA, 36 - *I always sought comfort in food. I slathered bread with peanut butter, ate whole cakes, family-size chocolate bars and entire multipacks of crisps. I told myself that I deserve these treats because I was upset, especially about my weight. It became a vicious cycle when I started to put on even more weight because this would upset me even more, so yet again I'd seek comfort in food. It's only now that I can see the irony in that situation.*

ROSE, 28 - *If I hit a setback on one of my diets, I'd get so annoyed with myself I'd go and have a pig out to make me feel better. Then I'd feel so guilty I'd start to cry and the only way I could think about feeling better, was to eat more. I desperately wanted to make changes to my life because I didn't respect myself. It's difficult to describe how elated I felt, when I could finally look at my reflection in the mirror and be proud of what I saw.*

If like them, this is how **you** deal with emotions and issues in your life, then it just has to change.

It has to stop. Obviously when you've finished *'comfort eating'*, you feel anything but *'comfort'*, it just makes you feel more depressed instead.

Food will not love you.
Food will not hug you.
Food will not make you laugh.
Food will not take you down the pub.
Food is not the answer.

You have to make sure that the stuff you do to feel better about yourself doesn't make you feel worse, so stop rewarding yourself with food, you're no pooch. Although having said that, when you start to take my advice you'll give that black dog a run for its money because you'll be considerably fitter... and thinner... and happier.

READER: *How do I know it's gonna work?*
Well, I'm typing these words over a decade after trying to top myself, so yep, it works alright. And if it works for me, it stands to reason it can work for **you** too.

Look, I've been there and I know what it's like. Depression is a horrible illness and unless you've had it in your life, it's difficult to fully empathise with people who suffer from it. Depression can take your soul, it can make you feel worthless and it can take any ounce of joy or feeling from you. You're not you anymore; instead you become a spiritless version of yourself.

That's why so many sufferers find refuge in a slice of cake, a tub of ice cream, a bottle of wine, shopping, fighting, watching porn, injecting drugs or internet gambling, anything really in order to just numb the pain and experience some temporary elation.

But rather than, 'why me?' how about, 'what can I do to improve my life?'
'How can I get out of this fuzz?'
'How can I be me again?'
'What will make me a happier person and still have time to watch Netflix?'

I don't think that GP's deal with depression in the best way because the first option is always to medicate. This seems to me like using gaffer tape, to fix a sinking ship. It's a bit of a kop out and it doesn't exactly help the individual attempt to combat the fundamental problems in their life, which are responsible for the black dog and the deep, dark abyss.

And one of the major problem with anti-depressants is they become addictive. And irony upon ironies, trying to come off these pills leads to withdrawal symptoms, such as headaches and more depression... **Kerching!!**

Yes, people that consistently suffer from depression *'may'* have some chemical imbalance that creates this funk but on the flip side to that, exercise, good food, fresh air, sunshine and laughter can reverse this condition, by helping to release endorphins.

And when you start adopting a positive mindset, you take a pragmatic approach to problems; you begin to see the best in any situation and as a consequence, become happier. Your mood improves. You gain a healthier perspective on life. The depression lifts.

Therefore why don't Doctor's look for lateral solutions to this psychological issue, rather than just prescribing medication?!
Ah!! What do I know?!
READER: *Yes, you're not a Doctor.*
You're right, I'm not. But I'm a fellow human being and whether you're thin, fat, ginger, bald, black, white, liberal, right-wing, blind, deaf, tall or even a Banker, we all experience life the same way.

We all have goals, we all get hungry, we all get upset, we all burp, we all pick our nose and we all have to urinate. There are no exceptions, it's just how we're packaged and presented to the world that differs.

LUCY, 26 – *Before I met you Paul, it was the worst I'd felt in about 6 months, maybe more.*
I was extremely upset, agitated, frustrated and snappy. Nothing could drag me out of this slump.
And if I'm honest, I was scared to be alone with my own thoughts.
Ok! I wasn't on the verge of doing anything stupid, but I was struggling emotionally at that stage. I knew my weight wasn't helping but after trying every diet under the sun, I just couldn't see a way out.
It still took a few months to turn my life around and I had the occasional bad day but after you replied to my e-mails and we chatted in person a few times, you offered a completely different perspective to my issues that I'd not even considered.
Nowadays, it's such a relief to go from waking up feeling miserable, unable to drag myself out of bed, to starting each morning excited about the day ahead.
Thanks Paul, I really appreciate your help.

Medication is not the answer.

The answer is within you... it's all in your head. At the end of the day, you're actually doing it to yourself.

You make yourself think depressing thoughts thus equally you could think of positive, happy thoughts instead. You have the power to change your thought process, so why don't you do it? Why don't you try to change?

Unless of course you want to be depressed, then it gives you a label, a convenient excuse for your problems.

- I can't do that, I'm depressed.
- I can't wash up, I'm depressed.
- I can't go to work, I'm depressed.
- I can't go to the gym, I'm depressed.
- I need to eat a whole packet of biscuits, I'm depressed.
- I need to drink these two bottles of wine, I'm depressed.
- I can't deal with my kids anymore, I'm depressed.
- I can't lose weight, I'm depressed.
- I can't go on, I'm depressed.

Cod psychology perhaps, or is it haddock now that we're over fishing cod stocks?

I just think it's much better for your health, for your sanity, for your wellbeing, that rather than finding comfort in a pill or food, you try to find it in exercise, music, comedy, or with your family and mates.

Shit happens in life but things can change in an instant, so you have to keep asking yourself, *'does it really matter?'*

It can only hurt you, if you let it.

When you allow positivity to take over your life, self-enhancement becomes the norm and you focus on becoming a better person, rather than wasting your valuable time on this planet moping about, bitching about people, fretting and feeling sorry for yourself.

I mean, it's so easy for us to spend our lives worrying and stressing about stuff which never even happens, that we actually struggle to remember what's truly important. Family, mates, new experiences, laughter, sex, travel, living and just bloody enjoying ourselves. Now **THAT** is what life is all about.

So let me help **you** achieve this better life.

I don't have any ulterior motive apart from a genuine desire to do something good, something worthwhile with my life.

I'm not trying to promote a DVD, or entice subscribers to my blog, Instagram page or *'You-Tube'* channel. I'm not allied to any gym, and I'm not a spokesperson for a so called *'miracle'* diet pill or food substitute. I won't try and bamboozle you with scientific gobbledygook either, it'll be straight talking with no added **bullshit!! Although it would be nice to sell a couple of books and hear your success stories…**

Okay, I may have lied in the past but I want you to trust me, so I'll be open and honest with you now.
No, I didn't lose my virginity at fourteen, or have trials for Leeds Utd.
Phew!! Nice to finally get that off my pecs.

All I'm trying to do is help **you** become the best **you** that **you** can be.
I know that sounds a bit cheesy but don't worry, this book isn't going to be about placenta smoothies, cosmic ordering, or ritual chanting. It's about choosing a path that helps to alleviate depression, increases positivity, enhances confidence, improves your fitness and leads to a healthier life.
What's not to like?

Obviously, I can't do it for you but I'm going to try and guide you in the right direction.
Then it's up to **you**, to work it out.

I won't be showing you pictures of good looking bodies, with firm abs and bulging biceps because you already know what these look like. You're bombarded with these images on telly and in magazines, to shame you into buying more crap that you don't need.

READER: *What about you do you have a great body then?*
Oh Aye!! I'd put Michelangelo's *'David'* to shame, but I'm just not photogenic enough. I don't have chiselled cheek bones and a cute boyband face, I'm an old git and an **ugly bugger!!** I've got a hairy chest, mono-brow, big nose, crow's feet, caffeine-bleached teeth, salt n' pepper hair and more wrinkles than a sharpei dog.

All in all a great face for radio, so trust me, you don't wanna see my fugly mug.

But ultimately it's not about me or anyone else for that matter; you've got to concentrate on yourself. It's about **you** and what **you** could look and feel like. So get your own piccies by taking some of them *'selfies'*, then send me an e-mail if you like (birchygoober@hotmail.com), I'd love to hear about your story.

So have I got your attention? You interested?

Look, if your life is perfect and you're happy with your weight, fitness, lifestyle and state of mind, then be my guest, put this book down and carry on.

Go back to your *'fat-free'* yoghurt, couch-potato existence and negative outlook.
But if you're not and you would like to improve yourself, then get reading.

It's true that many books make wild, unattainable claims but I'm not going to do that.
I'm not promising miracles either but I can guarantee that if you *'Wake the fit up'*, it will add at least ten years to your life… or your money back*.

C'mon!
What you got to lose?
Apart from negativity, timber, suicidal thoughts, anxiety, love handles, panic, shyness, depression…

*Proof of purchase required

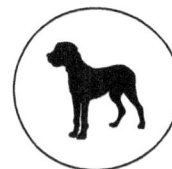

HELP

You've decided to go on a new type of diet. And this time, unlike the previous times, you have a fool-proof plan.

You've heard that this one definitely works.

Some bloke in the office told you about it, and he heard from Brenda that it's scientifically proven. Two boiled eggs for brekkie, tomato soup for lunch, and chicken with sprouts for tea. You do a detox as well, twice a day drinking kale juice with a sprinkle of cayenne pepper.
You can't fail.
You will not fail.

You're going to start running too. Probably join a gym, in fact, you might even sign up to do a half-marathon.

This time, it's going to happen, you're going to do it.

Your life is going to be so different.

You're gonna have loads of energy, you'll be happier and full of confidence. On your next holiday you'll look amazing, beach body in tip-top condition.

Watch out everyone, **Bowchickabowwow!!** It's going to be fan-tastic.

But then after a few days, you start to have doubts. The negativity kicks in. You don't know if you can do it, you constantly think about quitting. You become miserable, tired and irritable.

You fantasise about cakes, ice-cream, crisps, pizza and chocolate. Oh My God!! Chocolate, you need chocolate, you crave chocolate.

You must have **chocolate!!**

The odd bar won't hurt. You dunk a few biccies into your brew as well. It's not a crime, you know!?! So what if you miss a few gym sessions, you're still gonna do it. You'll do a long run tomorrow. And after a long week at work, there's nothing wrong with a couple of takeaways at the weekend.

You become stressed, agitated, desperate. You need some alcohol, a bottle of wine, beer, cider, **ANYTHING!!**

Sod this fuckin' diet!!

You know the rest because you've been there, you've done that, you've bought the XL T-shirt (or is that XXL T-shirt?).

So how do you change this cycle of failure?
What's the best way to be prepared for the hurdles, setbacks and inevitable excuses that you must overcome to be successful?

The first thing you need to do… is **stop dieting!!**
NEVER diet again.

Diets actually take the joy and pleasure out of eating, turning it into a punishing routine of calorie counting, portion control and forced restraint.

It's insanity. And the definition of insanity, *'is repeating a task over and over again, and expecting different results'*. Or voting as it's otherwise called.

Dieting for long-term weight loss is the equivalent of asking someone to repeatedly punch you in the face, so that you can donate blood.

Diets are like *'Rubik's cubes'**.

Only a few people can complete them successfully and most people get bored, frustrated or angry after a short time doing them and just give up.
* Gastric Bands and Liposuction are the equivalent of taking the stickers off and placing them back in the right order. You learn nothing, it's just cheating. And cheaters never prosper, so what's the point of that?!

Trying to sustain long-term weight loss by dieting is like trying to crawl up the escalator, on the wrong side. You might succeed eventually but it's bloody hard work, and you'll feel and look like an idiot doing it.

And when I say *'diet'*, I'm not talking *'slimming club'* diets (I will discuss those objectively later in the book), I mean the ones where you restrict your daily calorie consumption and don't get the requisite amount of nutrients that your body actually requires, in order to survive and exist.

You know the ones, the cabbage, cereal, parsnip, carrot soup, popcorn, maple syrup, Aloe Vera juice and meal replacement type of diets. Just stop doing them, they don't work.

Ok! They *'may'* work for some people but they do not, I repeat, **DO NOT** work in the long-term because they are short-term fixes thus completely unsustainable.

These *'diets'* lead to cravings and longing for foods that the dieter supposedly can't have therefore the dieter inevitably caves in, and has a massive blow out. This then leads to guilt, depression and frustration. Diet is over, weight piles back on and it's back to square one again.

A few months later the process starts again with another *'miracle diet'* but this yo-yo dieting just leads to more failure and misery.

If you want your weight to GO-GO,
then YO-YO is a NO-NO

Weight loss isn't complicated, it's extremely simple. A healthy balanced diet and some moderate exercise, that's all that you need, anything else is just a lie. If you're reading this book, no doubt you're sick of endlessly trying these weight loss fads?!

So what do you need to do in order to quit, quitting?! You need my help.

Naturally, you're probably sceptical, or maybe you're just one of those people who doesn't like to take any advice, out of sheer stubbornness.
Well, how's that working for you?
Yeah, exactly.

The only person you're punishing is **you** and where does that get you? Nowhere. Fast. Most people and that certainly includes me, give advice because they want to help. They care.

It's not about point scoring and even if it is, who gives a toss who wins, it doesn't mean anything. It's the drinks after the match that count, not the game itself.
So let's establish from the outset, do **you** need to *'Wake the fit up'*?

The following questions are based on honest and open discussions which I've had with some of my clients, and if any resonate or seem familiar, then you'd certainly benefit from my HELP.

1) Have you ever burst into tears after seeing an unflattering picture of yourself?

2) Do you worry about stuff so much that you actually become physically sick?

3) Do you refuse to get your legs out, even in hot weather?

4) Do you dislike your appearance so much, that you make up excuses and scarper whenever the camera phones come out?

5) Do you hate going out because you feel uncomfortable and think that you can't dress as well, or look as good as your slim, fashionable friends?

6) Do you yearn to feel normal, energetic and active?

7) Were School PE lessons such a nightmare, that you've avoided physical activity ever since?

8) Do you think you have no off switch and no self-control when it comes to food?

9) Is your self-esteem at rock bottom?

10) Did you think that taking diet pills and skipping meals would work but they didn't?!

11) Do you always seem to give in too easily?

12) Do you feel so lonely, even though you have loads of mates and a loving family?

13) Have you tried every diet going and none of them have worked?

14) Do you just want to feel comfortable in your own skin?

15) Have you ever caught your reflection in a shop window and couldn't believe how big you'd become?

16) Do you find it so challenging and difficult to face the world that you'd rather just stay in bed?

17) Do you simply feel, like a blob?

18) Have you ever asked if a dress makes you look fat, even though it's the fat that makes you look fat?!

19) Are you worried that you won't be able to shift baby weight, or lose some weight for a wedding?

20) If you're a bloke, do you think slimming is just for women?

21) Do you spend countless hours watching TV because it's the only way you can take your mind off your troubles?

22) Do you hate it when you open the fridge door and can't find what you're looking for, like perfect abs, sex appeal and happiness?

23) Have you been big since childhood and pretend you're not bothered about your size, even when deep down you feel miserable?

24) Are you trying to lose weight at the moment but take the elevator rather than climb the stairs?

25) Did you read that e-mail from Amanda and think that it sounded a little bit like you?

Okay doke. If you nodded in agreement to any of those statements, then I'm afraid you've got a problem me ol' mucker and you need help.
And you need it **now!!**

It's evident that your current lifestyle is not helping with your weight, state of mind or happiness. And if it's not working, it's not working. So, **you** need to make changes.
Whether it's weight-loss, depression, anxiety or loneliness, this is the specific help that you need:

H   E   L   P

is for   is for   is for   is for

HEALTHY EATING   **EXERCISE**   **LIVING & ENJOYING LIFE**   **POSITIVE MINDSET**

Each component of HELP is equally important and I'll discuss each strand in depth throughout the book. But what you need to bear in mind from the outset is that these elements work in harmony, not in isolation. Therefore you must apply and commit to each principle, because if you don't, this will hinder your chances of success.

For instance, it goes without saying that nutrition and exercise are extremely important regarding weight loss, but you also need to start making a conscious effort to really enjoy living and being alive.
Enough of the couch potato existence, you'll find that good things start to happen when you leave the house and switch off the box.
You have to make sure that your life is full, rather than just your stomach.

And if you *'Wake the fit up'*, you'll never have to do those dreaded diets again.

Look, keeping fit and healthy isn't a punishment you know but dieting certainly is. It should never be *'no food'* it should be, *'know food'* instead.

Whenever someone tries to learn a new language for example, they are completely immersed in the subject. It takes over their life. Yet when people try to lose weight or get fit, they generally go into it haphazardly. Buy some new trainers, a few punnets of fruit, a fitness DVD and then flap about a bit for a few weeks. Fail miserably and then get back to the old routine.

But you need to understand the basics of nutrition, or else this will limit your chances of long-term, weight loss success. You need to know which food types will boost your metabolism, which offer the most nutritional value and why certain food types actually improve your mood.

And don't worry you won't need to deprive yourself of any foods that you love either, as long as you only eat them in moderation. It's all about a sustainable balance.

Cakes, chocolate, pies, ice cream, even alcohol, a little of what you fancy does you good, and I'll be promoting that ethos.
READER: *Really?*
Yep, there will be no food restrictions at all but you have to be willing to make some lifestyle changes, especially if weight-loss is your ultimate goal.

READER: *Well I can't run, I'll never be fit.*
That's the spirit ☺

When I say exercise, I'm not talking extreme athlete here, moderate activity is more than adequate. You'll start slowly and then reach a level that you're comfortable with.

READER: *How? I can't, I'm just no good at exercise.*

You can and I'm going to explain how. But and if it's a big butt, you'll have to put some effort in.

One of my clients - **Jacqui**, that's not her name but we'll call her it anyway (I have changed the names of all the clients mentioned in this book, to protect their identities).

She was a 41yr old, single mother of two at the time and she wanted to lose three stone. Oh! And she absolutely detested going to the gym, or any other form of fitness related activity. She used to joke that the only exercise she ever liked to do, was five sit ups a day. Although there was only so many times she could hit the snooze button.

I encouraged her to change her attitude, and now she sends me e-mails containing links to her marathon finishing times. She chose to take action, she chose to put in the effort, she chose to take my HELP and she's never been happier.

Or fitter... or healthier.

! ! ! WARNING ! ! ! SPOILER ALERT ! ! ! WARNING ! ! ! SPOILER ALERT ! ! ! WARNING ! ! ! SPOILER ALERT ! ! !

Losing weight is no picnic, specific terms and conditions do apply and here's the spoiler, they're mandatory. It's gonna be really difficult therefore if **you** are going to succeed, you have to be prepared to put the effort in and you have to accept that it's going to be hard.

Not in an, *'Ooh-er Missus!'* type way, I mean that for the first few months it will be challenging.

It's not gonna be easy,
You will endure some pain,
But if you have a lot to lose,
You've got so much to gain.

You have to earn it with blood, sweat and tears. No less, nothing else, no more.
It can't be handed to you on a plate.
It can't be delivered to your door, donated, purchased, borrowed or stolen.
It doesn't come in a bottle, pill, sachet or cream.
And it definitely can't be downloaded in an App.

Success in any field is a by-product of permanent, habitual, gradual change. But the problem with today's society is we demand immediate gratification, we have no patience, we want everything faster, quicker, this minute, **now!!**

When you see some hottie who has a great body, you don't see the suffering and the struggles they experienced to earn it. Instead you judge them by different standards, assuming that they're just lucky, born like that. Then you look away and feel sorry for yourself, rather than asking them how they achieved it and how difficult it was for them.

When a great sculptor creates a work of art, they don't just chisel away for a few minutes and Hey Presto!! No, they agonise and labour and toil, and after months, sometimes years of endeavour, it's finally complete. And it might be their third, fourth, or twelfth attempt but you only see the finished article.

Your habits that have taken years to build can't be changed in a day, or a week. You're turning around an oil tanker, not a Pedalo.

And some of your habits have been ingrained since childhood but just like baldy, vest-wearing, wisecracking, Mister Willis, old habits die hard.

Think about how long it's taken you to put on the weight. It won't just disappear overnight.

It's a step by step process based on sustainable long-term changes, not *'get thinner-quick'* fads that are detrimental to your health and sanity.

Small, daily improvements are the key to achieving your weight loss goals.

If you expect virtually miraculous results, I'm sorry to disappoint you but it just doesn't work like that.
You need to have patience my Padewan because it will require dedication, hard work, sacrifice and a lot of willpower.

Throughout this book, I'm not gonna piss on your back and tell you it's raining, I want to be completely honest and upfront with you, it's going to be bloody difficult mate.

It'll be an ordeal. Aye, I'm afraid it's going to take a while and you have to accept that, there's no getting away from it. Or you can just ignore the problem and not bother trying. Up to you.

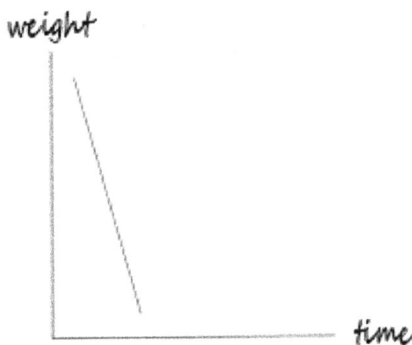

What people **hope** weight-loss success is like

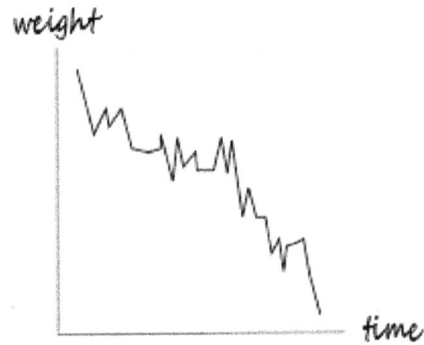

What it's **actually** like

Choices, choices, choices
Every second of every day, you make choices that change your life. It's up to you to decide whether these changes are for good, or for bad. You can choose to finally lose that lard, knowing that it will take time but it will be worth it in the end. Or you can choose to be overweight.

Now then, don't be thinking of loads of excuses as to why you can't do it. I know that you want to, so c'mon, let's go!!

Too many people talk a good talk but talk is cheap, unless you're ringing one of those sex lines of course, then it's really expensive.

Apparently!?! I've heard… sorry, I digress.

Less talk and more do.

Successful people are doers and those that do, *'do'* and those that don't… whinge and bitch about those that *'do'*.
Doers *'do'* stuff, talkers *'talk'* about it.

So don't go on and on to your family and friends about your plans to make changes, show them the results instead.

And don't be a *'gunner'* either...
READER: *What, an Arsenal fan?*
No!! I mean...

———

I was gunner do this,
I was gunner do that,
I was gunner get fit,
And get rid of my fat.

That type of *'gunner'*.

Look, we're all *'gunners'* at some point in our lives, we're all *'gunner'* do things and we're *'gunner'* see some stuff... eventually.

I mean, I was *'gunner'* take over the world this morning but unfortunately I overslept, so I'll do it tomorrow... maybe, perhaps... possibly.

Even when I made the decision to actually write this book, I still procrastinated. **A lot!!**

At some stage I'll get round to telling you about my procrastination issues but not yet. Suffice to say, I can completely empathise and understand how difficult it is to start a new goal.

For me it just seemed to click into place one day and after that, the process of writing seemed easier, although it still took about nine months to complete. And looking back, perhaps I needed that time to fully immerse myself in the project. Or I'm another lazy git trying to justify my excuses.

Regardless, at least I finally got off my glutes and got it done.

And my advice to stop you from procrastinating so much too, is simply to take some bloody action, in anything you want to achieve... **get on with it!!**

I'm a big fan of wordplay and granamas and if you unscramble the word *'action'*, in a roundabout way it sort of describes what **you** need to do – ON I ACT.

Not enough?

Ok! I get it, you need something else that motivates and inspires you to start.
Birthdays and the New Year are often the perfect opportunity to take stock of your life and make resolutions, chase dreams and take some action.

You could wait and do it then but why not just start now?

READER: *What, this second?*
Alright smarty pants, once you've finished reading this book but you know what I mean.

If you're waiting for a sign…this is it.

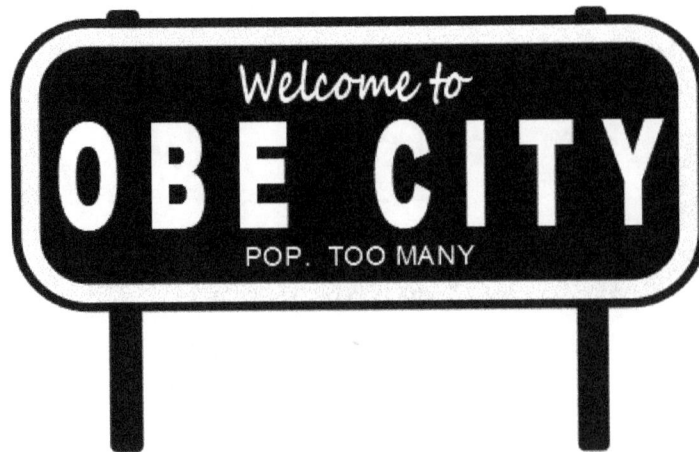

READER: *I'm probably too old to start.*
Don't be ridiculous, it's never too late.

If you're reading this sentence that means you haven't kicked the bucket yet, you're still breathing. Now isn't that something to be happy about?!

You're alive, so act like it before the very Grim Reaper gets you in his sights.

READER: *It's not the right time at the moment. I might do it next year.*
Yes but the longer you wait for the future, the shorter it will be. Don't live for tomorrow, you might not see it.
C'mon, three months from now you'll thank yourself for starting today, well once you've finished reading this book.

READER: *I'm a smoker.*
Ok! Well, erm… stop.
READER: *Yeah but if I stop, I'll put on extra weight.*
And…
So…
WHAT?

You'll just have more to lose.

I appreciate it'll be a challenge but stop using it as an excuse. Anyone can give up smoking; it's the starting again the next day that's the problem. It's not my area of expertise because I've never smoked therefore I can't really help on that score but if you can finally work out how to stop starting again, happy days.

READER: *Well that's not very helpful.*
Ok! Ok! It's all about willpower and I'll broach that topic later in the book. The principles outlined can be adapted to target any problem, including how to stop smoking.

READER: *I don't know if I want to stop though, smoking is cool.*
Oh aye!! Weirdly thin pursed lips, yellow fingers, bad breath, coughing, bringing up mucous, lung cancer, its cracking. Up to you fag ash…

READER: *But it helps me chill out…*
Well, you'll have loads of time to relax once you're in that early grave.
Look, I'm not gonna keep lecturing you about the dangers of smoking, it's fairly obvious, so do what you want they're your lungs. Next excuse…
READER: *I'm not sure my partner will be on board.*
If your partner won't support you, you're onto a losing battle. So sod 'em, get rid, dump the selfish **bugger!!**

16

It's better to be moderately happy and single, than miserable but in a relationship. One of my clients lost nineteen stone in the first few weeks of her weight loss.
Do you know how she did it?
READER: *No, how?*
She got divorced.

READER: *I've got kids*
Congratulations! Good for you.

READER: *Yeah but it's really hard to lose weight and exercise when you're a mother and have kids.*
I know, I completely understand but don't worry I'll give you lots of tips to help. You've got to be smarter, use time efficiently and alter your routines. Get 'em involved too, it can be fun and weight loss should be pleasurable, not purgatory. Up to you lass, just don't use them as another excuse.

READER: *I lack motivation.*
Translated as – *'I can't be arsed'*.
C'mon, no-one lacks motivation.

You know **what** the issue is; you know **why** you need to make some fundamental changes to your life. It's possible, that you could end up like Amanda. I'm not saying you will but it's entirely feasible. I mean, I'm only here typing these words 'cos I made some drastic changes to my life, and embraced fitness to such a degree that I became a qualified Personal Trainer.

It's up to you.

You can carry on the way you are and get bigger and bigger, health deteriorating and more at risk of developing asthma, cancer, heart disease, strokes and diabetes.

Or you can say *'Fuck that, I ain't doing it anymore'* and make some drastic changes to become healthier and fitter… and happier… for good.

At first, people will ask you **why** you're doing it but when they see the results, they'll be asking you **how** you're doing it.

Look…

- Do it because you have too many chins.
- Do it 'cos you can't fit into your nice clothes.
- Do it 'cos you're sick of wearing granny pants.
- Do it 'cos people that care for you, are worried about your health.
- Do it 'cos everyone tells you, you won't.
- Do it 'cos it's the right thing to do.

READER: *Ok! Ok! I'll give it a go but I've heard all of this before you know.*
You might think that but I can assure you that the guidance contained in this book is completely original and unique. I only wish that Amanda had given me the opportunity to share it with her because if she did, I'm convinced she'd still be alive today.

And she wouldn't be wearing baggy cardigans.
READER: *Are you sure about that?*
I'm sure.
In fact, I'm bloody positive.

And when you start adopting a positive mental attitude, you'll find it's a weight off your stomach **and** your mind.

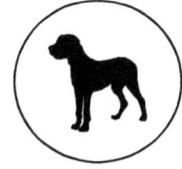

POSITIVE MINDSET

READER *(tutting)*: *Oh! God, here we go.*
Look, without a positive attitude, you're just pissing in the wind regarding weight loss or depression.

You won't embrace the changes that are necessary, to improve your diet. You won't attempt to perform the low-level exercise that is required to improve your fitness and health. And you certainly won't be able to live and enjoy the rest of your life.

When it comes to weight loss and depression, most people look for solutions in the wrong place but you're not gonna find them in celebrity magazines, social media posts, or day-time Telly. The solution is within **you** and it always has been and it always will be.

When you try to lose weight, you'll find that it's not just about exercise and food choices, it's also about your mindset, your approach to life, to other people, to yourself. It's a doctrine for living, not a hobby and you've either got it or you're unhappy. And overweight.

You must get into the habit of adopting a positive attitude. You have to believe that you will succeed and with such a passion that it becomes a reality. You have to be convinced, that you will definitely lose weight and you will get fitter.

No matter what, you will... not... fail.

Don't worry, I'm not asking you to walk around constantly grinning like some weird loon. But being positive isn't just a fluffy cliché, it's not psycho-babble. When you approach life with positivity your creativity improves, your motivation increases and you become more productive. You're happier, you're healthier, you worry less and you feel more confident. You approach your goals with vigour, not nagging doubt.

However, if you think something can't be achieved in your life then there's no way you will take the necessary steps required, to make that dream a reality. It becomes a self-fulfilling prophecy, and they are considerably difficult to overcome. This could explain why Amanda refused my help; she'd failed so many times before that she probably didn't think it would work another time, so just didn't bother trying.

She'd always struggled to lose weight in the past, so the positivity had been squeezed out of her like a used teabag. However, the problem with negativity is it feeds itself, and it grows and grows but a negative mindset is like a flat tyre... you won't get anywhere, until you change it.

HERE COMES THE SCIENCE

Getting stressed out, actually leads to weight gain.
READER: *Huh?!*
Yep! When our bodies are under stress we constantly churn out the hormones, *'Adrenaline'* and *'Cortisol'*. These hormones prepare the body for the *'flight or fight'* response. Blood supply is diverted away from processes such as digestion and diverted to the muscles so we can prepare to scarper, or have a scrap. This causes the body to

use glucose and not body fat as its primary fuel source, which is why stressed people crave sugary treats during times of stress because their bodies require it for fuel.The release of cortisol increases the bodies' capacity to store and cling onto fat, which as a consequence, increases your appetite. If you constantly feel anxious and stressed in your daily life, this means you will have elevated levels of cortisol. And studies have found that people with high cortisol levels tend to stockpile fat around their middles (the dreaded spare tyre).

Doctors will always advocate that obese patients try to lose some timber in order to reduce stress but the process of attempting to drop the pounds, could actually intensify stresses upon the body.
READER: *But… but… I want to lose weight, so you're telling me I'll be stressed out?*
Not necessarily but if you ever diet again, then yes.

Although if you incorporate all four elements of HELP you'll have minimal stress, so it won't be an issue.
READER: *Oh!*

I just want you to be aware of one of the many reasons why you and people you know who have tried to lose weight, have failed in the past due to stress.
READER: *Okay doke!! Carry on…*
Thanks.

The Science geeks have also discovered that fat cells actually have special receptors for the stress hormone cortisol, and there are more of these receptors contained within our abdominal fat than anywhere else in our body. Studies have shown that belly fat is actually an active tissue and responds to the stress response, by actually welcoming more fat to be deposited.

So how do you think you can stop this ongoing cycle?
READER: *By adopting a positive mindset?*
Bingo!!

Depending on your state of health, fitness and sanity, dramatic weight loss can increase cortisol levels. Your hormones directly contribute to every function in your body, and your hormones are negatively or positively impacted by what you eat, and how active you are.

Your body is a delicate, responsive machine, so it is important to eat in a way that prevents excess cortisol surges. To lower stress, get involved in low-intensity activities such as yoga, swimming, walking or Pilates. These are great exercises that actually lower cortisol in the body, whilst also promoting calorie burning and weight loss.

Your diet should consist of mostly protein, greens, healthy fats and low glycaemic starches.
READER: *What are low glycaemic starches?*
I'll mention these in the food section later in the book but to give you an idea, starchy foods are often referred to as *'carbs'* (short for carbohydrates), which include foods like bread, pasta, rice, couscous, potatoes, breakfast cereals, oats and other grains, like rye and barley.

When starchy foods are digested they are broken down into *'glucose'* which is the main fuel for the body, especially for the brain and the muscles. Starchy foods can also provide fibre which is important for digestive health, as well as a range of nutrients including B vitamins, iron and calcium.

The *'Glycaemic Index'*, or GI, measures how a carbohydrate food type raises glucose in your blood stream.

Foods are ranked based on how they compare to a reference food (normally white bread), which has a rating of 100%. A food with a high GI raises blood glucose considerably more than a food with a medium or low GI.

Examples of *'low glycaemic starches'* include dried beans and legumes (like kidney beans and lentils), all non-starchy vegetables, some starchy vegetables like sweet potatoes, most fruit, and some whole grain breads and cereals (although a lot of wholegrain products are extremely high in sugar).
READER: *Well you learn something every day.*
That's what I'm here for.

When you begin to diet, the body will naturally adapt to getting less calories, so it will store fat more readily thus it becomes harder to lose weight. If you cut calories too low, your body holds onto every little calorie you eat, weight loss plateaus, which understandably causes confusion to the dieter.

As you know, losing weight can make you a touch moody, especially if you're coming off processed packet pap, refined sugar and junk food. Your body is literally detoxing from all those foods you were addicted to.

Refined and processed foods have been proven to be as addictive as heroin. And we all know from the film *'Trainspotting'*, how moreish drugs can be. You're effectively undergoing *'cold turkey'*, so you're likely to endure headaches and migraines, which inevitably lead to more stress.
The joy of dieting… not!
READER: *Blimey a 'Wayne's World' reference, you really are an old git aren't ya?!*
Guilty as charged.

Dieters often complain of being tired all day, then having trouble sleeping at night. Their bodies are in shock due to the dietary changes and calorie restrictions which affect cortisol levels, causing irregular sleep patterns.

Stress and weight loss go hand in hand, so if you can't stay positive and have lots of fun whilst trying to lose the flab, you will undoubtedly fail.

I accept that it isn't always easy to let things go. We put too much pressure on ourselves, trying to meet unfeasible demands, taking care of others, trying to do well at work, and to make everyone around us happy. But when we forget about ourselves and don't take care of our bodies, the stresses will appear as extra pounds.

CONCLUSION: Enjoy life, or you'll just get more fatterer.

Are you positive?

At some time or another, we've all woken up in the middle of the night. We take a glance at the clock and realise that there's only five hours left until the alarm goes off.

As trivial as this situation may be, how you look at it dictates your entire outlook and attitude to life.
If you're a negative person, you'll instantly fret about losing sleep. You'll be so annoyed that your mind has had the temerity and nerve to actually wake you up from slumberville; you begin to get angry with yourself.

You'll slowly count down the hours, minutes and seconds until that annoying alarm starts a-beeping. You'll start to worry so much, that you'll struggle to get back to dreamland. Yes you'll nod off eventually but you'll be a right grumpy sod when you finally wake up.

And then all day at work, you'll be yawning and moaning to your colleagues that you've had another crap night of sleep.

However, if you're a positive person, you'll invariably fall back to sleep within minutes. You might not even bother looking at the clock but if you do, at least it's in the safe knowledge that although you've woken up, you'll be chuffed to bits that you've still got the reward and bonus of another five hours of blissful slumber to enjoy. Brilliant.

Snoozetastic!!

Rather than focusing on the negatives, you immediately look for the positive angle instead. You'll wake up in a decent mood, get to work with a smile on your chops and then have the mental dexterity to ignore that whining git at work who's complaining **yet** again, 'cos they didn't get a good night's kip.

Which one are you?

Yep! I thought so but you don't have to be, it's just a choice.

HEE! HEE!

I want you to think about the last time you laughed? And no, I don't mean when you typed *'LOL'* at the end of a text, or Facebook message. I mean really laughed. Guffawed, chortled and maybe even an uncontrollable snort or four. So much so that you had tears rolling down your cheeks and your belly was literally aching.

I bet you can't remember can you?
That's quite sad really but not uncommon.

Apparently, the average child laughs three hundred times a day and an adult, just six. Now I'm not sure who's counting, or how accurate that stat is but it seems apt based on the fact that sprogs have no worries at all. Apart from who can scream and shriek the loudest, what colour crayon to shove up their nose and selecting which toy they're going to break after nap-time!?!

Adults clearly have loads to worry about. Work, family, the mortgage, credit cards, Lecky bills, petrol prices, straightness of hedges, colour of crockery, whether their wallpaper matches their shoes and which vacuous moron will be kicked out of *'Big Brother'* next.

Do happy people not have these types of problem? Of course they do but happiness is not the absence of problems, it's the ability to deal with them with a grin on your boat race.

People who over-eat are not happy. People who drink alone in the house, are not happy. People who self-harm are not happy. People who watch hours and hours of porn, are not happy. People who sit on their arse of an evening, scrolling through their phone whilst watching the box, are not happy. Therefore these people need to change their mindset, adopt a different ethos, find a different path.

Under our meaty coats of flesh, we're all the same really. At some time or another, we've all been a little bit jealous. A bit short with someone. Embarrassed. Annoyed. Frustrated. Rude. Upset.
And we all get miserable at times too and I'm no different I assure you. I still get depressed now and again but these days I endeavour to spend the majority of my time enjoying myself. In fact, I can prove it, 'cos I have more laughter lines than the scripts from *'Blackadder'*.

Don't get me wrong, in the past I've been a right mardy arse, angry and full of self-pity as to how my life has turned out. But nowadays I try to not let things bother me so much and generally look for the positive in any situation.

Happy, chilled out, mellow individuals very rarely suffer from high blood pressure and stress related disorders. However, they do have loads of friends and an active social life, 'cos people want to spend quality time with them. No-one ever thinks, *'Oh, I must invite that grumpy, angry, sullen git to my party, 'cos it'll be a right blast then'*.

Ok! Ok! I appreciate that no-one can be happy 100% of the time, life just isn't like that but time flies whether you're having fun or not, so if you're the pilot, fly with a smile on ya grill.
C'mon, it's time to uncage your fun monkey.
Stop fretting so much and chill your designer boots!!
Relax, enjoy life and calm the flip down!!

READER: *Easy for you to say, you don't know what my life is like.*
Of course, you're absolutely right.
I understand that it's not as simple as me just telling you to be happy because it's up to you to find the way. But just like exercise, the more you laugh the better you feel about yourself, the more you want to do it and the more positive you become.

At the moment there are probably loads of excuses rolling around your noggin, as to why you're not such a positive person and this possibly explains why you've failed to lose weight in the past. And why you find it almost impossible to fight your depression.

So let's take a look at some of these alleged *'hurdles'* which are obviously a barrier to your levels of happiness, to see how they can be addressed with positivity.

BARRIER - AGE

Maybe you think you're too old in the tooth to keep trying to lose weight?

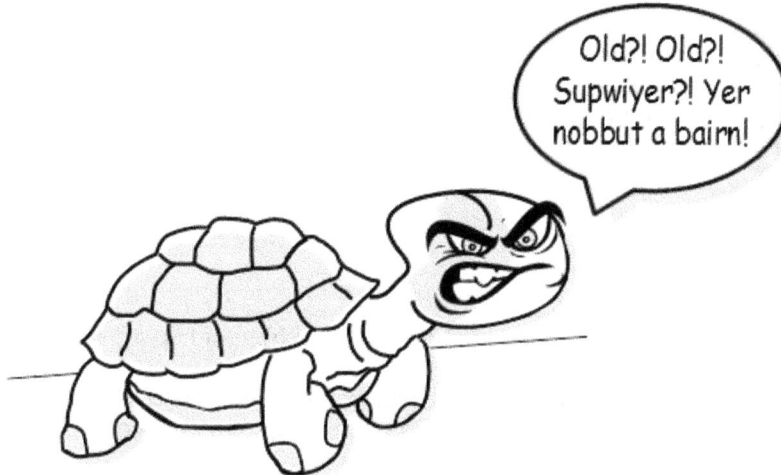

Old?! Old?! Supwiyer?! Yer nobbut a bairn!

How old would you be, if you didn't know how old you were?

READER: *I haven't got bloody Alzheimers you know, I know how old I am.*

I know you do, look, what I'm trying to say is that our age shouldn't define how we act, how fit we are and how we live. Age should **never** be construed as a hindrance to beginning to lose weight, or achieving any goal for that matter, as long as you're passionate and determined about succeeding. And if you're supported and encouraged by family and friends, you'll be fine, no matter how old you are.

We're all getting older but it's better than the alternative and to put a positive spin on it, at least you're not as old as you'll be this time next year.

Life begins at forty,
What a load of crap,
Your sex life's non-existent,
'Cos you'd rather have a nap,
Your hair it is receding,
You've had a better day,
And if you look inside your pants,
Your pubes are turning grey.

Unfortunately, the above poem is the norm for a lot of people but who wants to be normal? It's the magnolia of personality traits, and the most interesting folk in life are those that are definitely not.

I tried to be normal once, worst ten minutes of my life.

My advice is never conform to the norm. There's nothing wrong with getting old, just don't grow up.

And don't ever be one of these…

A **DULL**t

READER: *Yes but you need to act your age when you have responsibilities.*
Bollocks!! You were only young once but you can be immature for a lifetime.

And have you noticed that the word *'immature'* is used by boring people to describe the fun ones?!
The more enjoyment and laughter you have in your life, the more positive you will become and it will become far easier for you to lose weight, get fitter and be happier.
And that's what you want, isn't it? Isn't it?
READER: *Well, yes.*

I'm mature or immature?

It seems that our personalities are determined by punctuation, apostrophes and spaces.

But it's just a choice. You can choose archaic punctuation rules, or you can choose to be a grammar vandal. You can choose to be a boring, miserable, dour faced twonk; or you can choose to mess about, enjoy life and be a right laugh. Choice is yours.

'Young', 'old', 'middle-aged', these are just words, indiscriminate labels, it's how you act that counts.

There's an old Yorkshire saying that seems prescient regarding this topic:

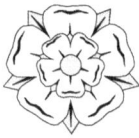

Tha dunt stop laikin', 'cos tha grows old, tha grows old, 'cos tha stops laikin'

READER: *What's laikin' mean?*
Oh! Sorry. Laikin' means *'to play'*… makes sense now doesn't it?!

Old people don't always die due to disease ya know, they pop their orthopaedic shoes 'cos there's no life left in 'em. Physical activity, at even a moderate level puts some pep back into the ol' folk, helping them to age gracefully, not decay like rotten fruit.

How many times have you heard about some ol' dear that's *'had a fall'*?
READER: *Ooh! Yeah, you do.*
Aye!! Too many times for my liking, it's a crying shame.
But physical exertion can strengthen joints and improve balance, reducing the chances of broken hips and hospital trips.

If you ever mentioned to me that you were too old to do summat, I'd slap you round the head with me tweed cap. Then I'd call you a *'Daft Apeth!'* and I'd be well within me rights too.

If you think you're too old to start jogging for example, let me put your mind at rest:

If you can walk, then you're never too old to run

I mean, bloody hell, you don't know how lucky you are; some folk are confined to wheelchairs so don't even have the privilege, and would no doubt swap their little pinkies for the chance to have a stroll or a jog. Look, use 'em, 'cos one day you never know me ol' cocker, you might lose 'em.

In this world today there are seventy year old Tri-Athletes, rowers in their eighties, marathon runners in their nineties and centenarian cyclists. Age and personal bests are just numbers therefore it doesn't add up that age should **ever** be seen as a hindrance.

'They' say that youth is wasted on the young, well I think old-age is wasted on the old. With more energy, just think what could be achieved with all that free time?!

Life has got **nothing** to do with how old you are, it's how fit and healthy you are that counts.

And if you think you're too old to join a gym, think again buttercup 'cos you're completely mistaken.
They'll let anybody in, even **you!!**

You should **never** use your age as an excuse to prevent you achieving any of your goals, there's always a way and a positive mindset is your Sat Nav.

BARRIER - ANGER

Perhaps you're too much of an angry person, to be positive and enjoy life?

In life, you can only control the controllables. So don't blame anyone else for your anger, your mood, and your frustrations. The common denominator is **you!!**

You get angry, **you** get upset and **you** get stressed.
Therefore **you** have the power to change that, it's just a choice.

You generated that negative emotion because you've programmed yourself to deal with situations in that particular way. So if you're angry that's your fault and not the person, or situation you're directing your anger towards.
READER: *Yeah but what if I'm driving and someone cuts me up or...*
Look, you can't control anyone else's driving on the road, unless you're a driving instructor and I don't have you down as a lecherous Perv, so that's out of the question (*only kidding, I love 'em really'*).

There are idiots everywhere and often driving cars with four entwined rings emblazoned on the front bumper. Or they're a taxi driver, who is under the illusion that the Highway Code is merely for other drivers to adhere to, but all you can control is how you react to their lunacy.

What good does it do, screaming at your windscreen, apoplectic at their blatant disregard for other road users? No good at all, they can't hear you so you just get spittle on your dashboard and that's not nice for anyone. Ultimately you want to be safe and secure in your vehicle (especially if you have kids in the car); therefore you need to be calm and composed. Ignore the behaviour of other road users, laugh to yourself and delight in the fact that no doubt they'll be getting a speeding ticket or another three points on their license before the day is up. Where's being angry ever gotten you anyway? It just makes you feel in a right strop for the next few hours and increases your blood pressure.

Did being angry change the person or the situation?
READER: *No, not really.*
No.
Because you can't go back in time and change the past, you're not from Gallifrey, you don't have a *Tardis*...
READER: *What?*
Ask your nerdy brother. Whatever it was, it is over, it has gone. LET... IT...GO.

READER: *But what if someone insults me?*
Ignore it, calm down and chill out.
READER: *But what if someone gives me the finger?*
OMG! An outrage, call the President.

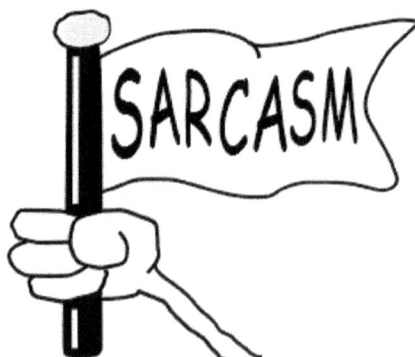

Woop-de-dooby-do. If someone displays their middle finger by extending it and thrusting it in your direction, they're the angry one, they're the one with the issues. There's no law that states you have to respond in kind.

Get a life, it's just a finger, we've all got 'em.

READER *(angry)*: *You get a life, you sanctimonious git!!*
Ooh!! Handbags at dawn. Chill out, tubby!!
READER: *There's no need to get personal, that's mean.*
I'm also sticking two imaginary fingers at you now, what do you think about that?
READER: *Erm… This has got a bit weird, I don't know what to say now?!*

Did that get us anywhere? No.
Are we both flustered? Yes.

It's a complete waste of energy having tit for tat, verbal volleys. Sticks and stones n' all that. It's just not worth it. Count to ten, laugh, take some deep breaths, shake your head, whatever you can do to avoid confrontation. You'll be far happier in the long run. I'm positive about that.

Bureaucracy is often the cause for anger and frustration. But no matter how much you whine and bitch and stamp your feet, they're not gonna change their policies just for you.
So smile.

Thank them for their assistance and politely accept their proposals. And as you walk away smug in the knowledge that their incapacity to adopt common sense has not riled you in the slightest, you can quietly hope that karma gets them instead and bites them on the posterior.

If you don't like something and you have no power or control to change it, laugh about it, you can't do anything about it, so ignore it and let it go man.

There's more to life.

Does anger make you happier? No.
Is it good for your wellbeing? No.
Is it good for your health? **Hell no!!**

If you want to succeed in losing weight, getting fitter and relieving stress, then you **must** change your mindset. You have to accept that loads of stuff will happen in your life that you don't like but because you have no control of the situation, you have to forget it and just move on.
Whatever it is, it's not worth getting angry about.
READER: *What, never?*
Never.

READER: *What about…*
Nope.
No exceptions.

When I was conducting research for this book, I met a personal trainer called Vito, who organised fitness sessions for a very close-knit community in New York City.

He was a lovely bloke, a real stand-up guy, a wise guy, he was a good fella.

His clients were these huge Italian-American men who worked in the Waste Management industry or something, and there seemed to be a lot of issues with contracts.

And I think because of their size, they'd get really tired due to the exercise, 'cos they'd forever go on about *'being whacked'*.

Anyway they had this great mantra that they'd use which would really calm them down whenever they had a beef, or something pissed them off. Vito would overhear these conversations at the gym and he'd use this anger-management technique with his other clients.

It goes something like this:

> SILVIO: *The Boss is really bustin' my balls, man!*
> ANGELO: Hey but Silvio, he's the Boss so wotchagonnado?!
> SILVIO: *Yeah, you're right Angelo. Ah! Fuhgeddaboudit!!*
>
> JUNIOR: *Yo! I'm freakin' out over here, I clipped Jimmy Two Bellies!*
> FRANKIE: You talkin' to me?!
> JUNIOR: *Well I don't see anyone else here.*
> FRANKIE: Alright, alright. But you do know he's not a made guy, right?
> JUNIOR: *He's not connected?*
> FRANKIE: No!!
> JUNIOR *(laughing)*: Hey!! Fuhgeddaboudit!!
>
> VINNIE: *That goomah of mine overcooks the lasagne, every time. She's a piece of work.*
> MARIO: Enough with the complaining, already!
> VINNIE: *Va fa Napoli!! Fuhgeddaboudit!!*

Apparently this method really works, so try it sometime.

All they need now is a solution to their high-carb diet and heavy drinking, then they'll be set.
It was a really tough ask for Vito to encourage healthy nutrition, so I created some tips in the form of inspirational rhymes to really hit home and promote the message for him.

Here's a couple of examples:

ENOUGH WITH THE MEATBALLS AND SPAGHETTI, CAPICHE?
Eat greens and fruit and tuna and quiche.

I'M GONNA MAKE YOU AN OFFER YOU CAN'T REFUSE.
You wanna get healthy? Cut down on the booze.

So wotchagonnado the next time **you** feel yourself getting angry?!
READER *(in best Noo Yawk accent)*: Fuhgeddaboudit?!

BADA BING, BADA BOOM!!

BARRIER - CHANGE

Maybe your capacity to accept change is a contributory factor to your negativity?

Ooh! No-one likes change do they?

We like things the way they are.

But if that was the case we would still be living in huts, hunting deer and painting indecipherable graffiti on cave walls.

Luckily, the times surely are a changin' me ol' mucker.
Everything ch-ch-ch-ch-changes... Oops! Sorry about that, my keyboard's sticking.

Yeah, everything changes, evolves, improves and **you** have to accept that because if you don't move forward, you'll just stay in the same place... and probably go mouldy.

If you're looking to alleviate depression, lose weight or get fitter, naturally there are going to be changes and you must accept that or else you will fail.
Because if what you did before isn't working...
READER: *It isn't working?!*
Exactly!!

Habits have to be adapted or created from scratch, it's not going to be easy, it will be tough, tough, tough but if you stick with it you will succeed... eventually.

The best way to embrace change, is not to do too much too quickly. It's far better to create a new habit than amend an old one because you invariably fall back into your previous ways. The common consensus by psychologists and the like, is that it takes about four weeks for a new habit to kick in and be accepted as a part of your daily routine. So you've gotta stick with it.

And rather than trying to change your entire lifestyle in one day, you should make small amendments instead.
Then the next day assess how that went, could you do it another day and if not, why not?
How can you adapt to make it work?
Are you trying hard enough?
What else can you change?
Are you getting the support you deserve?

If you can look yourself in the mirror and go *'yep, I did EVERYTHING I possibly could today to help me lose weight',* then great.
You can ask no more.
But if you can't say that, you're not doing enough and you need to ask questions of yourself.

If you do have a bad day or even a week, don't get your knickers in a twist, chill and look at what you're doing wrong and what you can adjust so you won't make the same errors again. But if you approach any change in your lifestyle in a negative manner, I guarantee that you will fail.

However, if you adopt a positive approach from the outset, accept that there may be the odd glitch now and again but you're confident that you can deal with it, you will succeed.
READER: *Easier said than done, what if it goes wrong, doesn't quite work out, there's just no point trying.*
Hallo!! What if it works?!

If you relax and don't fret about it, everything will be fine.

Positivity will help, I'm sure of it.
READER: *I'm too old to change.*

29

Absolute nonsense.
People that waffle on saying that a leopard can't change its spots, are off their head. You're not a leopard.

You have the ability to change, no matter how old you are. If pensioners can embrace the culture of social media for example, then you can make some teeny-weeny lifestyle changes.
READER: *What do you mean?*
Well, I've seen the old dears on *'Instagran'* and *'Snap-your-hip-chat'*; they've moved with the times, they're evolving with the Zeitgeist.
So if they can do it, you've no excuses regarding your ability to change.

Change is necessary and **you** need to change.
Change will improve you.
Change will help you lose weight.
Change will help you get fitter.
Change will allow you to actually enjoy life.
Go on, give it a go, at least **try!!**

C'mon, you know what being overweight is like, how about knowing what being thin is like?!
You know what being unfit is like, how about knowing what it's like to finish a half-marathon or an advanced spinning class?!

You know what being lonely is like, how about feeling what not being lonely is like?!

You know how depression makes you feel vulnerable, how the stresses manifest in illness, mood swings and frustration, how about knowing what positivity is like and how you laugh about situations you'd normally fret yourself silly about?

When people ask, *'how are you feeling?'* and you respond and state, *'I'm fine'*, how about actually meaning it?!

Think about it, if you start making positive changes now, some of the best days of your life are yet to come.

BARRIER - Confidence

Is your lack of confidence getting in the way of your fun and positivity?

Maybe you have an inferiority complex and if you do, it's not a very good one.

This is what most people's internal monologue sounds like when trying something new, or making a radical change regarding their lifestyle.

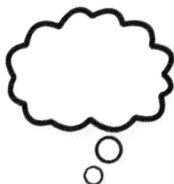

INNER VOICE: *I can do it, yes I can do it, err… no I don't think I can.*
Yes I can… I can't.
I can.
I can't.
Can, can, CANNNNNNNNNNNNNNNNNNNNNNNN!!

No I can't.

Oh my! Just imagine if you were full of confidence, life would be so much simpler.

But there's no magic formula, you can't just shout *'Abracadabra'* and suddenly you exude confidence like a teenager exudes *'Pound-shop'* deodorant.

No, it takes years of practice, self-reflection, self-evaluation and learning from your mistakes.

You have got to believe in yourself and it should be the loudest voice you ever hear. No excuses, no niggling doubts, just take some risks now and again or your life will never change for the better.

Most of us don't like trying something new, 'cos it makes us feel uncomfortable, uneasy. Tense. Nervous. Self-conscious.

So we make up some excuse that allows us to live safe and secure in our little comfort zone.
However, if you repeat a lie often enough it becomes a truth and as a consequence, you become imprisoned by the walls you build yourself.
READER: *No I don't, I'm not listening, Ner! Ner! Nerner! Ner!!*

The key to managing that fear is to do the very thing that frightens us. That's the best way to destroy **any** fear.

Do it until you're no longer scared, or the fear will own you because every time you choose safety, you just reinforce fear.
READER: *But I don't want to make a fool of myself.*
Hey!! It's never too late.
Anyway, what's wrong with looking foolish?
READER: *It's embarrassing.*

Bloody hell mate.

Who cares what strangers *'may'* or *'may not'* think about you?

It has no significant bearing on your life. Anyway they're probably thinking *'I remember when I started, I was just like that'*.

So rather than getting all shy and awkward, laugh about it instead but don't worry about it.

Who cares if you make a few mistakes anyway? That's how you learn. You do know that every expert was once a beginner?! That's a life lesson, my friends, **boo ya!!**

Please remember it.
Let yourself go, you'll enjoy life a whole lot more.

Have you ever just sat in the car trying to pluck up the courage to go to a slimming club, or take a fitness class but you became so anxious, worried that people might stare, you wimped out and drove off instead?
READER: *Yeah, I have done that.*
Well the next time I bet it was worse and so on and so forth, and it will be until you get out of the car, confront that fear and take a walk into the unknown.

We're all so worried that people are watching and judging us but in reality, they're thinking the same thing. Although having said that, most people at the gym are too engrossed on their own workout and their hair, make up, biceps, fake tan lines, cute girl on reception etc, etc to worry about you.

So don't fret, they won't be paying you any attention, 'cos they'll be so busy checking themselves out, to even notice the newbie.

MARK, 30 - *I used to pretend that the real reason I wasn't trying to lose weight was because it just didn't bother me. But that couldn't have been further from the truth.*
People in my situation, we tell ourselves that it's not worth the effort because the truth is, we're simply too scared of failing and then what?
Yes, we partially try it but don't put the full effort in, or we over analyse the situation to the point of paralysis... and end up doing nothing.
Luckily for me a friend gave me your number and after finally plucking up the courage to call, we met up for a chat, and I never looked back.
You once told me that a pessimist is so worried that people will gawp at them, they refuse to go to the gym but an optimist is already on the treadmill.
Well Birchy, now I'm a regular on that running machine. Cheers buddy.

I can guarantee that there will be people in gyms, fitness classes and slimming clubs who feel **and** felt just like you.
READER: *How do you know that?*
Because you're not unique, you're not some pretty lil' snowflake, there are **millions** of people who have similar doubts, issues and worries as yourself. Sorry to burst that bubble.

In fact, someone bigger than **you** in this world, has just this minute finished their workout.

They were embarrassed initially but once they realised that other people couldn't really give a toss and if anything, have huge respect for them for trying to change and take some action; they just got on with it.

It's never as bad as you think it will be... apart from burpees, they're worse.

If you don't like dogs, stroke a dog. Although select the right one first, so not those yappy, hamster types, they're like bloody animals them. Try a Labrador or a Terrier and you'll notice that they actually enjoy it and don't want to devour you limb from limb.

The more you stroke... Hey!! Behave yourself. The more you stroke these dogs, the less jittery and nervous you'll feel the next time you come across... erm, the next time you encounter one. And after a while you'll start to feel comfortable in the presence of these hairy, slobbering, beasts of Beelzebub.

If you're worried about learning to drive, just give it a go.

It's never as dangerous as you imagine and Mr Lecherous Perv has the ability to control the pedals too, so it's unlikely you'll cause an accident.

You might even pass when I did… seventh time lucky.
READER: *WHAT?!*
That's right, you read correctly. I passed on the seventh time, (long story, I'll tell you over a few drinks some day).

Each time I failed, naturally I got disheartened but rather than just quitting, I tried again… and again… and again… and again… and again and… **again!!**

So how's that for Percy Verance?! But it just goes to show that if you stick with something and keep giving it your best shot, eventually, you'll succeed. Remember that when you face any hurdle and start the long process of dropping those pounds, or salvation from the misery of depression.

If you're afraid of the water, forget about looking cool, strap some armbands on and learn to swim. It might even save your life and it's great for low-level exercise. We'll discuss it later in the book and I'll tell you about my swimming lessons.

If you're afraid of heights then get the elevator to the top floor and peer out of the window, or go balls out and do a tandem-parachute jump (not literally), or fly in a hot air balloon (awesome experience, just be prepared for an ungraceful landing). Never be scared of heights, be afraid of widths… especially around your waist.

If you're petrified of spiders, pick up a spider… Ok! Sorry, I realise I've gone too far now, there's always exceptions but I think you get the picture.

If you're anxious about screwing up or looking foolish, don't fret about it, these are common worries. No-one's infallible. Congratulations you're not a freak; you're just another human being, trying your hardest, giving it your best.

There's nothing wrong with being afraid, but if you challenge and face your fears with a smile on your face, these fears will eventually lose their hold over you and then you're finally free.

It will also give you the confidence to tackle other challenges, fears and negative concerns.
You'll go from self-conscious to self-assured.

READER: *Well it sounds like a doddle but I bet it's not as simple as that.*
Ok! I'll give you a perfect example.
Can you ride a bike?
READER: *Yes but so what?! It's easy and I was a kid.*
But think about the first few times you tried.

It's so scary when you first attempt to ride a bike, luckily someone helps guide you along, gently holding onto your side and then only letting go when they think you're in control. When you realise it's just you manoeuvring, you panic and start to flip out.

You wobble from side to side but then after you've pedalled a few times and managed to steer yourself in the right direction, you gain confidence, it becomes a lot easier and you let go of your fears.

You then forget what all the fuss was about. That epitomises perfectly what attempting something new is like, and we've all done it before in some way or another, and we'll all do it again.

Riding a bike, is actually a great metaphor for life. To get to any destination, you've got to keep pedalling and look forward. You'll fall off occasionally and it will hurt like hell but you'll have some great scars to show for it (chicks dig scars, man!!).

You might get a puncture or swallow a few bugs; but whenever you're freewheeling downhill, it's such a thrill that you won't have a care in the world. Sometimes you'll have to pedal uphill and it'll be tough, it'll be demanding, it'll be a struggle. You can take the easier option and get off the bike and push. Or you can push yourself instead and climb to the top.

It's a choice and it's up to **you** whether you decide to ride the rest of your life with the stabilizers on, or with them off.

Here's a little tip to improve your confidence, or what the young 'uns call... 'Swagga'.

tip   Have a theme song in your head whenever you're about to embark on a challenging situation.

READER: *Say what?!*
You've seen *'Saturday Night Fever'* haven't you? If not get it on Nowflix or Skynet, or whatever they're called this month.

The opening credits show Travolta looking the coolest that any man has ever looked, whilst holding a tin of paint.

He's not just walking; he's strutting, sashaying down the street.

He knows everyone's looking at him, checking him out... probably thinking, *'he is, isn't he, it'll be okay mate, just admit it?!'*

That bloke just oozes confidence, nothing is gonna faze that man. It's as if he's got the grooviest, funkiest DJ's in the world privately spinning tunes in his noggin.

You could do the same, well you don't have to walk this way, unless your song is by Run DMC.

Music releases endorphins, it improves creativity and raises serotonin levels (your happy hormone) but you've got to pick one that's upbeat and puts you in good spirits, so nothing by Nick Drake or Leonard Cohen.

READER: *Have you got one?*
Of course.
Mine is by The Stone Roses and gives you a wonderful insight into my musical taste and level of arrogance.
READER: *What is it then?*
It's the one about a deity coming back to life.
READER: *Don't know that one.*
Well, it's called, *'I am the Resurrection'*.
READER: *Oh! Nice one, Mr Narcissism, a bit of a messiah complex have we?*
Hey!! Don't besmirch the Birch... and I ask the questions around here.

Find a soundtrack that works for **you** and the next time you have a job interview, or a date, or you're starting a new challenge, just press play in your mindbox and visualise yourself succeeding as your theme song resonates in the background... although, don't mouth the words at the same time.

BARRIER - EFFORT

You're a lazy git and can't be arsed trying to lose weight?

1) RACISTS
2) LITTER
3) NEGATIVITY
4) LAZINESS
5) MANCHESTER UNITED
6) THE CONSERVATIVE PARTY
7) CURRANTS
8) DATES
9) RAISINS
10) SULTANAS

My top ten chart of stuff that I have personally encountered, which I absolutely despise and they are rated in order of annoyance.

I'll briefly mention each category throughout the book but let's take a look at the CBA brigade.
READER: *CBA brigade, what's that?*
People that utter the immortal words - *'can't be arsed'*.

It does my nut in when people act lazy. There's **never** a legitimate excuse for slothful behaviour. Unless you're a sloth of course, then feel free to indulge and enjoy your idle sluggishness, my little sloth-dudes!!

The most irritating and frustrating trait regarding anybody trying to lose weight or get fit, is the inane and moronic excuses they use to get out of putting in some effort.

- I can't be arsed going to the gym, I'm tired.
- I can't be arsed walking to school to pick up the kids, it's spitting so I'll drive instead.
- I can't be arsed washing up, I'll do it tomorrow, maybe, or the day after, if I can be bothered.
- I can't be arsed climbing those stairs to the second floor, I'll get the lift.
- I can't be arsed getting up early on a Saturday to go for a jog.
- I can't be arsed nipping to that shop down the road, I'll drive to the supermarket tomorrow.
- I can't be arsed cooking, so I'll order a takeaway.
- I can't be arsed trying to lose weight, it's too much effort, so I'll just moan to everyone instead about how difficult it is to actually take some action, rather than getting off my couch-potato-sore-arse and being pro-active.
- I can't be arsed typing another sen...

It's a wonder that these people actually have the energy for lethargy.

You don't have to strive for perfection or excellence, or to be the best, you just have to **try!!**

Look, if you don't **want** to lose weight that's fine but don't ever moan again when you're getting fatter and fatter, and you've got to buy bigger clothes, and your health is getting worse and worse.

But if you do, stop going on about it, get off your whiny, whingeing, saggy arse and do something about it.
READER: *That's a bit harsh.*
Well, the truth hurts. It's ugly. It's hard to hear and difficult to accept, but it's bloody necessary if you want to lose weight or change your life for the better. And you do. That's why you're reading this book.

When you or anyone else adopts the CBA attitude, you're just putting off problems, hoping that they'll magically disappear and life just isn't like that. You have to deal with issues head on, or else they get bigger and bigger and

BIGGER!!

Take some chuffin' responsibility for your problems. No-one can do it for you.

When you can't be arsed washing up, or tidying your house, or going for a walk, or cooking something nutritious to eat; not only does it reinforce your lazy mindset, it's also an indication that you have no respect for yourself. And that's not good for you. That has to change.

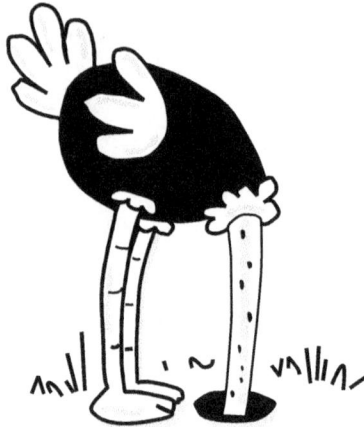

You want motivation? You want something that'll make you snap into action? Look in the mirror.
READER: *What?*
Look in the mirror. Spend a few minutes really studying your reflection.
Look at your face, then down to your body and really stare at those curves and rolls of flab.
If you're genuinely happy with what you're looking at, fine, no problem, just move on with your life and don't worry about it anymore.
However, if you're not, then it's about time that you started to wake up and make some positive changes.
No more excuses, you can't blame anyone else, it's entirely up to you. But you know this more than anyone else, so what's stopping you?
READER: *I've got an underactive thyroid, so I just get really tired all of the time and I have no energy.*
Ok! Here we go, this excuse is a beauty. Tiredness is a common symptom of having an underactive thyroid, I accept that but this doesn't mean you can't **try** and attempt to lose weight.

Your thyroid gland may be tiny, but yep it does play a big role in how well your body functions. That's because the thyroid produces a hormone that regulates your metabolism, the process that converts what you eat and drink, to energy.

When you have *'Hypothyroidism'*, or an *'Underactive Thyroid'*, your metabolism slows, causing you to gain weight more easily and feel sluggish and fatigued. Medical fact, I've no issue with that.

An underactive thyroid is usually treated by taking daily hormone replacement tablets (see your GP), and these will help you maintain a balanced and healthy metabolism. The majority of people feel back to their normal selves quite soon after beginning treatment.

Adopting a healthier diet that cuts out processed sugars and is rich in Iron, Selenium and Omega 3 will also help, as will low-level exercise and anything that alleviates stress.

It seems that laughter really is the best medicine. Ha! Ha! Ha!… **LOL**.

SALLY, 39 - *I used to love playing netball when I was a teenager, so much so that I actually represented my school and the County at national events.*
But as I got into my working life, I stopped playing and as a consequence my fitness depreciated. Then I had a child.
I'd put on about 3 stone during the pregnancy, I was forever tired and hungry but as a new Mum running around, I thought I'd lose it all.
I didn't.
I put on another 2 stone. It was so upsetting, I was constantly exhausted, I hated the way I looked and I felt incredibly low. After a visit to my GP it turned out that I had an underactive thyroid which had a considerable bearing on my weight gain. The takeaways, alcohol and cakes may have contributed too!!
I was prescribed medication but I was also advised to take up walking and make some substantial changes to my diet. Seeing you helped me get fitter and although it's been a slow process, I have managed to lose 3 and a half stone in the last year. I know that if I continue with your advice, I will lose the rest. I've also started to play netball again for a local team. I don't race around as much as I used to and I think the league might be out of the question but it's been fun nevertheless.

Next excuse…

READER: *I might fail, it's too hard, it might not work.*
I've told you, it's all about… **POSITIVITY.**

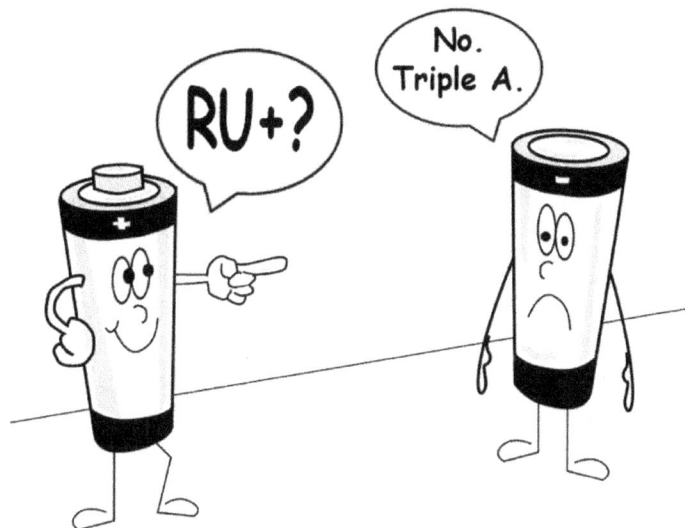

You have to truly believe that you will succeed. You have to relish the challenges, embrace the changes. All it takes is for you to implement one positive act into your daily life and you're on your way.

It will work. Believe it **baby!!** It worked for me.

But you have to force yourself to do things. Force yourself to get up out of bed each day and make changes. Force yourself to the gym. Force yourself to plan your meals. Force yourself to make a packed lunch. Force yourself to go for a walk. Force yourself to drink more water. Force yourself to act positively. Force yourself to turn the idiot-box off. Force yourself to learn how to cook. Force yourself to change your mind.

After that, it's all about repetition. It's all about repetition. It's all about repetition.
It's all about REP… ET… ITION.

The more you do any act, the easier it becomes and the less effort it takes.
It becomes a habit. It becomes part of your weekly routine. As a consequence, you boost and improve your self-discipline and it becomes your new way of life. However, the more you put it off, the harder and harder it becomes. Remember, you're doing this for **you** and no-one else can do it for you. You can't get a man in.

The only person stopping you from getting a healthy, fit body... is yourself.

And it's not about being better than everyone else; it's about being better than **you** used to be. Oh! And that bloke from work, I can't stand him.

Look, some people want it to happen, some people wish it would happen and others have just finished their workout at the gym.

Yes, you're going to struggle. Yes, you're going to have days where you'll want to give up. Yes, you're going to have weeks that make you wonder if it's worth it.

That's where the positive mindset comes in, and when you see the progress, no matter how slow it is, you'll realise it's the best thing you've ever done.

PARVEEN, 38 – *I actually lost 7.5 pounds in the first week* but this steadied to a pound, 2 pounds a week, sometimes staying the same. I knew if I had the patience, all the effort and hard work was worth it. After a month though, I could feel that my clothes were getting looser and I had more energy. When I saw my reflection, I could tell that I was getting slimmer, it was working. And when family and friends noticed too, I knew I had to continue. I actually started to look forward to the healthy meals you'd suggested that only weeks before I would've shunned. When I reached my first target weight it's hard to describe how I felt, I was so proud of myself, so elated and relieved but I didn't want the feeling to stop, I wanted more. I used to be greedy for chips and pies, now I'm just greedy for more success.*

*NB: There is a lot of water located in stored fat, which is generally the first to go in weight loss, sometimes quite rapidly but this slows down after the first week or so. This leads the dieter to doubt success because they're not losing the weight by the same ratio. Therefore the effort that is put in, seems counter-productive BUT this is not the case. I recommend that you gauge weight loss by your reflection, tightness of clothes, energy levels etc, etc **and not** just by numbers on the scale.

CHARLOTTE, 34 – *As you know, in the last few years I put on a good 3 stone and even though I knew it was a problem, I didn't really know what to do about it. You mentioned going for walks but I didn't really have the time and on an evening I just wanted to chill and relax, after being on my feet all day at work. My ex has the bairns on a weekend but I love a nice lie-in, so I couldn't go for walks then either. I'm fully aware that I eat far too much sweet stuff but it's really difficult to cut down, and I like a few glasses of cider on a Friday and Saturday night so I'm not stopping that either. I will do something about my weight at some point but it's just not the right time at the moment, what with the problems with my ex and my issues with work. I'll do it, I will, just not yet...*

Two different clients, two different outlooks and approaches to life.
Well, my advice to them both and to you is simple:

Weight loss is just like sex.
You don't stop, when it starts to get hard.

BARRIER - WORRIES

Do you moan and worry too much to be happy?

We all hate hard work and doing things in a different way than we're used to, but rather than gritting our teeth and just bloody getting on with it, we moan about it instead.
We just love a moan don't we?
We're a nation of moaners.
In fact, if moaning burned calories, you'd burn so much you'd have nothing to moan about.

Oh! No! It's gonna rain, it's a bit too cold for me,
It's not fair, it's too hard, are we having that for tea?
The sun's in my eyes, that just won't do,
Life is so difficult, boo fuckin' hoo!!

We're extremely molly-coddled as a society, so here are some inspirational words to help pull you out of your comfort zone:

Always look on the bright side of life & stop
being a whinging, mithering, mawngy git!!
If you've got yourself a kettle, then you can
always make yourself a brew.

Moaning about stuff is like lounging on a rocking chair; it gives you something to do but it gets you nowhere.

Whenever you think you have a problem or a worry, take a step back and assess it objectively.
There will always be a simple solution. You can sort it, so calm down. It's not the end of the world.

It's gonna be alright.

SO STOP FUCKIN' MOANING!!

Just watch the news for a few hours, then re-evaluate.

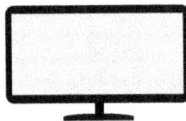

Terrorism, mass migration, tsunamis, unemployment, hurricanes, starvation, war, military coups, wildfires, earthquakes, rape, tax evasion, asteroids, revenge porn, grooming, debt, death, murder, death, bombs, death, beheading, death and more bloody **DEATH**.

But fair enough you've broken a nail, or someone's put that thing back in the wrong place, or you've misplaced a receipt, or you have to visit the dentist, or there's a scratch on your car.

Get… a… bloody… **grip!!**

Worries are illusions, tricks, just a mirage of the mind. We think we see them but they're just constructs of the imagination, not tangible, not real. Just temporary blips, nothing to fret about and there are always straight forward solutions to these *'alleged'* problems.

So stop being a bloody **drama queen!!**

And repeat after me – *'Women are like clouds and when they disappear, life is brighter'.*

READER: *WHAT?!*
Ooops! Sorry, I meant *'worries'*, worries are like clouds... WAHEY!! Only jesting!!
C'mon what's up with ya?! I'm only having a laugh, just turn that frown upside down, you're only winning when you're grinning... there you go.

Here's a few tips to help reduce your fretting (about some stuff anyway):

tips

Always try to plan for the morning, the night before. This enables you to stop rushing around in your sleepy pyjama state and lessens the likelihood you'll forget something.

Don't rely on your memory, write it down. It may seem daft but carry a small notebook on your person. If you're a bloke, put it in a coat pocket. If you're a lady then place it your over-sized, over-priced handbag. You can then write down all that important info your mind always seems to forget because you fill it up with status updates, celebrity gossip and weather info.

READER: *Nice one Grandad but SMART phones have a notebook facility on them, so I could use that instead.*
Ooh!! Look at you, technohead. Well why do you always forget stuff then, Hey?! Hey?! **HEY?!**
Whatever works for you, just be careful that the more you rely on scroll functionality, the more likely it is that one day you'll forget how to actually write.

tips

Make duplicate keys. This seems obvious but we never seem to get round to it, maybe if we'd written it down in a notebook perhaps.

READER: *Touché!!*
If it's for your house/shed/vibrator safe-box, hand the spares to your parents or someone you trust. Then those days of being locked out (and found out) are over.

tips

Always make copies of important papers. Same principle as the keys. Give someone you can trust the copies and you'll start to feel your worries disappear

Stop living for tomorrow when today is still around. Live in the **now** and stop regretting things that haven't even happened yet. If today isn't over, enjoy it.

Always have a Plan B, C, D, X etc, etc because this prepares you for a multitude of eventualities and allows you to make quick decisions, fret free.

Stop putting that thing off that you've been meaning to do for ages and **DO IT!!** Today.

Clean out your wardrobes/drawers and get rid of the clutter. This advice seems to be in every copy, of every female magazine I've ever skim read but it's actually great advice. If you've not worn it, watched it, read it or moved it in over a year, you're not gonna. So get rid.
This is such a cathartic experience that it declutters your mind too. Plus you can get into more debt, buying more clothes you won't wear. **Result!!**

How many times have you worried yourself sick about something and nothing bad actually happened?

Loads of bloody times, that's how many. You have to stop fretting, it's not worth the stress, so instead, try and spend your valuable time on this earth in a positive mindset, and you'll be a whole lot happier.

Not convinced? Ooh, you're so negative...

BARRIER - NEGATIVITY

You're such a negative ninny that you find it difficult to be positive

---

Person A: *Ooh! It's gorgeous outside.*
Person B: Yeah but it'll probably be raining later.

Person A: *Good win for the lads yesterday.*
Person B: Yeah but they'll no doubt lose the next game.

Person A: *That beer is lush mate you can really taste the banana.*
Person B: It should be at that price!!

Person A: *I'm having a really good time, you?*
Person B: It's alright, a bit late for me and it's a *'school night'* so I'm gonna head home in a bit.

Person A: *That's a cracking TV you've got there.*
Person B: Thanks but there's never anything on worth watching.

Person A: *Ooh! Those flowers smell delightful.*
Person B: They'll probably die soon.

Person A: *That jacket is nice, I really like it.*
Person B: Cheers but it's one of those that needs dry cleaning, so that'll be a pain.

Person A: *You ordered a lovely meal at that restaurant.*
Person B: Not as nice as yours though.

Person A: *Ooh! Your hair looks lovely.*
Person B: It should do… it cost a bloody fortune.

Some people are just miserable buggers aren't they?! They just seem to ooze moroseness. Mardy bums, the lot of 'em.

You probably know someone like that? Every answer they give to your questions seems to have a negative connotation.

Perhaps I'm actually describing **you?**

Well if that's the case, you've gotta sort your swede out. Rather than looking through turd coloured spectacles, start trying to smell the roses. Life ain't all that bad you know and if you want to succeed in losing weight and waving bye-bye to the blues, you must get rid of your negative outlook.

Maybe your partner's a misery guts, or your mates, or even your family? If that's the case then my advice is simple, stop spending time with them.
READER: *I can't do that…*
Look, it's true of any personality trait. If you hang around with negative people, you become negative.
If you hang around with people who order takeaways all the time, you're gonna put on the lard.

But if you hang around with healthy, fit, vibrant, funny people, it rubs off. And you'll change, for the better. It's no walk in the park trying to lose weight, it's an ordeal but like any challenge, negativity just becomes a hindrance.

You've gotta chuck those negative vibes away.

When a mountaineer climbs a mountain, they don't just jump to the top. It's a long and gruelling journey, each step carefully taken at a slow and controlled pace.

Yes, when they get to the summit the view is amazing **Blah!! Blah!! Blah!!**

But the real achievement lies in the incredible amount of effort, hard work and pain it takes to accomplish the ascent. And without a positive outlook, not only would they fail; they could even die, or put fellow mountaineers in danger. The constant agony they endure along the way can either be utilised for negativity, leading to frustration, fatigue and pessimism, or positivity, which can drive them on. It's a choice and you have the option to make similar choices too, when you attempt to lose weight.

With respect to all areas of your life, rather than focusing on the negatives, appreciate what you've got and how **lucky** you really are; try to see the positives and then you'll slowly start to find happiness.

When you find yourself about to say something negative in response to a question, or you're making an observation, take a few seconds and see if you can actually find something constructive, or optimistic to say instead.

The more you repeat this exercise, the more positive you'll start to become.

And then you'll start to notice this thing on your face called a *'smile'* and this warm, tingly, glowing feeling in your stomach, called a *'heart'*. You might even start to become *'happy'* and have some *'fun'*.

READER: *Aye but it won't bloody last long though will it?!*
AAARRRGGGHHH!!

I will keep banging on and on about positivity throughout this book, so **it's up to you** whether you embrace this specific outlook on life or not but as I keep saying, your chances of success are greatly reduced the more negative you are.

Don't be so glum, chum.

BARRIER – REGRET

Maybe you're just stuck in the past which doesn't allow you to actually move on?

As I've already mentioned, in this day and age, most people have some form of mild depression.

This clearly contributes towards feelings of negativity, which leads to weight gain in those people who deal with their emotions by eating.

But if you think you're depressed, you're probably reliving the past too much. If you're anxious, you're living in the future. If you're at peace, you're living in the present.
And if you're a Man Utd fan, there really is no hope for you.

Let me tell you now, the past was **never** as good as your mind lets you imagine it to be, it eradicates the bad stuff and just concentrates on the good. The Directors Cut, censoring the scenes we'd rather not think about and eulogising about the acts we long to replay over and over again.
Why do you think that is?
READER: *I don't know?!*
Well it's your mind, change it.
Your mind is who **you** are. Therefore if you change your mind, you can be anything you want. You can alter your mood, your perceptions, your feelings. But only **you** can change your mind.

With respect to the past, good or bad, every single thing that has happened in your life... has happened.

It can't happen again, you can't relive the past, no matter how hard you try. You can't go back and change it. It's gone. It's been laminated. The past is written, the ink is dry.

Hindsight is a wonderful thing but you can't erase the past, no matter how much you think about it, so stop fretting and move on. If you're wracked with guilt over some past event, then do your absolute utmost to rectify it and hopefully you'll receive forgiveness.

But if you don't receive forgiveness, even though you've tried your best to atone, move on. Just make sure you learn from your mistakes and don't make them again. You need to be aware that what you do today is actually creating your future.

The words you speak, your thought processes, the foods you eat and the actions taken are all shaping your destiny and what you will become. So don't keeping looking back, you're not going that way. You need to live in the present, in the **now!!**

You can't pause life	So stop moaning	Change the record	And stop rewinding to the past	Focus on the future	And always make time to play

What's the point, of internally chastising yourself about the bad stuff anyway? It's not just that bloke stuck to a cross with the great abs who can forgive you know. There's no point hating and punishing yourself.
What good comes of that?

Let other people hate you instead, 'cos you're happy, healthy, fit, positive and **smoking hot!!**

BARRIER - FAILURE

You've failed so many times before, so why will it work this time?

The reason it's going to work is because this time, you're going to get the specific HELP you need. You might be a little pessimistic now but once you've finished reading this book and started to make changes, you just won't fail. When you adopt a positive mindset, you'll quit the quitting.

Ok! You might have failed in the past but that just means you've found methods and ways that don't work. They're just blips, speed bumps on the highway to victory. All you have to do is learn from your mistakes and make sure you don't repeat them.

Adversity should make you stronger, not weaker, as long as you learn the lessons that were on offer and use them to grow.

Here are three possible reasons, as to why you have failed in the past:

Number 1 - You spent years filling those sacks of adipose tissue with extra fat calories, but for some obscure reason you expected them to empty in the space of a few weeks or months. And because you didn't get the miraculous results you hoped for, you decided to quit. What you needed was patience, patience, **PATIENCE**.

Number two - You got on the smoothie, kale and quinoa bandwagon but after you'd prepared a healthy meal you looked at it and thought eeuurrgghh!! It looked too bland, revolting even, and the only thought on your mind was to eat something taboo, something unhealthy. So you chucked the healthy meal in the bin and gorged on a full block of cheese, washed down with a litre of fizzy pop.

Everyone is allowed a bad day... or three. The secret is not to get het up about it and just make sure that the next day you get back to the healthy stuff. Or you incorporate a bad diet day into every week, so you can look forward to some treats. You don't just stop when you hit the first hurdle. You leap the bugger and head for the next challenge.

Number three - You decided to do an early run, you know, to get it out of the way so you could then enjoy your freedom. You hear the alarm blaring and decide you are just too tired, you can't be arsed. Then you decide running isn't for you, knock it on the head and get back to the old routine. Of course you failed you didn't enjoy it, so you were always destined to fail. You've gotta relish it, or you're onto a losing battle.

Let's get real. When you decide to get fit or adapt your diet, this is a new world to you. You've spent, I don't know how long living a certain way, so to just change and expect life to be plain sailing is just ridiculous. It takes time.

When you told your family and friends you'd quit another diet or fitness fad, how did it make you feel?
READER: *Terrible. I was... embarrassed that I'd failed... again.*
Exactly!!
You know what quitting feels like, so wouldn't it be nice to feel what *'not quitting'* is like?!

And if that unwelcome thought ever enters your melon again and you think about quitting, think about **why** you're doing it in the first place.

When an *'alleged'* obstacle is put in front of you or if you hit a wall, just try and get over it and forget about being graceful, smash right through. Bruised and cut shins are optional but that's why God invented plasters.

A major reason why people give up so fast, is because they tend to look at **how far** is left to go, rather than **how far** they've actually come.

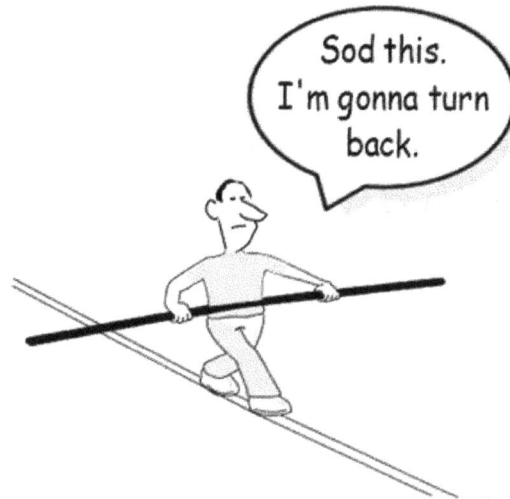

So the minute you think of giving up, think of the reason you held on for so long. You have to tell yourself that even though you might not be there yet, you're further than yesterday. Pain is temporary but quitting can last forever.

Long-term weight loss, fitness, happiness, positivity etc, etc is all about **U** and it's a simple choice:

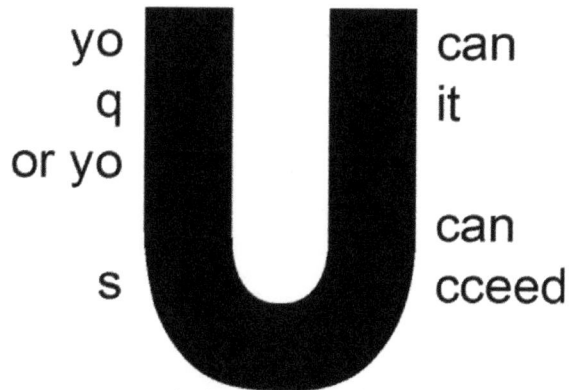

It might be a slow process; it might take longer than you hoped but as long as you're making progress, that's what really counts. I know you don't want to hear that, you want miracles but unfortunately you ain't gonna get 'em.

Anyway, I'm telling ya, I've a good feeling about you.

You're not a *'gunner'* and you're not a quitter, you're a *'progressor'*.

And progress is always a *'work in progress'*. So strive for progression not perfection because you'll never achieve that anyway.

Remember this time last year, well how did you feel about yourself and your weight then?

READER: *I didn't feel great about myself and I was overweight.*

If you start making changes once you've read this book, then this time next year, imagine where you'll be?

I'll tell you where you'll be, you'll be thinner, fitter, happier, healthier, sexier... So who gives a shizzle whether you've failed in the past or not.

This time, with a positive mindset and with my HELP, you won't fail again.

Okay doke! Now that I've nagged the negative knickers off you talking about positivity, the next chapter will deal with another key element of HELP... **Life.**

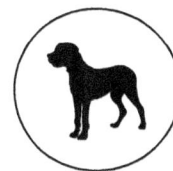

LIVING & ENJOYING LIFE

'You only live once' according to the young 'uns but they are... **wrong!!**

You actually **live** every day but you die only once, unless you're Jon Snow (ask your nerdy Brother again, although he is a character from the biggest, most talked about show on the telly-box so where've you been Grandma?!).

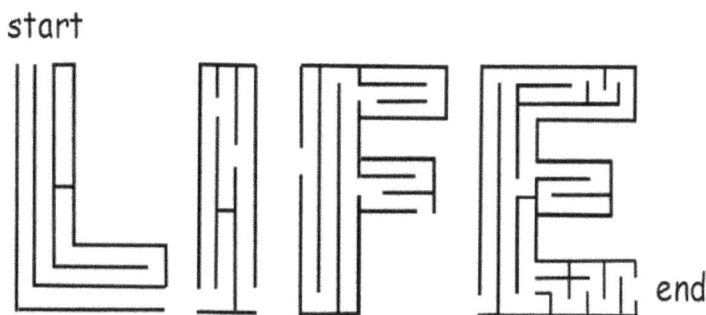

start

LIFE

end

Yep, death is certainly an obstacle to the fun life alright but do you want to know the secret to happiness?
READER: *Yes please.*
It's breathing.

If every day that you live is a day closer to death, then we've gotta start living now before it's too late.
Because death is just like premature ejaculation... it comes far too quickly.

You may be under the misapprehension that **money** is our biggest commodity but it's not, it's **time** and we waste it every single day. The well will run dry and then what? Eventually there is no tomorrow.
READER: *Blimey you're a right barrel of laughs you!*
Shut Up!! I'm trying to make a point, so just like your weight loss goals, have patience.

I'm not a religious man but there's a Jewish prayer which is extremely apt regarding the subject of mortality, and when translated states;

Let me not die, whilst I am still alive.

Therefore if you're just surviving from your late twenties onwards, then that's not living, it's just existing and where's the fun in that?! You don't want to have peaked already.

Dude just 'cos you're breathin, that doesn't mean **you're alive!!**

In the last few minutes in this Country alone, someone has just had a stroke and died, someone else has been involved in a fatal car accident and another has just committed suicide because they couldn't cope with their depression (Hey! Some of us have been too close for comfort on that score).

But rather than focusing on enjoying life and undertaking new experiences, too many people worry about trying to find themselves, trying to get the answer to one of life's eternal, pointless questions:

?   *Who am I and where am I going?*

If you're one of those types of people trying to find themselves, I have something to say to you that will help you answer this quandary.

You're right bloody there mate reading this book and you're **going** to die. You're nowt spesh either, just a regular, run of the mill, normal person.
Okay?! OK.

Don't be wasting your time trying to work out the meaning of life; they'll just change it anyway.

Here's a ditty to honour your birth,
To celebrate your inception,
Let's raise a toast, to your Ma and your Pa,
'Cos they forgot to use protection.

I feel it would be remiss of me not to inform you of this important fact, but you're just an accident of nature. You're only here because of a split condom, or your Mum didn't take the morning-after pill, or England actually won a football game at a major tournament.

You're actually very lucky to have the pleasure of living on this amazing planet.

So how do you show your appreciation to the angels of providence? You spend your days in jobs you hate and then your evenings glued to the idiot box.

C'mon!! Life's too short to live the same day twice.

When old fogies in Nursing Homes are interviewed regarding their lives, no-one wishes they'd made more money, had more possessions or spent more time at work. The vast majority (irrespective of which country they are from or their ethnic background) say they wished they'd spent more valuable time with their family and friends, looked after themselves better, encountered new experiences and travelled more.

Soooooooooooo…?!!

!!! THIS IS NOT A DRILL !!! THIS IS NOT A DRILL!!! THIS IS NOT A DRILL!!! THIS IS NOT A DRILL!!!

We're all dying you know, it's from a virus that is eating away at our bodies **every** single second.
It's called **life** and the only cure is death, and the Reaper's glistening scythe is remorseless and inevitable.
Just ponder that thought, I know I have many a time and frankly it's scary.

And because I passionately care and want to help you, here are a few paragraphs to really stamp that thought to your noggin'. It's not for the faint hearted but read them a few times so you truly understand the gravity of what's in store.

If it doesn't inspire you to take some action and make some positive changes, then nothing will.

Whether you're skinny, blonde, left-handed, unemployed, a tax-avoider or a tally-ho-mo-fo-fox-foe, your body is likely to die in exactly the same disgusting way as everyone else.

Once the last bit of oxygen in your body is used up, the brain stops secreting hormones that regulate bodily functions and starts the brief process of shutting down. The last of your energy stores are used and you stop breathing, which means each cell is then starved of oxygen. The sphincter begins to unclench and starts to relax, causing the body to release urine and excrement. Don't be embarrassed by the disgusting stench, after all, you're about to die.

Between 15 and 25 minutes after death, the lack of blood flow to capillaries causes the skin to go pale. Tan-Fantastique isn't going to help you then.
The heart stops beating, so blood is no longer being propelled around the body. As a result, the blood pools in the lower parts of the body. After about 12 hours, the skin will have reached maximum discoloration and turns a reddish purple, 'Fergie-nose', type colour.

Calcium leaks into muscle cells, binding to proteins which are in charge of muscle contraction. This leads to stiffness (no Viagra required) which is commonly known as 'rigor mortis', and sets in three to six hours after death, lasting for between 24 and 48 hours.

Dead cells and carbon dioxide causes the PH level of your skin tissue to rise. This makes the cell membrane weak and it bursts, releasing proteins and enzymes which further break down the surrounding tissue. This is your body decomposing and boy does it whiff.

Micro-organisms start to break down your entire body and bacteria in the gastro-intestinal tract eats through the abdominal organs. This process is called 'putrefaction', and the body starts to pong even more.

The breakdown of amino acids creates strong-smelling acids which attract insects that lay eggs in the rotting tissue. The eggs hatch after 24 hours and the maggots eventually consume 60 per cent of the body tissue, over a number of gluttony-filled weeks. Hmm!! Yummy yum-yum!!

Finally if you're buried, the maggots create holes in the rotting flesh, which allow decomposition fluids and gases to escape. After a month and a half, beetles and fungi further consume the remains.

This is called 'dry decay' which can take up to one year. Eventually, every part of the body will have been broken down and used, leaving just your bones behind.

The end.

Amen

READER: *Thanks for that, I've just eaten.*
Hey!! What can I tell ya?! Reality bites my friend, so enjoy your life to the max, before you become a maggot, all-you-can-eat buffet meal.

If you're reading this, you're still alive; you've survived another day on this planet…

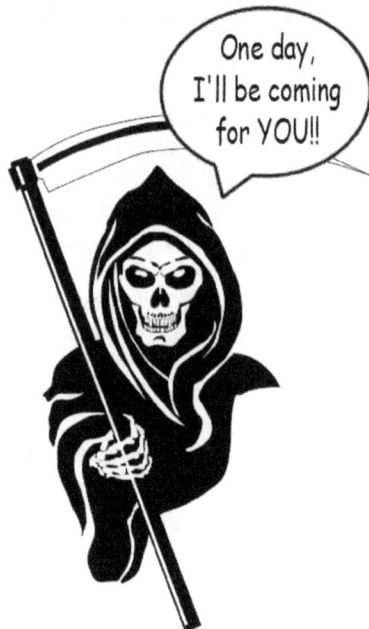

…now act like it, before you see this guy.

Life isn't an App or a computer game, you can't download cheats. You can't turn it on and off again like a reboot. Maybe the lifestyle you ordered is currently out of stock. Well, unfortunately your birth certificate isn't a receipt; you can't use it to exchange your life for something better.

Only **you** can make the changes.

When you think of it, life is like a piano, with all the keys in the wrong order. It's up to you to find the right melody.
READER: *I can't play piano.*
It's a metaphor, you've missed the point but you could always learn.
READER: *I don't want to play the piano.*
Ok! Ok! Here's another one for you.
Life is like the programme *'LOST'*, it's a bit of an anti-climax at the end but full of opportunities and possibilities until then.
READER: *I never saw it, was it any good??*
AAARRRGGGHHH!!

Ok! Here's one that's more up your street. Life's a cheesecake and you're the fork…

So stop waiting for things to happen, excitement doesn't arrive like a bus. There's no timetable for enjoyment, you have to search for it yourself.

Don't be so afraid of life that you're scared to actually live it. But on the other hand, if you don't expect much from life, you won't get much out of it either.

C'mon, everyone wants fulfilment in their lives but for some reason, most people are too afraid to do anything about it.

We aspire to be something, something successful, as long as we don't get our feet wet, or miss the X Factor results. But when it's all said and done, will you have said more than you've done?

And you can have as many inspirational posters on your wall as you like but if you don't actually get off your arse, use the words as motivation and do something amazing with your life, you'll just end up miserable.

Although your house will look nice.

Answer me this, when was the last time you did something for the first time?

READER: *I can't remember.*

It's a great question because we get so wrapped up in our menial, mundane, routine-centric lives; we forget that there are so many experiences we've never tried.

READER: *What about you then?*

Me?! I baked some flapjacks for the first time ever – here's the recipe for *'Birchy's Banana Jackflaps'*:

Ingredients

- Dishful of Oats or sugar-free Granola
- 2 x Eggs (free range if possible, I mean who buys eggs from battery hens, **you fowl git?!**)
- 1 Banana (riper the better, easier to mash)
- Butter or Margarine (your choice although don't get the *'fat-free'*, chemically enhanced shite)
- Chocolate (Dark chocolate is better for this recipe and about 8 chunks is more than enough)
- Maple Syrup (I'll leave it up to you how much but a good squirt works for me, **Ooh-er!!**)
- A teaspoon of Baking Powder (gives it some **Oomph**)
- Oven dish, covered with some greased proof paper
- Optional extras – add blueberries/walnuts/coconut or anything you want really, experiment and have fun with it

Instructions

1. Pre-heat oven (gas mark 7 ish)
2. On low heat, melt butter (a generous slab of), sliced banana and chocolate in a pan
3. Turn heat off and add eggs, maple syrup and baking powder, then mix the oats/granola in too, to create a sticky, gooey, mess of goodliness
4. Add mess/goo to oven dish and slap in t'oven
5. Heat for 8-12mins (checking after 5 mins or so to see whether the gooey mess is not overflowing or worst of all, burnt)
6. Remove from t'oven and cut cakey goo into sections (up to you how many, I'm not a slice Nazi)
7. Leave to cool for an hour or so, then remove from dish and place in *'Tupperware'*
8. Pop the *'Tupperware'* in the fridge (sample 1 or 4 if you're greedy like me)
9. Eat when you want a snack or treat, and revel in the fact that they're quite good for you and best of all, **bloody lush!!**
10. Offer to me when I come round and have a brew.

READER: *What's all this got to do with weight loss?*

Woah there Leslie.

Calm down, I'm getting there.

A lot of people eat snacks when they're feeling lazy or depressed but especially when they're bored, so they need to be active. You need to keep yourself occupied because the more you're doing stuff, the less likely you'll be shoving goodies down your gullet.

And although there's nowt wrong with having a nap, or lounging on the sofa watching the box now and again, it doesn't have to be accompanied by three packets of crisps, six biscuits and a slab of pork pie every time. Nor should it become part of your daily agenda.

Therefore and I'll say it again 'cos it's a great line I'm sure you'll agree?! If you want to lose weight and keep it off in the long-term:

You've got to make sure that your life is full,
rather than just your stomach

Too many people remain in relationships they know aren't going anywhere. They work at jobs they hate. They endure a weekly routine they absolutely despise. They do stuff every day of the week, every week of the month and every month of the year, which they actually detest.

But rather than taking the initiative to change their lives for the better, they remain stagnating in their conformist, comfort blankets. Yes they have some semblance of security but the lack of adventure, the lack of risks taken, is slowly eradicating what joy and happiness they could have in their lives, if only they had the gumption to just **try** and achieve their goals, or any of their dreams.

So the next aspect of my HELP relates to how **you** could achieve your goals, how **you** can be happier, how **you** can stop conforming and start... **living!!**

BARRIER - WORK

Is your job a major reason why you're so depressed?

Getting that dream job

The worst four-letter word on the planet is not the *'C'* word it's *'work'*.

Kids play and play and play and play and play until they're bored, and then they play something else. Yet we're supposed to do the same job for the rest of our lives. Sod that. Not for me, Clive.

Unfortunately, at work I suffer from a disease known as, *'attitude problem'*. Apparently, because I couldn't give a flying frig about sales targets, performance figures, synergy leveraging, hot desking, joined up thinking, benchmarking, unleashing my think rhino, team bonding and other such shite, they think this is a problem.

I disagree but hey that's me, I'm just a maverick.
EX-WORK COLLEAGUES: *You're definitely a word that rhymes with maverick. Starts with a 'P'…*
I prefer maverick.

Look, all I'm doing is whoring my time away and trying to get through the day without smacking someone. You can't choose your family, or your workmates and they both drive you mad.

The terminology in today's work place is enough to send anyone loopy.

Management speak is just jibber-jabber,
A way to climb up the corporate ladder,
To be honest with you, it's not for me,
So I'm gonna have to leave your company,
Drill down, touch base, whilst the workers make hay,
Let's move those goalposts at the end of the day,
Run them numbers up the flagpole for fun,
Blue sky thinking, when it's all said and done,
Review that agenda on a conference call,
Try and square the circle but don't drop the ball,
My colleagues think I'm jealous, 'cos this jargon rocks,
Oh! Shove your dirty-data up your messy inbox!!

'They' say, *'do what you love and you'll never work a day in your life'*. Now where can you get a job masturbating and watching box-sets?

Apparently, **doing** what you like is freedom, **liking** what you do, is happiness. So there you go. If you like your job, you've got a greater chance of losing weight and banishing those blues.

If you don't, then you've got to do something about it, or it will hinder your weight loss goals and continue to make you miserable. Sorry, that's the rules I'm afraid.

55

If you've always dreamed of being a Web Designer, Physiotherapist, Jockey, Geography Teacher, Undertaker or Lifeguard, now is the time my friend and the time is **now!!**

Or don't bother trying, 'cos you might get lucky. Yeah forget it, just work for someone else instead, who followed their dreams.

C'mon, there's no legitimate excuse whatsoever, for not **attempting** to get yourself a job which you've always wanted to do.

Some of my mates base their tolerance of a job on their personal *'hateometer'* scale. They despised a previous job so much, that subsequent roles are assessed comparatively and if they are mediocre on the *'hateometer'* scale, they continue to endure.

How is that living? It's not right... I hope you don't do that?!

You can imagine yourself doing any type of job in the world but imagination doesn't pay the rent, improve your sanity, or put waffles on your fancy china plates.

So get doing some research, tidy up your C.V. and start applying.

Alternatively, there are loads of specialist *'Recruitment Agencies'* that might be able to assist and help you find that perfect job. If there's a chance they can make some commission, they'll **definitely** try and help you. But be warned, Recruitment Consultants are just like politicians; you can't believe or trust a word they say. And they'll ignore you when there's nothing in it for them.

Running your own business

Rather than working for some faceless conglomerate, perhaps you want to work for yourself instead. Well give it a go, although if you steal any post-it-notes or A4 paper, just remember it'll be your profit margins that take a hit, not theirs. **Soz!!**

Admittedly this type of dream is a toughie; otherwise we'd all be doing it. However, thousands of people in this country run their own business and if it's good enough for them, it's time that you got a piece of the action and gave it a go. Although, if you're one of those that wakes up in the morning and you actually **look forward** to going to work, then it's the right thing for you and you don't need to make changes. You're set... **spawny git!!**

However, if you're thinking: *'Pffft! I don't think this is for me, I can't stand it here',* then make a bloody change. Either look for a better job that you'd feel more comfortable at, or bite the bullet and attempt to start your own business.

Greeting Card Designer, Fishmonger, Hairdresser, Florist, Landscape Gardener, Carpenter, Antique Dealer, Taxi Driver, Scuba-Diving Instructor or whatever... all achievable.
READER: *As if, how can I possibly achieve that?*
You know those people that are currently doing those jobs?
READER: *Yeah...*
Well they're human, just like you... if they can do it, then so can you. Maybe there's a course you can go on to help **you** get the necessary qualifications required to start, and your current company 'may' even pay for you to take it.

Get in touch with *'The Prince's Trust'* or the Local Government to establish if you're eligible for some funding. Have a word with your Bank, speak to the *'Citizen's Advice Bureau'*, get yourself on to the web and do some research. Create a *'Business Plan'* and just **try**, see if it's feasible, search and explore as many options and avenues as possible.

Pitch to the *'Kickstarter'* website, or get yourself on *'Dragon's Den'*, you never know, they might be in a charitable mood. I'll help on that score, here's an idea for you and I'll be happy with just taking 10% of the royalties.

POPPING BUBBLE WRAP

READER: *What you on about?*
Everyone loves to pop bubble wrap, right?
READER: *Err… yeah!!*
Of course they do, 'cos its cathartic, it's fun, it's a joy.
Sooooooooooooooooooo, create a shop that provides this as a service. You can charge per pop, or by roll, or by the different bubble sizes. And don't just stop with a shop.

Imagine the scene, emergency vans delivering bubble wraps to a stressed and frazzled nation. What a world, it could be.

You in?! C'mon, it's a money spinner. You'll be coining it in.
What do you mean, you're **out?**

Ok! Back to your *'winning'* idea, whatever it is. Ask your current employer about the possibility of taking redundancy. You never know, that could be the lucky break you've been waiting for.

Actually a friend of mine took redundancy at the same time as me a few years ago. I mooched around a bit, umming and aahing about what to do next, did a bit of travelling and then trundled back onto the office treadmill. But *'Deli-Dave'*, he had the stones to start his own business and it's still thriving to this day.

So if you're ever in Sheffield, get yourself over to *'La Coppola'* on Oakbrook Road for the best espresso and sarnie, this side of Italia.Deli-Dave gave it a go, he chanced his arm and it worked for him. What about you??

You can do it, I'm certain, you've just got to be…
READER: *Positive?*
Damn right baby!!

There are countless opportunities out there, you just have to find them and then give it all you've got.

Paul Birch

LA VIDA LOCA

What do YOU do for fun?

Most people don't realise how boring their lives are, until someone asks them that killer question.

If you can answer without mentioning *'watching telly'*, *'surfing the internet'* or *'scrolling through your mobile'*, then perhaps there's hope left for you after all.

But if you're struggling to come up with a suitable answer, then once again you will definitely benefit from my HELP.

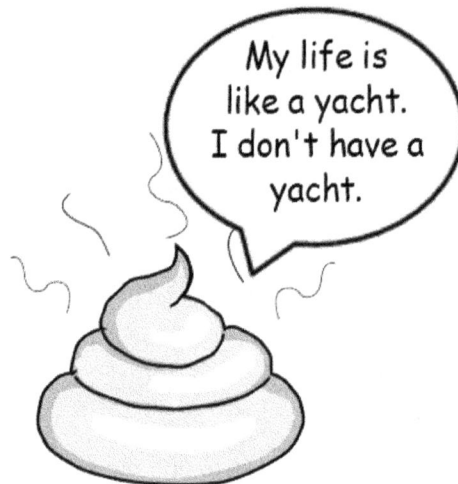

The joy of life comes from our encounters with new experiences.
READER: *Yeah! But I like things the way they are.*
For the love of all that is holy... Let yourself go.

In fact, I bet you're one of those people who wears *'shower socks'* and once you find a holiday destination you like, you go there every flippin' year. To the same hotel. Doing the same ol' stuff. Eating the same ol' meals, and booking it for the same week of every year.

Ooh! Imagine if you veered from this path and went somewhere else and it wasn't as good, hey?!
READER: *Exactly.*
Yeah?! But what if it was... better?

If you repeat something over and over, it loses its appeal. It's allure.

It's like going to a restaurant and selecting the same dish every time you go. Yes you know what you're getting but it'll never be the same as that first time. C'mon, where's your sense of adventure?

Happiness makes people more sociable and altruistic, it increases self-confidence and as a result, you become, *'friendlier'*. It strengthens your immune system and best of all, increases your chances of losing weight and getting fitter.
What's not to like?
READER: *I can't be happy all of the time.*
Of course not and statistically it's just not realistic. I mean, even six out of the seven dwarves weren't happy.
Look, no-one is permanently happy for the rest of their lives, it just doesn't happen but you can try.

Happiness should be measured in laughter, joy and fun but instead it seems to be measured in money, and I'm sorry to inform you but there's not enough to go round. **Soz!!**

Happiness is often temporary, it's far too fleeting therefore what we equate to happiness needs to be modified and not determined by footy results, alcohol, gambling, TV programmes, greed, social media, consumerism and bitching.

The reward centre of the brain is stimulated by sex, food, sugar, alcohol etc, etc but also good deeds, laughter, exercise, new experiences and *'Sunshiii-innnne!!'*

There are so many simple pleasures in life that we just take for granted, rather than savouring the joy.

So what gets in the way of your happiness? What stops you from living and enjoying life?
READER: *Money?*
No!! It's your attitude, simple as.

There are so many alleged *'barriers'* to the good life, so we'll take a look at some and see how they can be addressed with a positive and fun outlook, rather than the pessimistic, conformist stance that so many of us adopt in our daily lives.

Yes it's a cliché but if you've only got one life why not try and make it a long, moderately happy, fulfilling one.

Don't be so bloody serious all of the time, because life's clearly too short for that. And if you can't laugh at yourself, give me a call and I'll do it for you.

Some might say (actually a decent Oasis song) that the definition of hell, is that when you die, the person you are meets the person you could've been. That's nonsense probably but it's a thought isn't it?
So what could **you** have been?

Ponder that thought for a few minutes. Go on, I'll wait for you... and we're back.

What have **you** always wanted to do but haven't quite accomplished yet?

Me? I've always wanted to write a book.
READER: *Well maybe one day* ☺
Exactly!! It wasn't easy and it's taken me aaaaaaggggggeeeeeessssss to write but finally after years of endeavour, I've only bloody done it. Irrespective whether people think it's any good or not, I've accomplished another one of my dreams.

If I can do it and I'm just another regular Joe, then **you** can certainly achieve your dreams too.

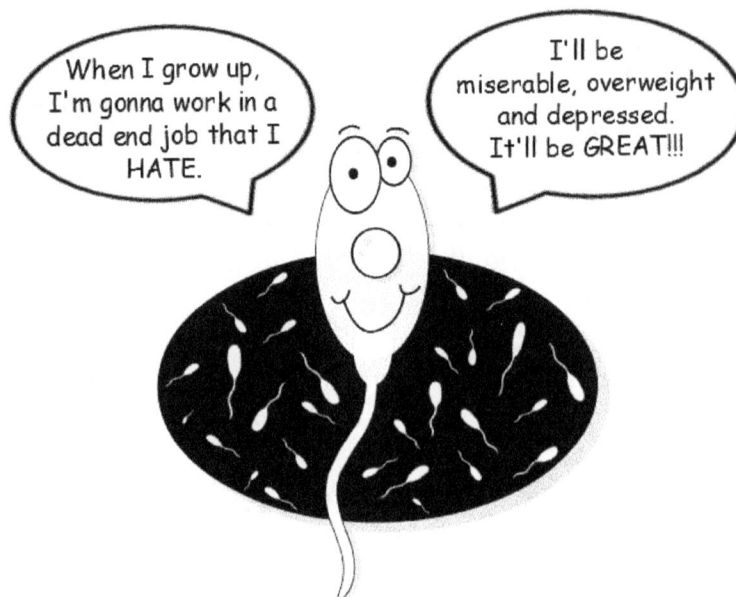

When you were a kid, I very much doubt that you dreamt of working in an office, chained to a computer in a job you despise, and your evenings spent slumped in front of the box.
READER: *Well, of course I had goals and ambitions but it's too late now, those dreams are over.*
Bollocks!!

I bet the next sentence from one of my clients sounds familiar to you because most people feel this way, regardless whether they admit it to everyone else or not:

*I wanted to believe I was capable of **more**.*
Life so far had been alright but I had this nagging feeling that there was something better out there for me.

What's the point in having a dream, if you're never going to try and make it happen?

Yes it's a risk to chase a dream 'cos what if it doesn't work? … But what if it does?!

You don't want to have this engraved on your gravestone, do you?

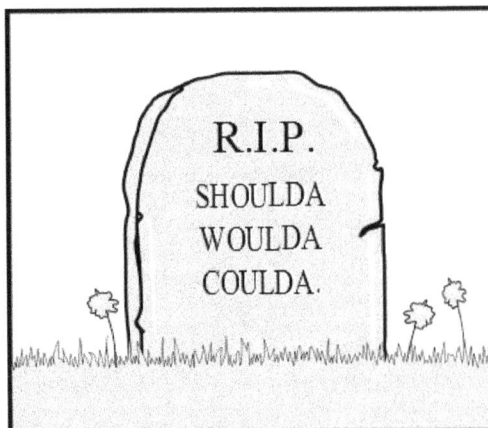

Maybe you attempted to chase your dreams years ago but it didn't quite go as planned?!
You failed so thought, *'Oh well, at least I tried'* and then **quit!!**

Look, don't become **someone** and **everything** you didn't want to be.

I believe it was Churchill, Mr Bulldog Cigarman himself, who uttered summat about:

'Never give in, never give in, never, never, never, never gonna give you up, never gonna let you down, never gonna run around and desert you...'

And that dude was leathered most of the time but even so, he hit the nail squarely on the proverbial, with relation to not bloody quitting.

Failure should not be an option. So stop saying the *'F'* word, all the F'in time and F'in get on with it.

As I've mentioned before, I've been trying to write this book for twenty years and failed, so many times. But did I give up? **No!!** Because it was my dream, my passion, my goal.

I know that I'll never be taller, my winkie ain't gonna grow again (Ooh! Er Missus!), I'm stuck with this boat race and the day that I'll need a hedge trimmer to sort out my ear and nose hair, is coming quicker and quicker. But I have specific goals and dreams and I will **never** stop trying to accomplish them, irrespective of which direction my life goes.

I'm not a success story by any stretch of the imagination and *'may'* never well be, but I will keep trying and trying until the day I die. Otherwise what's the point in living?

Just surviving, just existing, is **not** living but passionately chasing your dreams, is.

The most successful people in the world are all human, just like you and I. But rather than letting failure overcome them, they find a way to rise up again. What separates them from the rest of the planet is they seized their opportunities, they took risks and they worked harder.

Ok! Not everyone, I mean some inherited the silver spoon life (like Royalty or Members of the Tory Party for example) but the majority of successful people hit obstacles and had to smash right through them. They failed and failed and failed... and then failed again but they kept on trying.

Eventually they got a lucky break, or they were so passionate about succeeding that the Universe had no other choice but to allow them to achieve.

READER: *How can I chase my dreams, I have kids, I'm married, I work...*
Excuses, excuses, excuses.
READER: *Yes but...*
Excuses.
READER: *But...*
Excuses.
READER: *B...*
Excuses!!

If you don't **attempt** to go after what you want, you'll never have it. So my advice to **you** is don't just follow your dreams, run after them, then stamp on them until they're stuck to your sole.

Mate, the only time you run out of chances, is when you stop taking them.

And there's no such thing as spare time, free time or down time.

All you have is lifetime.

I've always said:

> *If you want something in life,*
> *stop mithering about how hard it'll be*
> *and just give it a go.*
> *Just try!!*

If I want to open a door, I don't just sit and **wish** it would open, I grab the handle and pull.
Ok! Sometimes it says *'push'*, so I look stupid but you know what I mean.

And don't listen to those folk who tell you that you'll **never** achieve your dreams; they're just people that failed at theirs and have quit trying. Ignore those people. You don't need that negativity in your life.

You need a goal, you need a porpoise in life, otherwise you're just surviving and if you haven't got a goal or purpose, why do you get up in the afternoon?

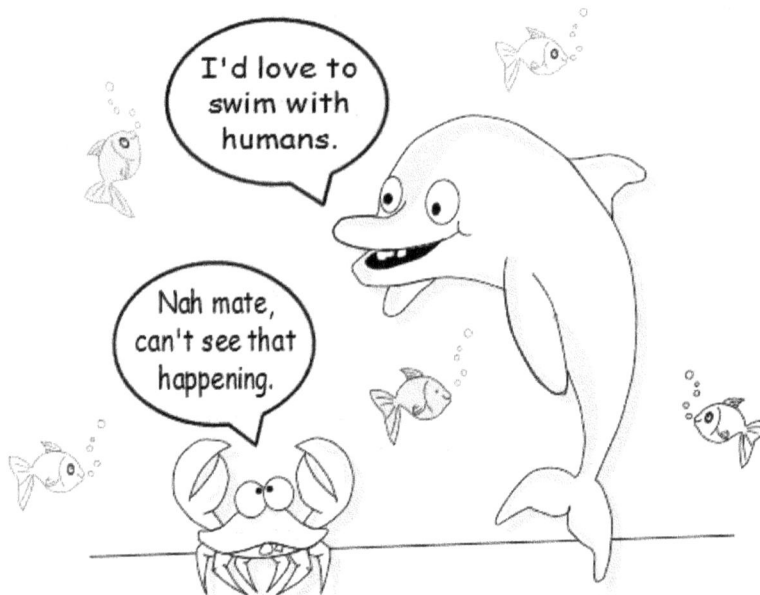

On your next birthday, you will look back at the previous year and be more disappointed by the things you didn't do, than the things you did.

Life is just not worth living until you've found something worth dying for, normally kids but could be a dream job, running your own business, travelling, art, writing, acting, knitting, sculpture, freecycling, up to you.

Ask yourself *'what do I want to do?'* and then contemplate if this *'dream'* is feasible, irrespective of the barriers your mind creates.

You don't want to spend the rest of your life looking back and thinking *'WHAT IF?'*

But a dream without a plan is just a wish and genies aren't real my friend... luckily, the pedantic **gits!!**

> GENIE: *What is your wish?*
> STEVE: I want to be rich!!
> GENIE: *Very well, your wish is granted.*
> RICH: Cheers.

So wake up, have lots of goals and aim for them all.

Challenge yourself and try to get out of your comfort zone but don't set impossible goals, make them smart instead.

S M A R T

is for	is for	is for	is for	is for
SPECIFIC	**MEASURABLE**	**ACHIEVABLE**	**REALISTIC**	**TIME-BASED**

For example, don't state that your goal is to just *'go on holiday'* next year. Actually pick a destination, choose a date, how much it will cost, who's coming with you etc, etc, and then aim for that precise location.

Don't be vague.

It's the same with your weight loss. Actually choose a realistic and manageable figure that you want to lose, allocate a time–frame, select a method and **GET ON WITH IT!!**

I'll tell ya now, losing weight is easy... keeping it off that's the difficult bit.

You can measure success by using the scales but you can also gauge it by the fitting of clothes, your moods, your social life and how much you're getting on the wick of everyone, by being so damn **positive** all the time.

Maybe you want to run a marathon? Twenty six miles, three hundred and eighty five yards of pavement, road, grass, puke, spittle, discarded water bottles, cheering supporters, crying, fainting, heat exhaustion, blisters, chafing, nipple sores, twisted ankles, jelly babies, pulled groins, bloodied toes, stiff knees and millions upon millions of money raised for Charities.

A brilliant, amazing, never to be forgotten experience.
You in?
READER: *Oh aye I'm sure, as if I could run that far.*
Look, in any goal it always seems impossible... until it's done.

Obviously I'll be discussing fitness in more detail later in the book, so I'll explain how this particular goal is entirely feasible. But let me tell you something, those people that finally complete a marathon after six, seven or nine hours, they have so much guts it's unreal. They are winners, irrespective of their times because they accomplished it.

And I know how hard that is from personal experience. It's tough. It's bloody tough!! Therefore I have the utmost respect for these people and if they can do it, then so can **you!!** So stop with the excuses and lace up your trainers. It doesn't matter how long it takes you to finish, as long as you finish.

On second thoughts, forget all that. Life is hard, so don't bother following your dreams, there's bound to be something good on the telly instead.

BARRIER - TV

Does TV get in the way of you achieving your goals and enjoying life?

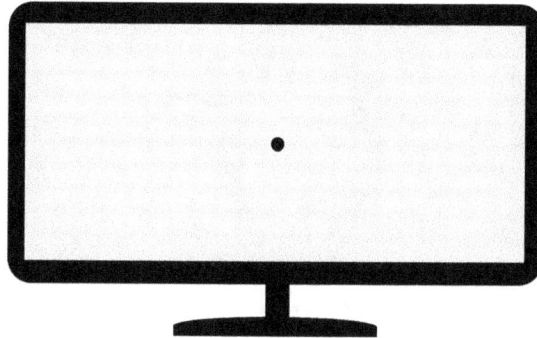

Let's try a little experiment.

Just stare at the dot on the above TV screen for **two minutes** and contemplate its significance.
After a while you'll start to realise that nothing is happening. It's like life. It will only get better once you look away from the box.

As short as life is, we make it shorter still by our careless waste of time. We spend so many hours, of every day, watching television. But you'll never get those hours back, they're gone. Erased. Defunct. **Wasted!!**

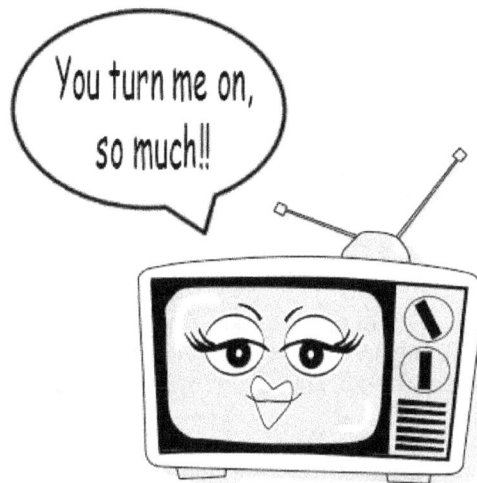

Our lives seem to be governed by it.

What we eat, what we wear, what we buy, who we like, what we think, what music we listen to, who we vote for. We are manipulated by distraction pixels every single day. And do you know what?
READER: *What?*
We seem ok with it.
Madness!!

But you need to think for yourself, form your own opinions, make objective conclusions, go your own way but this is impossible when you are controlled by the beaming rays of the sparkly, rectangle of wonderment. You don't **have** to do what everyone else is doing you know, go your own way.

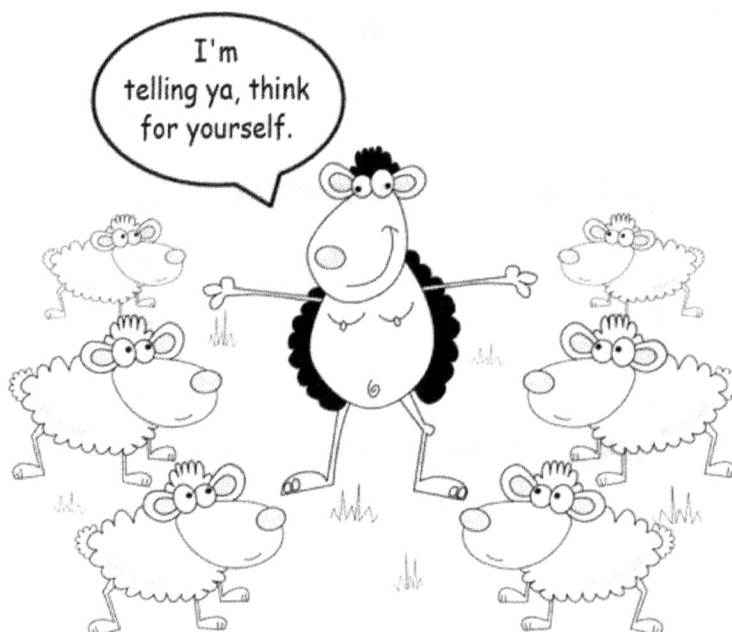

I have overheard my Mother and Sisters discussing people who've committed atrocious and outrageous acts. They speak about these people with such passion, spitting vitriolic abuse regarding their actions, but it turns out that the subject of their heated debates aren't murderers, or rapists, or Tax avoiders, or even Tory Politicians. They're soap actors. Merely acting out a part that is written for them.

Hallo!! These events are not really happening, it's not real life.

If you're similarly enthused by these repeated story lines that go round and round and round and round on a loop every single year, I offer the same advice I give to my family… **get a fuckin' grip!!**

Don't get me wrong, I love to watch the telly-box and I've wasted many a night through to the early hours, gawping at the screen as a coping mechanism for my depression. So much so, that when my life finally flashes before me, at least I'll be able to relive some classic TV episodes.

> Seinfeld, Curb Your Enthusiasm, Friends, The Sopranos, Peep Show, Spaced, The Mighty Boosh, The Office, Breaking Bad, LOST, Bo' Selecta, The Big Bang Theory, Frasier, Game of Thrones, The Trip, Big Train, Newswipe, How Not to Live your Life etc, etc join me after the break etc.

I've watched **every** episode of the above series, twice sometimes three, four, ten times…

Yep, I can binge watch like the best of 'em but I now know that the real meaning of life, is adventure. And the only way to really experience it… is by stepping out of the living room.
READER: *What, into the kitchen?*
Ha! Ha! Ha! Ha! I hope that was a joke?!

I love to watch comedies more than anything else (as you can see from the above list), or perhaps an inspiring documentary. I believe that if you're gonna veg in front of the box, you need to take something worthwhile from the experience. If you're laughing, then this improves your happiness and we know what increases as a result?
READER: *Positivity!!*
10 points, **Yay!!**

Watching miserable dramas and soaps will make you feel sad. Watching comedies, makes you feel happy. It's just simple mathematics. Or as the Yankee doodles say, *'y'all do the math'*.

I know that the boob-tube is just escapism but too many people take it far too seriously and would rather stay in watching another episode of some rehashed pap, than go out and speak to the real people, or actually try to achieve some of their life-long dreams.

Therefore if you're one of these types, I have some great advice for you that will **definitely** help you achieve your goals.

The next time you're lounging on your sofa, flicking through the hundreds of channels trying to find something that is worthy of your evening's attention. Put the remote down and then actually turn the telly off. Just walk outside to the garden and stand there in complete silence.

Look up to the stars and for a few moments just contemplate how amazing life is, and the endless possibilities that are out there.

Nip back into the house, open a bottle of wine, or pour yourself a beer and toast the fact that you're still part of it.
READER: *As if.*
Why not? What's wrong with appreciating the true wonder of life and being alive?! Thanking the flying spaghetti monster that you're a part of this wonderful planet, and have the freedom to achieve **anything** that you put your mind to.
READER: *You're a bloody fruitcake you.*
Aye, you're probably right. Although I am fit, healthy and moderately happy though **:P**

Living and enjoying life will **definitely** help you lose weight, but the longer you lounge and laze in front of the TV, the harder it will be. Ultimately, it's back to choices again. Flat telly or flat belly? Goals or near misses?

Television is just another addiction and extremely dispiriting but the less you have it in your life, the less you miss it.

Just like pizza.

Why not read instead?
READER: *Eeuurrgghh!! Reading?!*
Aye! Reading is so rewarding and you can actually *'learn'* stuff too.
If you're trying to lose weight, get fitter or achieve any goal for that matter, then *'reading'* will definitely help. Just like any project, the more you read and research about a subject, the more knowledge you obtain and thus the easier the task becomes.

The alphabet for book lovers:

A B C D E F G H
I J K L M N O P
Q R S U W X Y Z

And when you think about it, knowing how to read and not reading, is almost the same as not knowing how to read.
READER: *Nice try.*
Ok! One great advantage of reading rather than gazing open-mouthed at the box, is the lack of adverts.
And I for one welcome a world where I don't have to observe polar bears drinking Cola. Or those sofa adverts featuring tiny actors to make some leather number look bigger. Or Banks pretending they actually **care** about their customer's wellbeing.

Ok! Another angle for ya.
TV is just a law n' order mechanism, designed to keep the electorate chained to their couches.
We pretend we have total freedom but we're locked in our houses, too afraid to actually live. So we put on the box and rejoice in a safe, comfortable world, watching others live instead whilst we decay, slouched on the sofa.

Is this your concept of freedom?

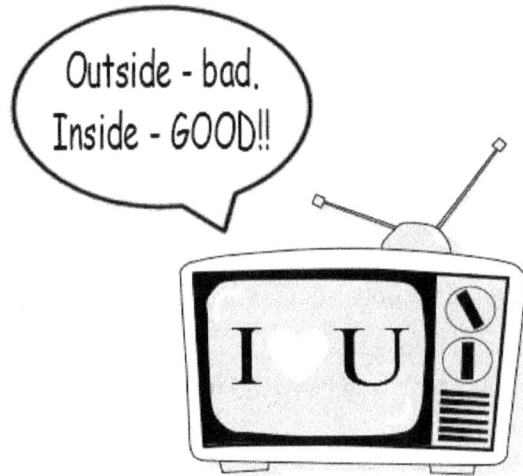

Obviously it's up to **you** how much TV you endure but the next time you find yourself watching some pap on Telly and you think, *'why am I watching this?'* well there's a way out.
A simple solution.

Turn it off.

Live your life, and chase your dreams... it's why God invented Sky+

BARRIER - SOCIETY

Is society to blame for you not living and enjoying life, or chasing your dreams?

These days, people are a bit, you know, erm… thick.

Not **you** obviously, I mean them other people. It's probably down to the excessive consumption of fast food and E-numbers but above all, it's down to society, **the zeitgeist**.

There's a great comedy created by Chris Morris (comedy genius), called *'Nathan Barley'* and the premise of that show revolves around *'The Rise of the Idiots'*. It's more a reflection of media and fashion in that there London, centring on the moronic gullibility of these *'sheeple'* but could easily be describing the country as a whole.

Art imitating life or Vicky Versa? It's hard to tell but I can tell you this, society these days is proper shite. We seem to be regressing as a nation and the values, principles and ethics that created this alleged *'Great'* Britain are being eroded on a daily basis.

Do you remember politeness? Do you remember respect for your elders? Do you remember community spirit? Do you remember kindness to those less fortunate than ourselves? All vanishing before our very eyes.

It's criminal how much dumberer we appear to have become. Certainly TV, Radio and the Print media assume we have very limited cognitive and analytical ability, and thus need to be spoon fed complete and utter tripe, to keep us sedated. Sorry, I mean entertained.

It's a real eye-opener to watch some of the political, scientific, and documentary programmes from the late 60's to early 80's (check 'em out on *'You-Tube'*). These programmes took it for granted that the audience had a proficient level of education and aptitude, to think about what they were witnessing. To debate, to ask questions, to contemplate, to challenge. That would be way beyond what today's audiences are drip-fed.
READER: *That's a bit condescending.*
I'm not trying to be but have you ever watched any *Freeview* channel on a weekend for instance?
READER: *Point taken.*
'No likey, no lighty' – a modern day catchphrase for the waxed, fake-tanned, goggle-box generation. The lights might be on but nobody's home.

Is it parenting? Is it politics? Is it education? Is it the media? Is it food? It's probably all of them and more but rather than *'evolving'*, we're just getting stupiderer by the day.

One of the major problems with society is the unrelenting message that you can only lead an idealistic life, if you have pots of cash. As a result we all want more money, more spondoolies, more moolah! We want money **NOW!!** And we don't care how. It seems that our principles have flown out of the window.

We even take out ridiculous loans, irrespective of the scandalous interest rates. We need as much as we can get hold of and we actually believe that life will be just dandy with loadsa dosh.

That right?

So you'll be healthier, fitter, have more friends, different family? Happier?
No!! It doesn't change anything really, it just means you can afford Lipo and you'll have shiny new cars and a bigger house to clean. Wellbeing, peace of mind and contentment can't be won by scratching a lottery card, or maxing out your Visa, you need to embrace positivity and fitness to achieve that type of happiness.

There appears to be limited compassion and empathy for other folk less fortunate than ourselves.
This is the tag-line for society nowadays:

LIFE IS LIKE AN ORGASM
Mine is more important than yours and
I don't really care if you have one or not.

What about Billionaires as well? I mean how much money do they actually need? Last time I looked they only had one arse, so why are they buying so many sports cars, yachts and houses? Insecurity and plain, simple, *'couldn't give a toss about anyone but myself,'* greed.

It's an addiction and I'm sure you're fully aware of how **greed** can harm your chances of success regarding weight loss. It's a sickness and it encompasses society perfectly.

Look at the opulence and lifestyles of the rich and famous. These people could do such good, promote a more humble life, helping others, setting up charitable foundations and paying the correct tax. But no, instead they flaunt their excessive, extravagant, superficial world to *'lemmings'* all over the world who seem happy enough to lap it all up.

Why? It makes no sense, we're like a race of budgerigars, *'look at the shiny baubles, they're so pretty'.*
READER: *OMG!! You're just a hippy...*
I suppose I am really but I don't see anything wrong with that, I just like helping other people.
When you've been brought up to care and respect other folk, you seem to be denigrated for this ethos. It's like there's a stigma attached to people that show compassion.

We live in a, *'I'm alright Jack, so up your trumper'* type world, which I believe is why we're buggered as a society.

But if positivity helps you to lose weight, and the happier you are in your life, the more positive you become, and helping other people makes you feel happier, then... do you see where I'm heading with this?!
READER: *I think so...*
The sun does not revolve around **you**, it orbits the **entire** planet.

Rather than focusing everything on yourself, think of others instead because this will make you forget about your own problems and your depression will lift.

So c'mon, see how you can help your family and friends, or better still, your fellow man, them folk we don't know... strangers.

Do some good with your life, rather than spending the majority of your time scrolling and swiping on your smart phone.

Take social media sites (please, someone take them):

@

> *"Look at me, look at me, please lavish attention on me because I've taken a picture of my lunch, or a meal in a restaurant, or a cocktail in a bar, or my child in a funky outfit and I don't get satisfactory attention anywhere else which makes me deeply sad, emotional and clinically depressed. Please validate my life choices"*

@

These sites are a cesspit of neuroses and complex emotional needs, which should be dealt with by professional therapists. Not that bloke you went to school with who just adds a *'like'* and a smiley face to your updates.

It's just a sanitised version of the world which appears to revolve around one-upmanship. You look at the uploaded pictures of one of your *'friends'* and then assume that they're living this idyllic life. Secretly, that pisses you off, so you compete by uploading piccies of your own, highlighting what a wonderful life that you're having. They get jealous too and the merry-go-round continues.

This perception that there is such a thing as perfection out there in social media-land, is just another illusion because folk only upload their highlight reels. The mundanity that takes place for the majority of their lives is well and truly hidden. Left on the cutting room floor.

As a consequence, these sites create a very unhealthy mind frame, the user chasing a dream-state of reality that doesn't exist.

Look, I'm not condemning you, it's a major part of life these days and you should embrace it, enjoy it. But all I'm saying is don't let the fake, fickle, shallow world of social-media take over your life so you can't accomplish your goals. And talk to your kids. And have fun. And live.

You'd like to lose weight and get fitter right?
READER: *Erm, yes...*
Well if you've time to waste scrolling around FB, you've obviously got time to exercise. Yeah?
READER *(in stunned silence)*:...
U ok hun? X

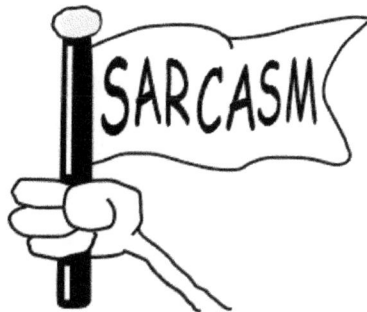

Don't get me wrong, the concept of *FB, WhatsApp, Instagram* etc is great if you want to see photos of family and friends you haven't seen in a while, or you're celebrating some fantastic achievement like finishing a marathon, scaling a mountain, or losing half your body weight.

But it's not just used for that is it?
No, it's full of links to videos of dogs playing the piano, pictures of your new dress, outrageous insults, xenophobic news articles, Selfies, Belfies and Velfies, or your ankle biters in fancy dress.

With respect to social media, I get it, I get it but it's just not for me. I prefer to actually *'talk'* face to face to people that I know, rather than conversing over the digital highway. Human interaction. Laughing together. Having fun.

Anyway, back to society.

I know that some people **need** to conform to the zeitgeist but the reward for conformity is that everyone likes you, except yourself. By all means follow the crowd but only if it's going to be a laugh, or a queue to a gig or it's a half-marathon (you don't wanna get lost).
READER: *Yes but I don't like to do anything too different because people might judge.*
So what?! Let them judge.

Whatever anyone else **says** or **thinks** about you, it means diddly. They have no direct or positive influence on your life whatsoever but if you continue to live your lives based on other people's perceptions and thoughts and internet feedback, your life will be shit. **Guaranteed!!**

If you don't want to fit in, then don't. It's entirely up to you, your choice.

But when you embrace positivity and fitness, you won't care about being tagged, or fret about FB comments, you'll be more concerned with PB's and the status of your weight.

And finally, one last thing, believe nothing and question everything by doing your own research.
READER: *Why?*
Because you'll never learn otherwise, you'll just follow… and I see what you did there.

BARRIER - SUPPORT

Are you getting enough support from your partner?

Whatever you are trying to achieve in life, be it weight loss, getting fitter or trying to complete your bucket list. Integral to your chances of success is the support and encouragement from your family and pals.

And most importantly, if you're in a relationship, your partner too.

When you hit a bump and you will, you'll hit many, you'll need a lift and everyone goes through phases of feeling discouraged, of feeling despondent. For far too many people, the *'winter blues'* become the mood for *'all seasons'* blues.

Sometimes your family and friends won't be around but your partner will be, so they **must** be on board with ALL of your goals, otherwise you'll probably fail. Without their support you're onto a losing battle.

If you're married, no doubt you both spoke some vows at the ceremony and they probably went something like:

...to have and to hold, from this day forward, for better, for worse, for richer, for poorer, in sickness and in health, to love and to cherish, till death do us part...

If your partner truly loves you, they'll abide by those principles and **support** you in whatever goals you try to achieve.

And it works both ways, so you should respond in kind too.

But if you're single, don't let that insignificant matter hinder your chances of weight loss success.

As I've mentioned, I'm single at the moment or as I like to call it, *'between girlfriends'*.
Granted it's been a long, long, long, long, long, long time since the last girlfriend but it's fundamentally true. If I ever get another girlfriend that is.

But I'm great at relationships; it's my exes that are the problem. When we break up I'm always told that it's **them**, not me. It's just not the right time apparently. So even though our relationship may have been stale and uneventful, it wasn't my fault.

It was all down to chronology. Time was to blame, not me. **Shame!!**

Yep, I'm useless at the old dating game...
THE ENTIRE FEMALE POPULATION of the WORLD: *You don't have to tell us mate!!*

Yeah, well anyway, the only thing I seem to pull these days is the odd muscle after a long run.
READER: *Aww!! I'm sure you'll be fine, there's plenty of fish in the sea...*
Oh aye I'm sure. But what if you haven't got the right bait?
What if the fish just aren't biting?
Or you catch a fish but have to throw it back because it belongs to another? Or the fish just doesn't want to be part of your net? Too many holes. Not well made. Equipment, not expensive enough.

READER: *But if you try to be more positive, surely you'd do better with the girlies?*
Bloody Nora!! You have been listening, nice one.
You're completely right of course and maybe this is just an elaborate bluff to guide you into accepting that a positive demeanour will help you achieve anything or I'm just **a pathetic saddo!!**
Either way, I haven't got all the answers, I'll admit but guess what? I'm gonna let you into a secret. No-one has.

Anyway, back to the point.

It's great when you're single.
In fact, the best thing about it is you can sleep around.
READER: *Behave, I'm not like that.*
Go on, you'll **love it!!**

Left, middle, upside-down, spread-eagled, star shape, in a ball. You can sleep anywhere you like on your bed, without the danger of feet in your back, snoremageddon, or an over-zealous duvet hogger.

KATHY, 29 – *When I split up with my boyfriend, I took it really bad because he cheated on me. I stopped caring about how I looked and started to use food as a crutch, something to make me feel better about myself.*
Whenever I pondered the relationship, I'd have some chocolate, or a pizza, or a full pack of family-sized crisps. Before long, I'd put on 2 stone.
I despised how I looked, felt so unattractive and actually thought I'd be single for the rest of my life. After bumping into the two-faced, lying scumbag, I could tell he was shocked to see how big I'd become and no doubt relieved that he'd moved on.
But rather than getting more depressed, I used this as motivation to lose the timber and get fit again. As you said to me during our first training session - if you're an X, you don't have to be an XL girlfriend. Sometimes that's easier said than done. But you're right. I'm finally back to my normal size, feeling happier and in another relationship. Thanks Paul.

VERONICA, 31 – This woman came to see me after she'd had a relationship break-up. Similar situation to Kathy, she'd put on a few stone after splitting with her partner. She was full of enthusiasm initially but after losing a few pounds quite quickly, she got complacent, thought that it would be easy losing the weight and slipped back into previous habits. She started cancelling the fitness sessions and after a while I stopped hearing from her.

Positive results often fool people into believing that weight-loss is simple, therefore commitment wanes and effort is reduced. Invariably the weight piles back on again and the cycle continues.

With respect to Veronica, were her failings down to loneliness, support, effort or ignorance?
Who knows?
But don't be like her.

Yep, there will be times when **you** are not 100% positive and things aren't going so well but these are just blips not legitimate reasons to quit.

And whenever you hit a wall, reach an impasse or things get on top of you, your partner needs to be there to hug you, comfort you, encourage and support.

But if you're single, or your partner is a selfish pillock, then you'll have to look for this help from your family and friends instead.

BARRIER - SUPPORT

Are you getting enough support from your family and friends?

Your friends are like boobs

Some are real, some are big, some are flat, some are bubbly, some are small, some are melons, some are firm, some are fake and some are tits but we all need them, even if they're hard to get to when you want them the most. But they've been around for years and we've shared some great mammaries between us.

As you grow older, people come and people go, a bit like working in a brothel but even though your circle may decrease in size, it's likely to increase in value, as long as you've put in the time and effort over the years. Because mates are like bank accounts, the more you put in, the more interest you'll get. So if you know more about Ross and Rachael than your real friends, you've got a problem. Although, any type of relationship is just like a fart. If you have to force it, it's probably shit.

Never take your friends or family for granted, no matter how bad you're feeling because they don't deserve your wrath. Like you they have issues, setbacks, doubts and worries.

Like you, they want to share joy with those that they love and respect. Therefore you have to make the effort to be respectable to them. **Always!!**

And remember, **respect** is how to treat everyone not just those you want to impress, or get into their knickers.

So try to treat strangers with respect too because even though you don't know them, they're just like you and have problems, fears, passions and hopes. But if you respect them and actually talk to them, get to know them perhaps, you *'may'* get a new friend and we all need as many as we can get.

It only takes a second to show someone how you feel about them. The Police call it *'Indecent Exposure'* but whatever.

I'm not a religious man as I've said before…
GOD: *Thou can say that again matey.*
But one of the stories in the Bible mentions the phrase *'Do unto others, as you would have them, do unto you'*, which seems a decent approach to life if you ask me. If you treat your family and friends in this way, you should always receive the support you deserve. If you don't, then you don't deserve the support.

When you ask for advice from your family and your mates, initially, all you're really looking for is validation.

You want support and kudos for reaching a particular conclusion because you're afraid of the consequences. But **you** know **you** more than anyone else knows **you**, so **you** know what **you** need to do, therefore it **you** must do.
READER: *Que?*
Subconsciously, you've made the decision already but when one of your closest friends or family members agrees that what you're doing is right, only then are you ready to make that commitment.
However, it's not them that will be putting in the effort but the support from family and mates, will be invaluable and spur you on when you're struggling and help keep you focused. Yes, your family members and mates can be like haemorrhoids sometimes…
READER: *Excuse me?*
Oh! a pain in the arse.

But you'll definitely need their assistance when you adopt a new diet, start a fitness regime or maybe require a bit of help putting down the dark pooch of despair. Therefore you need the right people around you and if they're not prepared to encourage and assist you, stop wasting energy and time on them.

They're not worth it.

Paul Birch

TOM, 37 – *I put on a considerable amount of weight after I broke up with my ex, but in the last year whilst trying to get rid of it, I've finally realised who my real friends are. As you recommended I've tried to become more active and as a result I've played 5' a-side, gone swimming, been walking and attended boxercise classes at the gym.*

I'm a bit shy, so having a mate with me has really helped boost my confidence and get me out of my shell. The problem initially, was that a lot of my pals simply wouldn't come along. They'd rather stay at home watching the box with the wife. Fair do's it's their life but a bit of support would have really helped in the first few months of my weight-loss programme.

I used to call, leave voice messages but get no answer.

Or I'd text and not get a reply. These were my mates, yet they seemed so wrapped up in their own little worlds, that they really didn't give a shit about my problems.

I know people are busy with stuff but I needed them and they actually let me down. Having said that, two of my good mates really came through and we've become like the Three Musketeers these days. Organising footy games, country walks, having a jar after we've been to the gym and just being good friends really.

All three of us have issues and having someone to confide in, really helps sort you out. These guys keep me grounded, fill me with positivity and have helped me lose the lard 'cos we share a common goal.

We've become a lot closer as a result of keeping active together and I have to say, it's been a really enjoyable year.

There will be times in everyone's life when your back is up against the wall, so you'll need someone to call… luckily I've got two really great friends to call upon.

The bestest family members and friends are those that are always open minded, they're positive people, who won't actively judge you. Everything is about empathy and understanding, offering objective solutions and encouragement.

They'll accept **you** for who you are but won't pussyfoot around regarding the truth. They want to help you, because they **care** and that's what mates and family do, they care. You might not like what they say sometimes but they always have your best interests at heart.

These are the type of people you need around you when you're trying to lose weight. In fact, these are the type of people you need in your life, at **all** times.

Hold onto it, if you can get it.

Did you know, that some people actually hurt others, to feel better about themselves?
That's right, some people don't want **you** to succeed, 'cos if you do, they won't have any excuses left for their own issues. So if one of your pals or family members starts to criticise you and belittle your plans to change, lose weight, get fitter, or chase a goal, it's a reflection of them, not you.
Bullies need to find control somewhere but their opinions aren't facts. So stop worrying what these types of individuals think of you.

You **do not need** these people in your life, **you deserve better**.

Stop swimming across oceans of mud, for people who wouldn't jump puddles for you. If they are willing to encourage and support you, great, but if not, stop spending time with them, **ditch 'em!!**

You don't need that type of negativity ruining your life.

Get rid, and move on to move on.

BARRIER - AGE

Is your age getting in the way of your goals?

Maybe you want to have a go at spelunking, or Zorbing, or bopping about on a bouncy castle but you think you're far too old to mess about doing things like that?
READER: *Yeah, maybe.*
Perhaps you want to get back into the world of education and fancy going back to College, or even do it for the first time and undertake an *Open University* course? But 'cos you're knockin' on a bit now, you think you're too old to fulfil your dreams and goals?
READER: *Well, yes.*
If that's the case, I want you to know that someone cares… not me but someone.
Only teasing, of course I care, that's why I'm typing these wonderful words of wisdom and trying to help you lose that lard, embrace positivity, get fitter and wash away them blues.
If you'd like to attempt any of your goals, there's one important factor you need to take into account.
READER: *What's that then?*
If you're still breathing, you've no excuse… **you old wrinkly git!!**

My mate's missus has just finished studying for her degree. It took her **eight** years to finally pass the course because she studied on-line, was a working mother and also took care of her elderly, infirm parents. She's fifty-four years old.

Did she let her age get in the way of her goal? Did she **buggery!!** It was her dream and she did not want it to go unfulfilled.

Was it tough? **Ab-so-bloody-lute-ly!!** But just like long-term weight loss, no-one said it was going to be easy.

Can you imagine how she felt when she finally found out she'd passed?
Let's ask her, how did you feel Debbie?

DEBBIE: *Well, when I opened the letter that confirmed my exam results, I think I shouted something like,*

'YEAHHHHHHHHHHHHHHHHHHHHHHHHHHHHHHHHHHHHHHHHHHHHHHH!! GET THE FUCK IN, WOO-HOOOOOOOOOOOOOOOOOOOOOOOOO!!

So yes, I was quite pleased.

BIRCHY: Was it worth all the sacrifices and hard work?
DEBBIE: *Definitely. If you're desperate to achieve your dreams, you just have to give it a go otherwise you'll regret it for the rest of your life. If you're full of determination and positivity, then anything's possible.*

So there you have it, conclusive proof that age is no obstacle to achieving your goals, even if you want to study. Oh! And if you want to improve your education, I strongly recommend you study Food Science… I've heard that the courses are great.

Age should **never** be construed as a hindrance to beginning, or achieving **any** goal. As long as the clock is still ticking you can try anything, it just means the batteries might need replacing now and again. And you're never too old, to dream big. Look at Susan Boyle.

Ok! Not too much but you know what I mean.

Paul Birch

She finally plucked up the courage to belt out her warblings. She was probably nervous as hell but by gum, she give it a go and now she's living, not dreaming the dream. She's also making her and the hirsute, big cheeked, square-headed, high trouser-wearing man, richer and richer. In our superficial world, she may not have the looks but she's a proper inspiration, a true role model.
Good on her.

In your youth, you were crazy and wild,
But now you're happy with a pint of mild,
At footie you used to score with ease,
But now you can't play because of your knees.
You used to go gigging and play music real loud,
But now you can't stand to be in a crowd,
In the bedroom dept you were kinky and naughty,
But not anymore 'cos you're turning forty!!

So let's knock this on the head once and for all. Age is **NOT** a legitimate reason to stop you achieving any goal, or enjoying life. Yes, know your limits but never stop trying to exceed them.

I don't want any more excuses coming from **you** regarding age because you know the deal now.
READER: *Ok!*
And what is known, cannot be unknown, studies have conclusively shown. For example, we've all heard the crazy frog, we can't go back.

Your past is gone, it's over but the best of **you** is yet to come.

Right, you've got support covered, you know your age isn't stopping you achieving your goals, so no excuses, it's time to sort out that bucket list…

BUCKET LIST

What do YOU wanna do?

It's a bit of a cliché these days but writing a bucket list should be part of everyone's life. I mean why wouldn't you? It's a list of things that **you** want to do before you die. Therefore writing the list allows you to plan **how** to accomplish them.

Win/win.

Write down what you'd like to do in life, assess whether they're feasible, do some research, take some action and then tick them off one by one when they're completed. You'll feel so good achieving each goal, a real sense of accomplishment. And you can always omit some if you decide you don't want to do it anymore and write a new list if you want. No-one else will know, you won't get told off.
It's your list.

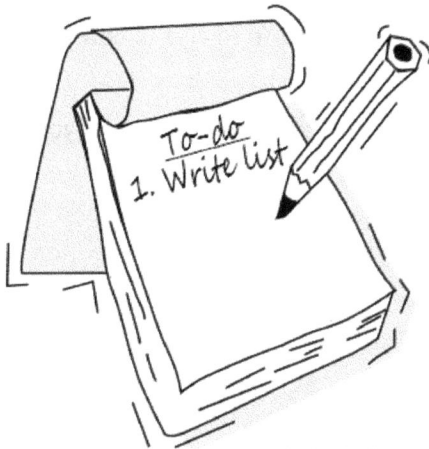

READER: *I'm not sure what to write.*
Ok! This might help. What would you like to do if you only had six months left to live?
READER: *Ooh! I'm not sure.*
No doubt you'd panic initially and cry… a lot.

But then you'd probably calm down and assess the situation rationally. You'd start to bemoan the fact that there's so many things that you wanted to do, see and experience before you passed away.

Let's pretend now.

You, the *'reader'*, yes **YOU**, I'm sorry but you've only got six months to live… so what you gonna do with that time?

Please, do yourself a favour and spend a while pondering that question. I mean, really, you should think about it every day 'cos it's happening whether you like it or not.

Go on, have a break for a few minutes… dooby-dooby-doo, dooby-dee, dooby-dah, dibbidy, dibbidy, doo… a few minutes later. Ok! We're back.

You don't want to be on your death bed and look back on your life and think *'if only'*.
You want to look back and say *'**Fuck yeah!!** I did as much as I could. It didn't all work out but I tried and I had a fun life, full of wild and enjoyable experiences'*.

So what have you always wanted to do but never dare attempted?

Write it all down and then think how each one could be achieved. It's up to you then to give them a go. Whether it's mountain biking over The Alps, bungee jumping over Victoria Falls, travelling on The Orient Express, running a marathon before you're thirty or losing four stone, every day you should be asking, *'What can I do **today**, that will get me closer to my goals?'*

For example, if weight loss is your goal, and you're about to buy a bacon sandwich or a cream donut, ask yourself, *'Will this action help me achieve my goal?'* If the answer is *'no'*, then don't do it.

If you decide to walk home from work and your goal is to get fitter, clearly that action **will** help you attain that goal. If you're saving up for a once in a lifetime holiday and you have won £60 on the work lottery, or you receive an unexpected tax refund; don't spend it on some meaningless tat, add it to your holiday fund instead.

Basically, every day you should be performing some act that contributes to accomplishing your goals. If not, then you've wasted another day of your life and taken a step backwards.
READER: *You make it sound so simple but life isn't like that...*
Of course it is.

If **you** want it to be that is. Stop being so defeatist and negative all the time and make some positive changes, do things differently. Remember, if what you did before isn't working, then it isn't working.

Ok!! Here are some other important factors **you** have to take into account when you're writing your bucket list.

You'll never succeed in something that you don't like. Whether that relates to nutrition, your job, exercise or trying to learn a foreign language. It's all about enjoyment. If you're not loving the experience, you'll quit. **Guaranteed!!**

You can't predict the future because it doesn't exist but you can start to shape it with the actions you take. So ditch the routines. Shake it up a bit because they just make you miserable.
Same ol', same ol', is not living. I hate routines and conforming, so have no idea where my life is heading but I can't wait to find out.

Also, you've got to be aware that everything happens for a reason and sometimes that reason is that you're an idiot and you make bad choices.
READER: *Charming!*
Nay bother. Look we all do at some time or another. Apart from her. Yeah, **her!!**
At least you bought this book though, that was a good choice, especially if you actually take on board the advice.

Like every goal, small daily improvements are the key to success. Step by step progress.
As the oft quoted Chinese philosopher, Lao Tzu said:

*The elevator to success is out of order
so you'll have to use the stairs, you lazy git*

I think he said that anyway.

And you've probably heard this one?

Aim for the stars and you may reach the moon

What a load of balls. Did Neil Armstrong do that? Of course not, he never went. Oops, wrong book.

You need a target, something **specific** to aim for but even though you may not achieve **exactly** what you intended, if you think so big *'they'* can't ignore you, you'll surprise yourself at what you can achieve. For instance, you probably won't score the winning goal in the FA Cup Final but you could play at Wembley in a charity match perhaps, or be a steward, reporter, mascot, photographer, volunteer, cheerleader etc, etc. Just do your research and adopt a bit of lateral thinking.

If you've always wanted to be on TV, well you might not become a famous actor but you could be an extra, make-up artist, runner, researcher or game show contestant.
Think outside the box.
Logic will get you from A to B but **imagination** can take you anywhere. The only limits are those that you set yourself and your refusal to take risks.

Do it, try it, give it a go,
'cos if you don't, you'll just never know

Or as my Geordie mate Keith would say, *'Jus' gan n' dee it man, fella, pet, man, but'*.

So now that you're on your way to achieving all of your dreams, what else will help you enjoy and live your life to the full??

Ah!! You need to de-stress, you need…

STRESS-BUSTERS

This section contains tips on how to have a laugh, enjoy life and let yourself go!!

You've just been dumped,
Now you're on your own,
Who ya gonna call?
STRESS-BUSTERS!!
Crap day at work?
'Cos you hate your job,
Who ya gonna call?
STRESS-BUSTERS!!
You've run out of dosh,
No dough in the bank,
Who ya gonna call?
STRESS-BUSTERS!!
You've put on a few stone,
Now your clothes don't fit,
Who ya gonna call?
STRESS-BUSTERS!!

MUSIC – There's no better sound

The food of love, yep music is a powerful medium. Not only does it make you want to shake your booty like a *Polaroid* picture but research has identified that when you listen to music you like your brain releases *'Dopamine'*, which is a *'feel-good'* neurotransmitter.

Thus by definition, good music makes you happy and being happy makes you…??
READER: *Positive?!*
You're getting the hang of this, well done. Patronising smiley face, coming your way ☺

So the next time you need an emotional boost, listen to some of your fave toons and make sure you sing along and tap your feet to the beat Grandma. You know, to get the maximum benefit.

As I've already mentioned, studies have shown that there are more than 350 million people on this planet who suffer from depression. In fact, it's believed that 1 in 5 people in just the UK alone suffer from the curse of this dispiriting illness. A whopping 90% of them also experience insomnia.

Well, music can help you sleep better too (as can exercise, we'll come to that later).

If you're having trouble sleeping or feeling a little low, try listening to some classical, chill-out or Irish folk music (Lisa Hannigan has the voice of an angel, and if she ever wants to have an affair, then I'm happy to oblige) before beddy-byes to help you catch some Z's.

Probably best to stay away from Rage Against the Machine, Public Enemy, Royal Blood or Sleaford Mods though. Mind you your dreams would be interesting and rather than sleep walking, you'd end up sleep-marching or sleep-protesting and want to fight the powers that be. Actually, sod it; give it a go, maybe you'll help change the world for the better.

It doesn't matter whether you're young or old, healthy or sick, happy or sad, music can improve the quality of your life in numerous ways. It reduces stress and anxiety, lifts your mood, boosts your health, helps you sleep better and it even improves your performance in the sack.
READER: *I'm sorry, what now?!*
Oh! C'mon!! If you haven't serenaded your loved one with a bit of Marvin Gaye or the Walrus of Love, you're missing out. I mean Bazza, he knew all about a deep throat... **Ooh!!** You dirty gits, behave yourself, I meant he had a distinctive, bass-baritone voice of course... ☺

To enjoy life, turn the volume button up to eleven and just press **play!**

THE WEEKEND

I'm gonna bust some more knowledge on your ass here. I don't know if you're aware but there are seven days in a week? Yeah I know, who knew? So c'mon, you shouldn't just live for the weekend and ignore the rest of the week. However, when it does come along you've gotta make it count and put in as much effort and energy as possible, into having a blast.

Here are my top ten tips, for having a cracking weekend:

1 - Do not worry about work - At all. If you're forever pondering about that report, personal development plan, e-mail, quarterly meeting, below inflation pay rise etc, etc you won't be able to R – E – L – A - X.

And that's what the weekend is for. To recuperate, recharge your batteries, chill them designer boots. You can't do anything about it anyway so just wait until Monday. If you feel chilled out, happier and more positive, that alleged problem will be addressed in no time.

2 - Do not spend all weekend watching the box - Go out, see your mates, catch-up with family but if you just slouch in front of the radiation emitter, you'll be zonked and definitely not refreshed when you drag yourself out of bed on the Monday morn.

tips

3 - Have a bath - Maybe this is one for the winter months but there are not many better things than a long soak in the tub. I don't know what your bath game is like but personally I'm a big fan of the soapy bubbles. I like to have some music playing too, and candles do improve the setting. Now this could be a solo adventure, or depending on the size of your porcelain basin, get your partner in too. Alone or intimate, the heat, sweat, aroma and ambience create a lovely, relaxing environment. How you towel down afterwards is up to you.

4 – Explore - Have a picnic, go to the seaside, get your wellies on and discover this beautiful country. Strap your kids into the 4 x 4 and head over t' countryside.
Get some **fresh air** before the Tory party start charging us for it. It's grand, you'll love it but you have to open your door and travel a bit to see it.

5 – Sunday - This should be the most relaxing day of the week. It bugs me no end when I'm out jogging and notice that so many people spend their Sundays driving on jam-packed roads going to D.I.Y. stores, Supermarkets, Carpet shops and the like. Why? They're just busy, crowded, hotbeds of consumer monkeys. How is that in any way relaxing? I would much rather go for a stroll in the countryside, or even just chill at home. I mean it is supposed to be the day of rest after all.

READER: *I thought you weren't religious.*

Far from it but me and her (Word is telling me this should be *'I and She'* but I write how I speak and I would never say *'I and She'*. Never. Ever. Sorry Mr Gates) definitely agree on this one, it should be a day spent recuperating, chilling and spending time with family and friends.

tips

6 - Read a book - Go to a quiet room, sit in the garden, or go to a park bench and just read for an hour or so. No interruptions, just you and a good novel, an autobiography, a holy book, or a weird, hilarious, fitness, depression free guide book.

And don't give me all that *'yes but I need a babysitter'* lark. I'm sure yer Ma, sis, boyfriend, lover, mate or Postman will look after your bairns for an hour so you can have a bit of peace and quiet. It's always excuses with you isn't it?

7 - Phone a friend - No I'm not referring to that quiz show which was actually quite good really, I mean pick one of your pals or a family member you haven't spoken to in a while and give them a bell. Have a natter, a chinwag, a good ol' catch up.

They will be chuffed to lil' mint balls to hear your voice I can assure you and you'll feel great too. Win/win.

Or and hear me out on this one. Write a letter…

READER: *What's one of those?*

A letter is like a text message or an e-mail but considerably longer and involves the use of a *'pen'* or *'pencil'*.

Yeah, I know that they're *'so last century'* but let's bring em back. It used to be a great feeling receiving a letter and you could add poems, doodles, secret codes etc, etc and make it fun.

Not sold? Oh well, I tried.

It's all mobiles and social media these days I suppose.

What's the deal now with mobile phones? Do foetus text expectant Mothers with due dates?! I mean, do we really need to be accessible 24/7?

What about a three hour amnesty and maybe have face to face conversations instead?
Try it one weekend, you might like it.

Don't worry… you'll still be able to breathe…

DIANE, 42 – *I took your advice Paul, no mobile phone after 9pm. I did it to gain some work-life balance because I was addicted to checking my work emails as well as Facebook, but also just to have a bit of quiet time before bed. It's made a huge difference. It was a bit of an irritant at first but after the first week it became easier. I didn't miss it one bit and I felt less stressed out. I also slept better, so much better. Some of my friends complained that I missed their text messages, but it was nothing that couldn't wait until the next day.*

Our fast-paced world is never unplugged. We rarely have time to disconnect from technology, what with our mobiles, t' Internet, email, tellybox, even our heating these days. We're so wired, is it no wonder we're so tired too?!

The amount of times I'm in a pub, on the bus, walking in the park or even with my family and **everyone** is just glued to their phone. Not paying attention to what's going on in the world… I said, not paying attention to what's going on…

READER: *Sorry, my mate just uploaded a picture of a panda wearing a dress, so I had to tag my sister and my cousin and my mate Steve and my Aunty Rose and the milkman and that bloke I met on that holiday but can't remember his name and…*

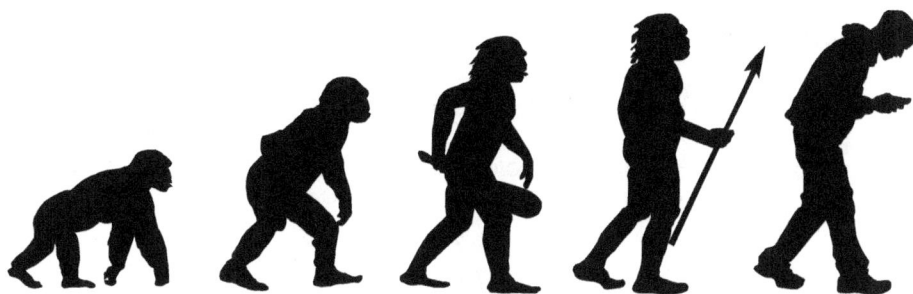

Maybe we should start again?!

Practice what you preach *'they'* say, but I can be just as bad sometimes. I admit that I've even rung a mates mobile **hoping** to get the voice mail so I can leave a message and forego all the usual unnecessary pleasantries. It's ridiculous really and I feel quite ashamed that I've done that… only a few times mind but nevertheless, it's like a phone box in a country village…
READER: *What?*
Out of order.

The majority of people now spend their days, alternating between staring at little black boxes in their hands, to larger boxes on their desks at work, and then to gargantuan boxes in their living rooms.
This pixellation-fixation has to stop. It's not good for you. For us. For anyone. **Stop it!!**

tips

8 - <u>Go for a Friday night drink</u> - Oop North, did you know that Friday neet is for the lads or groups of lasses and Saturday is couples night? Well it is. Madness right?
But you should respect these traditions and I've always found that if you go out on the Friday night, the weekend seems to feel that much longer.

A few shandies or glasses of vino will definitely help you unwind and de-stress. Just don't get paralytic, 'cos then your Saturday morning will be ruined. Or when you get older, it takes the whole bloody weekend to get back to your normal self.

A giggle, a bit of banter, a few sherbets, you can't go wrong. Back home early so you can enjoy the rest of your weekend safe in the knowledge you won't be puking your guts out and curled up in a ball, shaking and weeping uncontrollably in the bathroom. Cheers!!

9 - <u>Go to a Museum or an Art Gallery</u>.

READER: *Boring!!*
When was the last time you visited one?
READER: *Actually, I can't remember….. maybe when I was at school.*
They've changed loads in the last decade or so, they're awesome and you, erm, learn stuff n' that. Knowledge is power you know?!

Normally I'd promote the fact that although education is important, a healthy fit body is more *'importanter'* but we seem to be missing out on so much culture these days.

I mean it would certainly help society evolve, which ain't a bad thing. So take your kiddies, your mates, your Ma, your Aunty Carol and get them involved too, it can be a laugh.

Whether it's surrealist paintings, papier mache ornaments, dinosaur fossils, engineering wonders, or teapots through the ages, the UK is filled with amazing attractions. In fact, there's so much to do and see that you'll never be able to fit them all in. But you could try.

tips   **10** - <u>Get your leg over</u>.

Rekindle the romance, get them flames a-burnin'!! It's as good a time as any.

You've got from Friday night to Monday morning, so no excuses, there's plenty of time to get that bed A-ROCKIN'.

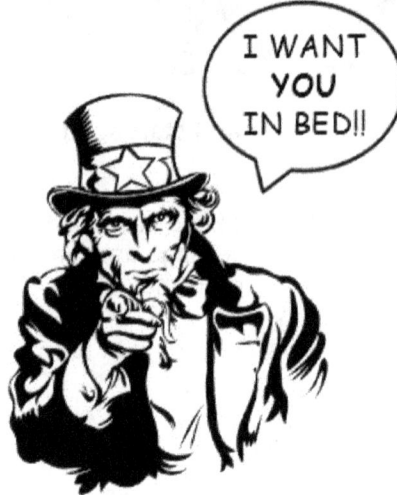

It's also been scientifically proven that sex alleviates and relieves headaches too.
Oops!! Sorry Ladies, you can't use that feeble excuse anymore.

Whilst we're on the subject, let's discuss *'the physical union of male and female genitalia, accompanied by rhythmic movements'* in a bit more detail.

COITUS

How's your father, bumping uglies, getting down and dirty, hiding the sausage, making the beast with two backs, knocking boots… doing it. The old rumpy-pumpy will definitely make you happier. Hands down. Or around, underneath, on top etc nudge, nudge, wink, wink, etc.

When you're in the throes of passion or laughing so much you nearly pee, are you concerned about weight, love handles, muffin top? **No!!** Because this is when you're at your most joyful therefore it doesn't matter.

And it doesn't matter.

You're so God damn beautiful,
I'm absolutely smitten,
I can't believe that you're my girl,
'Cos you're one hot sex kitten!!

Some people seem to get so prudish when it comes to sex, yet that's why we're all here. Let me tell you now, vigorous sexual activity is a fantastic, enjoyable, orgasmic calorie burner.

It gives a whole new meaning to the term, **'hot in bed'**.

Obviously I'm awesome in bed, that's why my ex-girlfriends used to nickname me *'Picasso Lover'*.
READER: *Why's that?*
It's because I was an artist between the sheets.
Oh yes!!
Ladies and gentleman, tip your waitress, I'll be here all week.

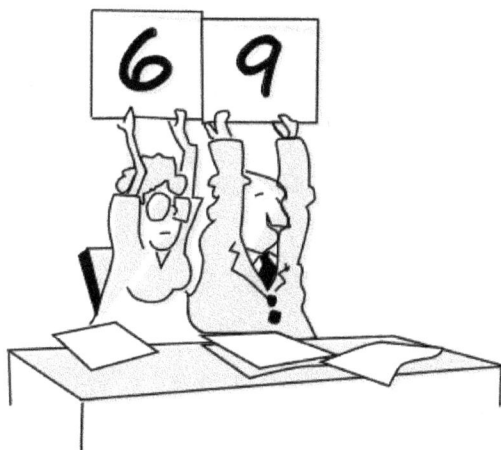

Perhaps I'm exaggerating slightly for comic effort but I always tried to liven things up a bit although I'll confess, I'm no Mr Grey.

Sex is so technical these days, it's as if every performance is being monitored, judged and assessed based on movie-sex.
Which isn't real.

It's make believe, fake, a fantasy.

There's so much pressure these days, especially on blokes but I'm sure you'll agree ladies that a minute in heaven, is better than a few seconds in heaven?!

Anyway, sex is not about quantity it's about quality.
READER: *Speak for yourself.*

Ok! Fair do's but it should always be fun, not nerve-wracking.

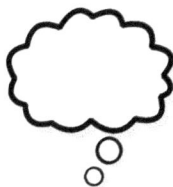

- *Am I big enough?*
- *I hope I don't come too quickly.*
- *I wonder what they're thinking about.*
- *Has he noticed my cellulite?*
- *Are my boobs symmetrical?*
- *Do I have a weird vulva?*
- *Is it in yet?!*

Its madness and it has to stop. The last one by the way, include the worst four words that any man can hear. Luckily it's never happened to me... **honest!!**

Sex should be fun and pleasurable, it's not a test but yet we seem to treat it this way. For me, if I can undo a bra first time without any help, I do a lap of honour around the bedroom.

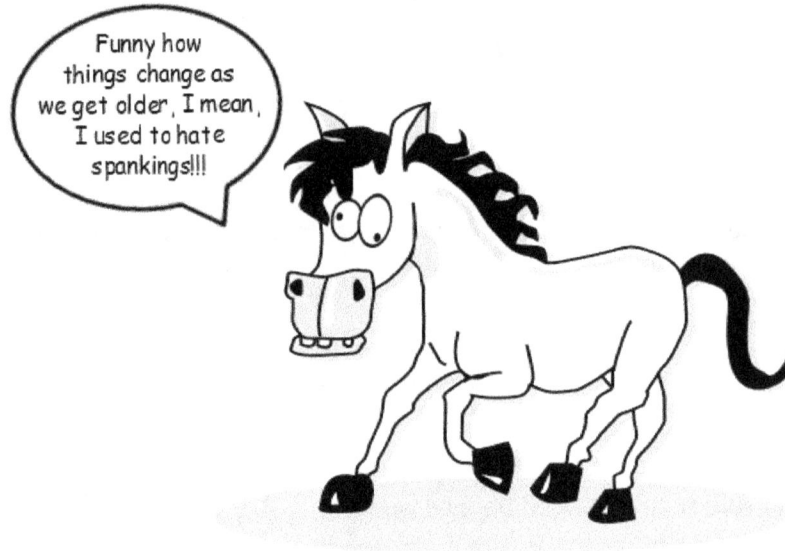

Sex is a great stress-reliever, so stop ruining it by making the experience like an examination, unless it's an oral one.
READER: *You're filthy you!!*
I'm sure you've grasped the fact by now that I just like to have a laugh. For over ten years now, I've begun not to take life too seriously and try to see the fun in everything.

That's what happens when you see the light and you find positivity; it's the only way to live.

Why do you always leave the toilet seat up?
And never clean out your favourite cup?
Why can't you ever just make the bed?
Or listen to the words that I've always said?
Why is football more important than me?
And why do you never cook my tea?
Why do I love you when you treat me this way?
'Cos you shag like a rabbit,
You're the 'World's Greatest Lay'.

!!! TIMEOUT!!! TIMEOUT!!! TIMEOUT!!! TIMEOUT!!! TIMEOUT!!! TIMEOUT!!! TIMEOUT!!! TIMEOUT!!!

I'm just gonna give it five, I've been typing for hours, I'm knackered, so talk amongst yourselves...(five minutes later) okay doke, back to it.

When you start to incorporate fitness into your world and it becomes an integral part of your life, you're in for an additional treat. A Brucey bonus!!

Exercise invigorates your sex life by increasing your libido.
READER: *What, really?*
Oh aye!! It gets you horny baby!! **YEAH!!**

> **LAURA, 38** - *Losing this weight has not only given me more confidence, more energy and improved my health; it's actually given my relationship a spark.*
> *I find my partner taking cheeky glances at me, checking my bum out when he thinks I'm not looking and I love it. Even the guys at work have started to notice me and not that I would do anything because I love my fella, but knowing they fancy me has given me a boost too.*
> *In the past, if I'm honest I've never really felt 'sexy' and I didn't always feel comfortable in the bedroom because of my size but nowadays I'm insatiable.*

To conclude this section on coitus, let me leave you with some sage advice. Cookies and porn are always better homemade.

The following pages contain additional suggestions to help you alleviate stress.
Firstly, you shouldn't get so stressed in the first place but I accept that it will take you time to evolve into a progressive, purveyor of positivity. Therefore the more you do the stuff I suggest, the easier your life will be and the happier you'll become.

Have a go at as many as possible and obviously, feel free to adapt and create your own.

STAND-UP COMEDY

In my opinion, the stand-up is the modern day preacher. And some of them deserve to be worshipped, especially the legends of the game like Billy Connolly, George Carlin, Eddie Izzard, Bill Hicks, Bill Burr, Richard Pryor and Mitch Hedberg to name but a heptade (fancy word for seven, sorry I'm showing off now, won't happen again).

These guys are all *'nearly pee my pants, they're so funny'* good but the way they observe society, makes you question reality and... **think!!**

Therefore I recommend, nay beseech you, to watch as many of their comedies as possible.
READER: *They're all blokes though... sexist.*
Yep, you're right. It is a male dominated industry but there are definitely some great female comics too. Joan Rivers was brilliant. Witty and acerbic, she set the tone for both male and female comedians with her rebellious take on life. Sarah Silverman is amazing too, really ballsy actually. In fact, not only is she hilarious, she also motivated so many people to vote for Barack Obama in 2008 that she should've been credited in his inauguration speech. Caroline Aherne was quite rightly described as a comedy genius and a hell of a talent. Her take on modern life with the sit-com *'The Royle Family'* was extremely sobering, especially as a fellow Northerner. Sadly missed that lass. As is the late great Victoria *'hit me on the bottom with a Woman's Weekly'* Wood, who was another fantastic writer and comedian. Katherine Ryan is very droll and the women that acted in *'Smack the Pony'* and *'Pulling'* are also **ace!!** Check them out too. And quirky Julia Davis off of *'Nighty-Night'* and *'Gavin and Stacey'* has me in hysterics. That woman can pull a face. But my favourite female comedy writer has to be Sharon Horgan. She is awesome. Funny as the proverbial and damn sexy too. Brilliant, brilliant comedian. Check out *'Catastrophe'*, it's gotta be one of the funniest programmes **ever!!** Seriously, it's brilliant, brilliant TV.

Hey if you're a funny lass, maybe you should be on stage, perhaps that could be your goal? The world could certainly do with more humour.

Anyway, there's loads of comedy out there and I advise you to watch as much as poss, either on DVD, through *'You-Tube'* or actually get yourself out to a local Comedy Club.

They will inspire you and they will help your personality evolve. You'll start to question life but from a quirkier perspective.

When I finally become a successful writer, you'll be able to watch my sitcom. It's about a Personal Trainer (obvs) and centres around one client who progressively loses weight as the episodes continue. Can you imagine it? The main protagonist actually getting thinner and thinner. Yeah, it'll be great, ground-breaking. Check it out in five years or so, it'll be on Channel 4 no doubt and be **hilarious!!**

Anyway back to the point. As I keep repeating, you need to **laugh** as much as you can. So whether the comedian is critically acclaimed or a tad mainstream, if they make you laugh, watch and listen to them as much as possible.

Because enjoyment begets happiness, which begets positivity.

So let's **begetting** more fun in your life.

CREATIVITY

As you've probably noticed, I do like a rhyme or fifty. I know that the rhythms are slightly off beat and perhaps don't scan like the pedants in the poetry world would desire but I don't care. I'm a grammar vandal and proud of it. So you can shove your *'iambic pentameters'*, where the gaseous ball of fire fails to extol its illuminating qualities.

I **enjoy** writing little ditties, irrespective of whether they fit in with the antiquated rules or not. It gives me pleasure, it makes me **happy**. I also like to doodle and draw because that fills me with happiness too. When I was younger I studied *'Advertising'* and *'Graphic Design'*, so I've always had a leaning towards the Arts and a certain talent. I know that I'm not as good as I think I am and I sometimes find it difficult to execute my ideas successfully but I still enjoy the process and so can **you**.

At junior school we were **all** taught to express ourselves creatively, no matter how talented we were but in our archaic and out-dated education system, this creativity is drummed out of us as we get older. Everything has to be quantifiable but art is subjective and always will be. You can't really give it a mark. It's like Marmite. You either love it or you want to chuck it against a wall and destroy the foul tasting, yeasty, pastey, mush. But who cares how good you are, it's a cathartic and liberating experience.

Therefore I recommend that you start drawing, doodling, painting and writing poetry. Who knows, this may lead to a new career in greeting cards, posters, t-shirts or novels. I can assure you that you'll get more enjoyment out of it than watching that rectangular harbinger of doom we've all got displayed in our living rooms.

C'mon, get your pens and pencils out for the lads!! On your marks, 1, 2, 3... **DRAW!!**

UP TO BEDFORDSHIRE

The early bird gets the worm but who wants to eat worms, so get up when you like. Although don't be misled, this isn't me suggesting you should be a lazy git but we all need a lie in... now and again.

Just don't let it become the norm but when you do get the chance, treat that duvet like you're stir-fry chicken and it's a tortilla wrap.

Not much beats being cocooned in blankets, all warm and toasty on a cold/rainy/snowy/windy morning (all four could happen at once if you live in the UK). In fact, don't worry I won't tell anyone but I reckon you should pull a sickie one day in the next few weeks and have a *'Duvet day'*. Hey, c'mon, that's why God invented the *'24hr bug'*. Do it. You won't regret it.

READER: *Ooh! I wouldn't know what to say.*

It's easy, ring up really early (set your alarm) and put on your best *'pathetic whimpering voice'*. Pretend you've been up all night, puking and shitting. Say you've got really bad diarrhoea.

Your Boss or Manager won't want to ask too many questions, 'cos folk don't like discussing the dreaded squits, so you're sorted. Then it's box-set, duvet day, **Yay!!**
Enjoy.
NB: This was a joke by the way, please don't take this literally ;)

FILMS

Have a movie night and eat some popcorn. Watching a great film at the Cinema is a brilliant experience. Super-dooper-whooper HD or 3-D, massive screens and ear-splitting sound, all combined with munching, crunching and slurping. It's a shame that other people turn up to ruin the fun. What is it with people? They're the worst aren't they?!

All you want to do is watch the exploits of *'Slothman'* and there's some teenagers virtually shagging in one aisle, a couple arguing 'cos she bought a £6 bag of wine gums rather than jelly-babies, and some blokes who just won't **shut the fuck up!!**

And the litter, what is it with cinema goers and litter? Whenever I leave the cinema these days the sole of my trainers are covered in chuddy, slush puppy juice and cheezy nachos. Just pick your fuckin' litter up and place it in a bin you fuckin' degenerates, have some fuckin' **RESPECT!!**
<u>60% of CINEMA-GOERS</u>: *Everyone does it, chill out, it's not my problem.*

And that Ladies and Gentleman is why we're so messed up as a race.

"I can't be bothered, somebody else will pick it up"

Anyone that litters, should be punished… severely and repeatedly.
For me, it's just as bad as assault, robbery or Corporate Tax evasion and anyone that commits any of those offences, deserves a custodial sentence.
<u>READER</u>: *A tad harsh, don't you think?*
No!! I bloody well don't.

Anyone who thinks it's okay to litter, is a TWAT and they have a personality defect known as *'selfish-buggery'*. They believe that everything is **owed** to them. They don't think anything is **their** fault and they are egotistical, brainless scum. All of 'em.

Have you heard of the *'broken window theory'*?
<u>READER</u>: *Nope, please enlighten me.*
Basically it relates to Communities and their *'quality of life'*, which is linked to the level of crime in that neighbourhood (successfully introduced to New York in the early 1990's). When a building window is broken and left unrepaired, the rest of the windows invariably get broken too. An unrepaired broken window is a signal that no-one cares, so more windows are damaged as a result.

In these types of environment where anti-social behaviour goes unpunished, more serious street crime then flourishes. The area becomes run-down and thus a *'no-go area'* for respectable citizens.

It's the same principle with litter. If people notice an area is clean, tidy and well preserved, they are less likely to litter. If an area has become a cesspool of mattresses, crisp packets, junk-food trays and dog poo, it will become a shithole.

The *'broken window theory'* states that maintaining and monitoring environments to prevent low-level crimes such as vandalism, public drunkenness and **littering**, helps to create an atmosphere of order and lawfulness, thereby preventing more serious crimes from happening.

<u>CONCLUSION</u>: **The more we punish litter-bugs, the less our green and pleasant land will be sullied with crap.**

And you thought happiness, health and fitness was all about designer clothing, legwarmers and pointless silicone wristbands. Well it's not. Anyway back to films, the sequel. This time it's personal.

To escape *'those annoying littering people'*, my advice is to take the afternoon off from work and go then. Yes there's a strong chance that *'Mad Eric'* may also turn up with his inappropriately placed popcorn bucket but generally speaking it's a quiet affair.

You'll be able to enjoy the experience with very little interruption and who knows; perhaps the film will be good too… as long as you like remakes and comic-book adaptations, 'cos that's all they seem to make these days.

Alternatively, use that fifty inch plasma you've got at home and test its surround-sound capabilities to the max by watching a DVD. To be fair, you probably spent so much on it that you can't afford to go out these days anyway, so it's bound to be the best option. You can pause the film when you like, turn the volume up or down and even eat a three course meal in the middle if you so choose.

Plus, if you get a little bit frisky, it's not too far from the boudoir if you know what I mean?! For our older Readers, *'and why not?!'*

HAPPINESS BEGINS WITH A SMILE

Look, the passport office don't control your life so you are **allowed** to smile when out wandering through this dark and dangerous world. Therefore find your perfect smile and use it as often as possible.

You can't waste a smile.

And how nice is it when a stranger passes you on the street and smiles at ya?! You get all warm and tingly. You actually feel that maybe, just maybe, you might be attractive after all. Well **you** could be that stranger. Imagine a whole day walking around a city, smiling at people. You'd make such a positive impact on their lives, plus you'd feel great too. Who knows, one of the recipients might smile back, you get chatting and next thing you know you've just come for the fourth time.

<u>READER</u>: *Saucy git!!*

That's right **baby!!**

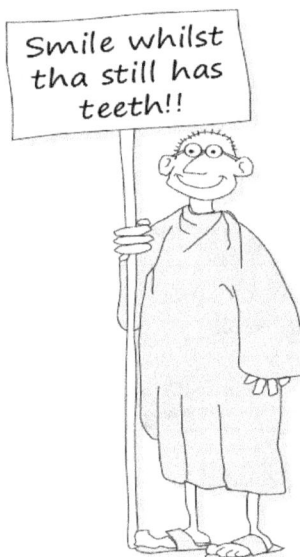

Smile whilst tha still has teeth!!

GUILTY PLEASURES

The phrase, *'guilty pleasures'* should be made illegal really, although I suppose it does infer a certain predilection for summat cheesy. But never feel guilty about pleasuring yourselves. Unless it's in public, c'mon there are kids about.

Saying *'that band is better than that band'* is like saying *'that orgasm was better than the last one'*. Just appreciate and enjoy it for what it is.

If you spend all your life trying to be cool rather than acting the fool, you will never be happy.
So let yourself go and dance like everyone is looking and you couldn't care less. Stop thinking you're some sort of *'hipster'*, you're fooling no-one, you're just a fashion **victim**.

Let me tell you something. *'HIPSTER'* is an anagram of *'PR SHITE'*, which perfectly describes the fickle, superficial world of fashion, music and media.

If you like it, don't apologise for it. Who cares if it's critically acclaimed or not, if you like it then watch it, eat it, drink it, wear it and love it.
READER: *Do you have a guilty pleasure?*
Glad you asked, probably Elvis but I ain't guilty about it, perhaps a little shook up. Thank you.
Thangyaverymuch!!

I do love to sing along to his greatest hits, although I draw the line at eating like he used to.

You can shove your peanut butter-jelly-bacon-cheeseburger and fried banana sandwiches where the fiery hot ball of plasma, refuses to express its self.

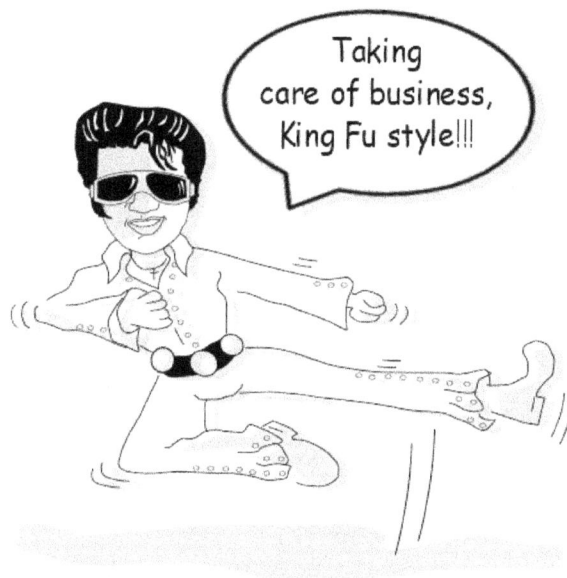

KINDNESS

As one of the greatest philosophers of our time contends, (Joey off of *'Friends'*... obviously) there's no such thing as a selfless good deed.
The reason?
The beneficiary will clearly appreciate the gesture and it'll make **you** feel good about yourself too. But that's brilliant and just like a smile you can't waste kindness, no matter how small the deed is.

It sort of goes without saying that you should be kind to your family and friends, but being kind to strangers is another thing entirely.C'mon, who doesn't love a random, good deed from a stranger?

Well **you** could be that stranger.

Whether it's paying for someone else's petrol, helping someone with their shopping bags, hailing a taxi, or allowing a car to pull up in front of you in a traffic jam. You'll get a warm buzz and you'll help their mood improve too.

I've been a selfish bugger for a lot of my adult life but after hitting rock bottom and nearly doing myself in, I've come to realise that helping others is such a rewarding experience. When I qualified as a Personal Trainer, rather than join a gym and charge people for my services, instead I offered to help people for free. I spent a considerable amount of time and effort helping *'strangers'* lose weight, get fitter and banish the blues.

I compiled a dossier of the common issues, mistakes and pitfalls that each client underwent in their quest for weight-loss and the result forms the basis of this book.

It was evident that the majority of my *'overweight'* clients suffered from low self-esteem, had a poor self-image and classed themselves as depressed. Yet once they started to embrace fitness and positivity, it was amazing how happier they became. This made me feel awesome too because I helped them achieve this fundamental change. This is why I had to write this book, to share these experiences and promote the ideology of HELP... because it works.

Ah! Enough blabbering on, back to the point.

Altruism isn't a new shampoo ingredient, it's a way of life...

Why not try some of the following ideas:

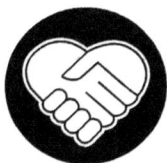

> - Ask you friends if they need any help with a project, or babysitting, or even paying the rent. Be there for them.
> - Buy some flowers for your Mother or Grandmother, for no other reason than just because.
> - Allow fellow drivers to merge into your lane or to turn into the road, without pulling a grimace all over your mug.
> - Rather than trying to sell your unwanted nick-nacks on *'E-bay'*, donate them to a local charity instead and even ask them if they need any volunteers.
> - Plant a tree in your garden.
> - Teach an ol' dear to use a computer, so they can surf the Internet for pensioner-porn, or write e-mail complaints.
> - Organise a family meal and just appreciate the time being together.
> - Collect stuffed animals or toys from family members, friends, and neighbours, then donate them to a local children's hospital.
> - Sign up for a First Aid course. And then you can be a superhero when you least expect it.
> - Don't just donate clothes, toys and old books, donate blood too.
> - Start to pick up litter that's been left in your street. Hopefully the neighbours will cotton on and they'll also get on board.
> - Swallow your pride and apologise for something you *'may'* or *'may not'* have done. C'mon it's not worth arguing about, let it go and laugh about it instead.
> - Return a text from a pal that you have been putting off. In fact sod that, call 'em. They've been your friend for years and there's a good reason for that... apparently you're mates.
> - Arrange a fun day at work with all proceeds going to a local charity. Fancy dress, bake sale, band t-shirts or maybe dress up as a zombie. After all, most people look half dead at work anyway.
> - Join a fitness class and befriend a classmate.
>
> - Volunteer at a homeless centre and then you might even have a deeper appreciation of food and waste, and your own greed perhaps?!
> - Don't ignore those *'foreign'* looking people. They're just like you and me. They have worries, concerns, fears and hopes. Be nice.

Alternatively, you can just be polite instead. Thank people you encounter at work and in your daily life. Open the door for someone, don't push into a queue, be respectful to your neighbours... you know, be nice n' that.

And with respect to work, by giving someone genuine praise you spread positive energy, you boost that person's self-esteem and their motivation, plus it gives **you** a few satisfaction goose bumps in the process. Also, being told you can leave work early and you'll still get paid, is one of the greatest events in life. So, if you're a Gaffer **you** can make this happen.

Just imagine, somewhere, somebody will be thinking fondly of you because of the kind and tremendous impact you made on their life. Not me... I think you're a knobhead but someone.

Become a good listener too. Whenever someone is chatting to you, rather than piping in every two minutes or talking over them, just listen. Once they've said their peace, take a few seconds to reflect. Have a bit of a ponder and then respond. It's called a conversation but people seem too inept to hold one these days.
That's because of our over-inflated egos and wanting to be right all of the time. We love being right. Even when we're wrong.
READER: *Huh! Coming from you!!*
Aye you may be right. Although in person I'm an empathetic, considerate, compassionate **hoot!!** And a good listener to boot.

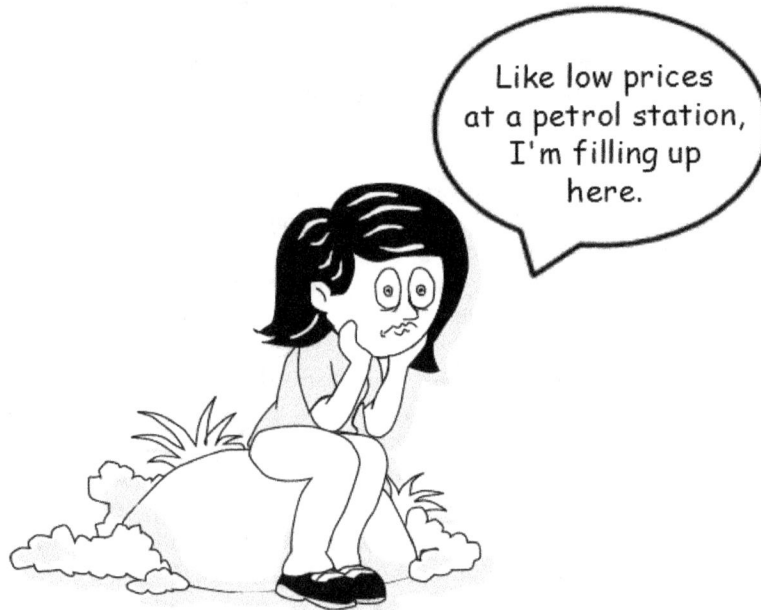

Like low prices at a petrol station, I'm filling up here.

A conversation should be a two-way process, you're not one of them dickhead MP's interrupting all the time and refusing to actually answer a question. You're a nice normal human being, with ears. And ears are made for listening... so I've heard.

HUGGING

Who doesn't like to be hugged? I'm a late bloomer to the concept of hugging. In fact, it wasn't 'til I was well into my thirties that I started to embrace the hug bug. I was never hugged as a child, you see.
READER: *Aah!! Explains everything.*
Shut up!!

When you haven't seen a mate, or family member for a while, give 'em a hug. It's a great way to show them you care. And you do you know, **you do care**, so show 'em. Just know when to stop.
Five Mississippi's is about right, any longer and it might get a little awkward.

LOVE

Where would we be without it? Alone, depressed and writing health & fitness books probably.
Only joking, or am I? Yes, yes I am... **honest!!**
Maybe...

With respect to your family and close friends, how about saying *'I love you'* every so often.
Hearing someone saying *'I love you'* when it's completely out of the blue and you know they mean it, is a wonderful, wonderful moment. Some might say, *'heart-warming'*. **You** could be that person to elicit that response.

Although these people that say it after every conversation, erm guys, it's gonna lose its meaning.

Pass me the salt – I love you.
Use a coaster - I love you.
*Piss off - **I love you!!***

Like most things, there's a time and a place. Oh! And if **you** are single due to unrequited love, let me tell you now from heart-breaking experience, it's a complete waste of time. If it ain't happening my friend, it ain't happening. Wake up and smell the restraining order.
Lots of love,
Birchy.

TREATS

Do something today that your future self will thank you for, like cake... **Hmm!! Cake!!**
READER: *I thought you were a fitness fanatic, do you eat cakes?*
I used to eat cakes... I still do but I used to, too.
Aye! I try to say *'No'* to cakes but they just don't listen.

Don't worry, when you adopt an active lifestyle it doesn't matter if you have an extra slice of cake, a few choccy biccies, or miss a gym session or three. You won't beat yourself up about it, 'cos it doesn't matter in the grand scheme of things and you'll work harder the **next** time you exercise.
Therefore treat yourself... but in moderation.

Although don't fall into this trap whatever you do, *'I've been good this week, so I deserve a treat'.*
You know the score, calorie restriction all week, then ruin all your good work by scoffing a days' worth of calories in one sitting... as a treat.

My family have a tradition that is known as a *'Half Seven'*.
READER: *A half what?*
Seven.
When we were kids and another one of my Step-Dads had sodded off and left me poor old Ma on her tod to fend for herself yet again, we didn't have much dough. We were brassic. Thus our sweet consumption was very limited to say the least but what me Mum did, was allow us to have a treat at 7:30pm ish when she made an early evening cup of char. This meant that we had something to look forward to during the day, and also reduced our overall daily sugar intake. Something the young 'uns of today, **desperately** need.

In hindsight, it's probably why I'm not totally obsessed with biccies, cakes and chocolate. Yes I've got a sweet tooth and the fillings to prove it. Thank you, wine gums and flapjacks. But I don't scoff them all day and all night, which is probably because even to this day I still try to have a *'half seven'*. Not every day mind, I'm not an animal. This enforced restriction has increased my willpower and saves my teeth looking like *'Black Jacks'*.

You should give it a go.

If you eat treats in moderation they don't lose their appeal, 'cos too much of a good thing... can kill you apparently!! Something like that anyway.

Less is always more, except when it relates to penis size.

Paul Birch

HERE COMETH THE SUN

Liam from Oasis might be an arse sometimes but he can belt out a tune and nobody can sing the word, *'sunshine'* quite like Mr Gallagher. You should try it, it's fun.

'Sunshiii-innnne!!

Did you know that half an hour of sunlight each day boosts your serotonin levels?
<u>READER</u>: *No I wasn't aware of that, thank you for informing me of this fact.*
You're very welcome.

Yep! The sun makes us happy. Who'd have thought?!

Although, there is a sun that is bad for you and it calls itself a *'newspaper'*, has Page 3 girls in it and would be more use wrapped around a cardboard roll in the toilet. Actually, here's *'the truth'*, I wouldn't even wipe my harris with that pile of crap.

✝ JUSTICE FOR THE 96 ✝

I don't believe in horoscopes or *'Horrorscopes'* if you will, which are so called 'cos it's **scary** if you actually believe they are true. The time of year you were born *'may'* have some miniscule bearing on your personality but don't **ever** put any stock in newspaper, or magazine articles based on your birth **day** because it's invariably bunkum. I just don't believe in star signs, it's all mumbo-jumbo but that's me, typical Gemini.

However, being a summer child, in fact I was born on the longest day of summer; I've always felt more comfortable in hotter climes. Then again, don't we all?! That's why we spend a fortune jetting off to the foreign seaside. But even in the UK we still get some decent rays and with global warming it's gonna get 'otter and 'otter.

So go for a walk, sit in the garden, get on your bike, go to the beach, get thissen some vitamin D.
<u>READER</u>: *Why vitamin D?*
We need vitamin D to help the body absorb *'Calcium'* and *'Phosphate'* from our diet. These minerals are important for healthy bones, teeth and muscles. And fortunately we can absorb vitamin D from sun exposure. **Praise the Lord!!**

A lack of vitamin D can cause bones to become soft and weak, which can lead to tenderness, fractures and even deformities. As we get older we are all susceptible to developing *'Osteoporosis'* which causes bones to become brittle and fragile, therefore it's imperative that we obtain both calcium and vitamin D from our diet and sun exposure.

KIMBERLEY, 29 – *Being plump, I always felt self-conscious about wearing a swimsuit. I used to love going to the beach but because I was insecure about how I looked, I'd just wear a long flowing skirt and a baggy top. And being big, I used to sweat so much, which made me feel extremely self-conscious in the heat.*
Losing weight has given me the confidence to wear a bikini on the beach and I go to the seaside as much as I can.
A bikini. Me!! I feel like a member of Baywatch now. Mind you, still got a face off Crimewatch, Hee! Hee!

So whenever you feel stressed and you're concerned your teeth might fall out or your knees might pop, get yourself out in the sun.
After all, that's why God invented beer gardens and cornetto's.

BAKING & COOKING

It's so rewarding cooking a satisfying meal. Especially one that doesn't involve popping a fork into some plastic and the whirr, ping of a microwave. Slap some music on, get stirring and mixing and slicing, make a mess, enjoy it, have a giggle.

And who cares if those snotty pedants off *'MasterChef'* and *'Bake Off'* wouldn't approve. Cooking isn't all about double entendres and soggy bottoms with a blackberry jus. It's subjective. Everyone has a unique culinary palette. Different tastes.

So, if you want to put burgers and beans in a pie… do it.

If you want to pour orange juice over your roasties, or put avocado and mayonnaise on a pizza, it's your choice… **barmpot!!**

I'll tell you now, it's so cathartic chopping up ingredients, dancing in your blue suede shoes and chucking stuff in a wok or baking tray, not knowing if it's gonna be the best meal you've ever had, or you'll be vomiting within the hour.

Just like life, if you don't try you'll never know. You have to experiment. I mean, that's why we sup coffee now isn't it? That's why we have eggs over easy and fish-finger sarnies. And those Monks who started breweries, well Amen to them. **Halle-Bloody-Lujah!!**

Some visionary way back in the times of yore, looked at a pig and thought *'I'm gonna eat that'*.
Their mates probably gasped in disgust but by the end of the week, they couldn't get enough of bacon butties. To be honest, I don't **want** to know what the first person did after they looked at a cow and thought, *'that white liquid would be ace in my brew'*. But without their foresight, Mr Kellogg would be in abject poverty, and my granola would be dry and still in a packet.

These days we have hybrid desserts such as the cro-nut, do-waffle and battered muffins (behave yourself) but as bad as they are for your gut, you've gotta admire the creativity.

I often hear the phrase *'I just love food, so much'*, yet whoever is saying that actually eats the most bland, tasteless, boring food imaginable.

- Garlic bread from a packet
- Microwaveable ready meals for 2, for 1
- Mounds and mounds of pasta
- Gargantuan plastic-cheezy-doughy pizzas
- Oven *'Oh aye, we're made from 100% potato, honest Guv!'* chips
- Smoked sausages, containing 90% pork and 10%, *'we couldn't actually determine from the autopsy report what type of animal it was'* – meat

All in all, it's a bunch of flavourless bollocks, really. And that's not good for anyone. Actually, I once tried some sheep's testicles and I don't advise you go down that veiny, rubbery, bulbous route. They were disgusting. The sheep was bloody furious, I can tell ya!!

Why not eat some gorgeous home-baked delights instead? Spend your free time learning **how** to cook a tremendous meal. Drink wine, listen to music, chat and giggle whilst you do it but actually **try** to get the full benefit of that fancy cooker you've bought. You know, the one that you got into more debt for. Use that smart cutlery set your Aunty Maureen bought you. Invite your friends round. Make it a special evening. You've probably seen *'Come Dine with Me'*, well do your own version. Add as many luscious ingredients as possible, attempt something new, think laterally and expand your culinary knowledge. Get the kids involved too, heck you can even let them lick the bowl.

A lot of folk love a roast, which ultimately is quite a healthy meal (bar the Yorkshire's, cauliflower cheese and six pints) but only have it on a Sunday. For God's sake, if tha wants a roast and it's a Thursday, have one. There's no harm in it. Meat and loads of veg is a cracking diet all in all, so get filling that gravy boat, whatever day of the week it is.

Did you know that playing music whilst you dine can actually help you eat less?
READER: *How? Sounds too good to be true.*
Some boffins did some research which showed that softening the lighting and playing music while people ate, led them to consume fewer calories and enjoy their meals more. So if you're looking for ways to curb your appetite, try dimming the lights and listening to plinky-plonky music the next time you sit down for your spag bol, lasagne or risotto.

SOCIALISING

You can say *'No'* sometimes, and decline the opportunity to spend quality time with family and friends but the more you say *'No'*, the more it becomes your default setting. And then eventually, people will stop inviting you. No-one's going to walk into your living room and ask **you** if you fancy going to the pub, or the cinema, or anything really, so try to get into the habit of saying *'Yes'*, instead.

It's also a great feeling when you've had reservations about going out but end up going anyway and you have an absolute blast. As I've alluded to in an earlier chapter, life is all about adventure but you only find it, once you open your front door and step outside.

THE SEASIDE

Psychotic seagulls, dogshit on the beach, paddling in sub-Arctic temperatures, skimming pebbles, the incessant rain, haggard donkeys hee-hawing for a break, that weird smell, over-priced ice-cream, wind that hits you from all angles, old-school arcades, litter, tonnes and tonnes of litter, what is wrong with this country and our distinct lack of respect for others and ability to actually place refuse in a bin? **Aarrgghh!!**

The good ol' seaside. Admittedly, a lot of seaside resorts are extremely run down these days (thank you, austerity cuts) but some are still magnificent and well worth the appalling traffic you have to endure and manoeuvre out of in order to get there. And when you arrive, you have to indulge in one of the Great British traditions. Fish and chips.

Now, if you're a Northerner like me, you'll smother this dish with mushy peas and vinegar.
But if you're one of those soft, shandy-drinking Southerners, you'll probably think you're far too sophisticated to get involved in the mushy-pea-madness. But you're wrong, try it.

Quite simply, if you need to de-stress, you should read as much as possible, never trust politicians, down turn down invites, try as many different experiences as possible and don't sup cola. **Ever!!**
No probs having a beer or three but if you're pouring it on your cornflakes… think about cutting down.

Oh!! And just be yourself… all the others have been taken.

Right then Ladies and Gentlemen it's time to unchain your activity cheetah, it's time to release your zestful zebra, your vitality vole, your motion monkey, your animate ape, your ebullient emu, it's time to… **WAKE THE FIT UP!!**

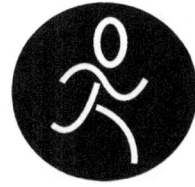

EXERCISE

On your marks, get set, 1, 2, 3   **GO!!**

The nuts and bolts, the name of the game, the essentials, the chapter and verse, the lowdown, the bedrock of weight loss. No, not *'The Flintstones'*.

FITNESS!! Eff to the eye to the tee to the ness!!

I hope you've brought your kit; otherwise you'll have to run in your pants. Sorry, I don't make the rules. You might want to do some stretches, touch your toes, a few arm circles, a couple of star jumps, jog on the spot and shake what your Mama gave ya!! It's time for some physical *'Education'*.

So you ready?! You warmed up?!
Okay doke!! It's time to get active.

Whenever I asked a client what they wanted to achieve regarding fitness, invariably they'd give the same answer:

                    Yeah, I want to lose a few stone, get fitter and be more toned

Easy peasy!!

It doesn't matter if you're posh, council estate chav, black, white, gay or even a Goth. In weight loss it's generally 20% fitness, 80% diet and 100% mental.

Now, this book is for those people that **want** to lose weight, not those that half-heartedly bang on about it and do nothing.

So my question to **you** is this, do you wanna lose weight, get fitter and be a whole lot happier?
READER: *I suppose…*
Blimey, that's about as enthusiastic as a sleep-deprived hostage in a ransom video.

Let's try again. Do you wanna lose weight, get fitter and be a whole lot happier?
READER: *Yeah, sure…*
What's up with ya, where's the verve?
READER: *I just don't know if I can do it, I've never really been fit, so…*
Let me stop you there.
Anybody can get fit.

ANYBODY.

Any…body.

That includes **you** as well.

So let's get rid of the inevitable excuses which you **pretend** are stopping you from getting fit.
READER: *I'm too old to start getting fit.*
Surely the message has filtered through by now that age is **never** a hindrance to any goal?!
But I'm trying to help you so here we go again.

For some reason, most folk believe that it's inevitable they'll get bigger as they get older, which is absolute bollocks!!

It's true that many people tend to slow down as they get older, especially after retirement, and as a consequence this inactivity results in poor fitness and leads to weight gain. But this is not the law!! There's no **rule** that states at a certain age you've gotta hang up your boots, and settle into suburban-sofa-sedentary.

This book is your fitness pension, and I can guarantee that it will continue to pay out until the day you die. So, irrespective of how old you are, start off slowly, don't get ahead of yourself and have plenty of rest. Take it step by step, week by week, month by month and so on and so on. After a while you'll be able to increase intensity, speed and effort.

But the first phase is simple, **get off your arse!!**

READER: *I haven't got the time to exercise.*
Did you know that a one hour workout is only four percent of your day? Four. Per. Cent.
Which means half an hour is?
READER: *Two percent?!*
Excellent mathematical skills there, I didn't realise you were such a brainbox.

Think about this. If you struggle to fit exercise in, you'll be struggling to fit into your jeans.

If you lie to yourself that you **can't** find the time to exercise, you will have to find the time to be sick and unhealthy. So don't **try** to find the time to exercise, **make** the time.

Someone busier than **you** is working out right now and if you're true to yourself, you know that you could be doing it too. Fitness is all about D.I.Y. and you can't just get a man in to do the job for you. The clock is ticking buggerlugs, time is running out. And every hour you live is an hour closer to death. **So, c'mon!!**

Look, don't worry, you've got plenty of time to exercise but if you just **long** to be fit rather than physically doing it, you'll be waiting a **long** time. And thinking about working out burns zero calories. So, if you're sick of the timber, then you gotta get limber.

READER: *It's too difficult, so why bother?*
What if being fitter is easier than you thought?
Unless you've been bitten by a radioactive spider, it's very unlikely you'll wake up tomorrow with a great physique and mental agility.

By the by. Surely Spiderman would just hang out in the corner of rooms or in the bath, rather than fighting crime? And why doesn't he eat flies and insects all of the time?
No? Just me?

Anyway, to get fitter you've gotta work on it. Evolve. Improve, step by step.

Get better and better. So it's over to you, you can keep fat or you can keep fit?

Your choice.

FIONA, 43 - *I never had a problem with exercise, until I started doing it. I just hated the thought.*
I found it so difficult to start off with and I'd nearly pass out bending down to tie my shoe laces. We used to go for those walks and whenever I saw a hill, I'd get really nervous that I wouldn't be able to walk up it. But with your kind words and encouragement, I realised it was far easier than I imagined.
Yes it was tough at times but certainly achievable and after a few weeks I started to look forward to it. Maybe it was because we used to chat and have a laugh so time went by a lot quicker.
Nowadays I go jogging with a friend. We're no athletes I can assure you but we run at a very leisurely pace which suits us both.
I feel embarrassed now admitting it, but I really enjoy it. You said I would, thanks Paul.

So what **you** worried about? What **you** got to lose? Apart from the fat of course!!

VICTORIA, 41 – *I tried to get fit but it was too hard. Whenever I went for a jog, I'd feel light headed, I'd get pins and needles and just felt miserable.*
I'd be forever stopping and resting on benches and walls, I couldn't stand it.
I hated running in the rain, in fact I hated running when it was sunny too.
I could only fit exercise in after work but all I wanted to do was veg and watch the box after a hard days slog. I used to get terrible blisters, my ankles were giving me grief and my back hurt too. It was bloody awful.
Admittedly, I probably gave up too soon but maybe I'm just destined to be fat all of my life.
Oh well, at least I tried.

Oh! Vicky, Vicky, Vicky!!
This woman frustrated the hell out of me. She'd arrange to go for a jog and then cancel a few hours before we were supposed to meet. It was clear she didn't like running so I suggested going for walks or cycling, but nothing seemed acceptable. I'd explain that being more active would actually **boost** her energy levels and **suppress** her appetite but she was having none of it. After a few months the excuses stopped and she quit saying she was going to join a slimming club instead.

All in all, she just didn't put in enough effort. She was lazy, simple as. And so negative. Forever moaning. If you could just give her a pill and she'd wake up thin the next morning, she'd sign up immediately. Mind you, she'd then get fat again and the process would continue.

She completely failed to adopt a positive mindset, which I'm afraid sealed Victoria's fate from the outset, and she was definitely destined to get bigger and bigger.
READER: *Maybe I'm like Victoria and just doomed to be fat.*

Perhaps we are all pre-disposed to live a certain way, destined to be this or that, thin or fat, big or small, skint or rich, positive or a whining, doom-monger.

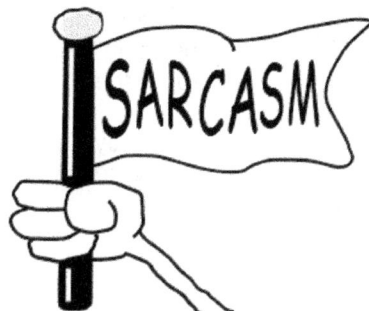

SARCASM

Or maybe that's total fuckin' shite and we have **absolute** freedom of choice, to live and act and **be** what we want.

There are three recognised body shapes according to the biology experts but because of the increase in morbid obesity, I've added an extra one.

ECTOMORPH

An ectomorph is a typical skinny individual, with the string bean, body type.
They generally have a light build, with small joints and lean muscle. Their shoulders tend to be bony with little width, and they find it very difficult to gain weight.
READER: *Why?*
They have a fast metabolism which burns calories very quickly, so they need to consume a huge amount of grub in order to gain weight.
Yep! Ectomorphs can lose fat very easily... **lucky gits!!**

ENDOMORPH

Their body type is solid and generally soft, a tad stumpy if you will.

Endomorphs gain fat very easily, are usually of a shorter build, with thick arms and plump legs.
Muscles are strong, especially the upper legs but unfortunately they find it very easy to gain weight.
READER: *Sounds like me, that.*

MESOMORPH

These people have a large bone structure, big muscles and a naturally athletic physique. Think of a sprinter... although not too much, calm yourself, but sprinters have the archetypal mesomorph body.
They find it quite easy to gain and lose weight, are naturally strong and are seen as the *'ideal'* body type... like there's any such thing.

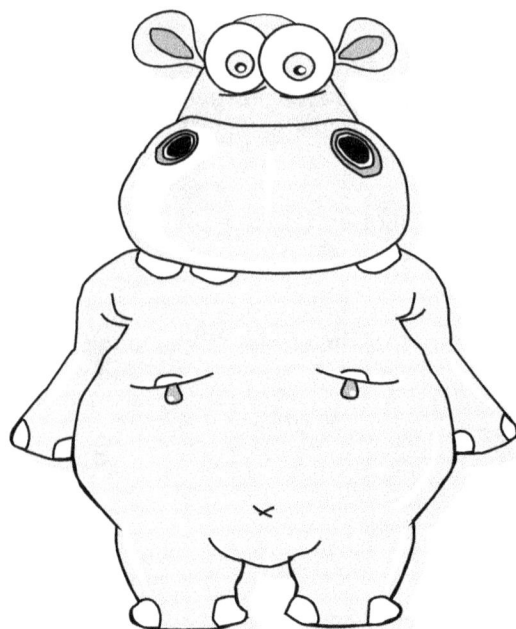

HIPPOMORPH

Due to the proliferation of cheap, poor quality food, processed junk, fizzy-sugary pop and the soft-cushiony absorbency of couches, the hippomorph is a common site in this day and age.

You'll find they have a muffin top, jelly bellies and the disturbing absence of a neck.

If you'd like to observe the hippomorph in its natural habitat, you'll find them waddling down most High Streets, either perched atop one of them motor-scooters, supping a jumbo-sized cup of diet-coke, or moaning relentlessly to some other hippomorph about their irritable bowel syndrome.

By the by, these people are not *'fat'*, they are just *'big-boned'*.

These body types and definitions have been created by the experts but that doesn't mean to say **you** can't change yours. In fact, most people are a combination of two body types, and it is not uncommon to find a pure mesomorph that gains weight like an endomorph for example.

But c'mon, experts know nothing. They base their limited findings on small sample sizes which can be skewed to fit any narrative, positive or negative, depending on which organisation is financing the study. Their conclusions invariably relate to the **average** because there are **always** exceptions to every rule. That's why we're all so different, although we are genetically designed to be a certain build or shape.

However it's not set in stone, but you do have to work harder to be, or maintain a different physique.
These little guys have a **lot** to answer for:

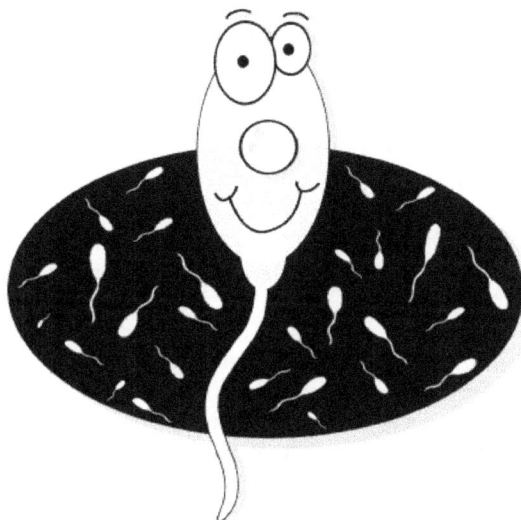

Yep, we're all mutts really, genetic mutations. **All** of us from distant parts of the globe, with genes that can be traced back thousands and thousands of years (even you Mr & Mrs Xenophobia, even you).
And like a Hells Angel, you can't change your genes. It's who we are and that comes from your Dad. And his Dad… and his Dad and so on and so on, primordial soup, big bang, infinite regression, OMG, too incomprehensible to contemplate, my head is about to explode – **KAPOW!!**

Back to the point. You're just like the *'Bionic Man'* and we can rebuild **you** with exercise, healthy nutrition and a brain that's programmed for positivity.

Please, I implore you… don't be a Hippomorph.

READER: *I'm just concerned I'll get bored or I won't enjoy it. I've tried before you know and it just didn't work, or appeal to me.*
Ok! Well those are fair points but it'll work this time because this time, you're getting my HELP. So put your negativity in a box, close it, sellotape it shut and then chuck it in the bin.

People conform so much when it comes to food and fitness, which is another reason why **you** and so many others have struggled to lose weight and get fit in the past.

I'll discuss *'food & nutrition'* in a lot more depth later in the book so for now, I'll just concentrate on fitness. The majority of people attempt the same fitness regimes as everyone else just because it's the norm, and are reluctant to try something… different.

For example, whenever someone decides they're gonna get fit, invariably the first thing they do is sign up to the gym. Even though they have never shown any interest whatsoever in fitness.

This then means they're stuck with a twelve month membership to a place that they're probably not gonna like. Try before you buy, don't just jump in, assess which areas of fitness you **enjoy** and base your entire fitness regime around that area.

Do some research. Although, sometimes you're so busy researching, buying matching shorts and tops, smart trainers, funky headbands, electronic *'I'm sorry but I can't do the fitness for you'* wristbands etc, etc that you forget to actually do the exercise.

But don't conform, I'm telling ya, its bad form.

Ok! Let's look at the intrinsic rules of fitness and some of the countless benefits.

rules

It's against the law to wear fitness gear and running shoes unless you actually partake in fitness. Sorry!! Don't shoot the messenger, I'm just telling you the rules. And it's not about the fancy new trainers; it's what you do in them that counts.

If you don't **enjoy** it, don't do it but if you don't try, you won't know if you'd enjoy it or not. If you hate going to the gym you won't get any benefit, so don't go. If you don't like fitness classes but sign up to do 12, you'll fail. If you despise running and have told your mates you'll do a park run on a Saturday morning, it's likely you'll be cancelling. Experiment with as many forms of exercise as possible but you'll only succeed in the ones you enjoy the most.

Strength is built in the mind, the body, just follows. And our bodies are capable of **amazing** things; it's our mind that gets in the way. So if you **believe** you can do it, you're half way there. Trust me, your body is amazing. Yep!! It is. Even yours. There are **no limits** to what you can achieve; the only barriers and obstacles are those your mind creates. Leap over them.

It's called a *'work out'*, cos it takes **effort** and if you're not sweating, you're doing it wrong. The most important element of *'work outs'*, is that they only **work out**, if you do them. Embrace the sweaty, smelly liquid of success. Become a *'Sweat Junkie'* and your chances of losing that timber will increase.

When you put money into a savings account, interest accumulates over time. The more you put in, the more you get out. Luckily no-ones taxing your exercise but it's the same principle. You don't just earn money; you **earn** your body too. And don't worry; no-one has ever drowned in sweat. Blimey can you imagine? The logistics behind that type of death are mind boggling. Fortunately it's never happened... yet.

Exercise is like laughter, you can't fake it but it's so much fun the more you do it and you miss it, when it's not in your life. Once you get the fit bug, you'll work out 'cos you'll **want** to take care of your body, not 'cos you hate it.

READER: *Oh! I'm sure...*
Believe me. No-one regrets a jog, Zumba class, gym session or countryside walk... once they're finished, that is.

Look after your body; it's the only one you've got. And once you start to take care of yourself, your weight will do the same. Your body continues to burn calories for up to 48hrs after your workout, which means even when you're recovering you'll still get the benefit. Therefore exercise is great for couch potatoes because every other day, is a rest day.

Fit hurts so goooooooooddd!

rules

Pain - that's just your body telling you it hurts like hell 'cos it's difficult, it's not easy, so embrace it, love it, endure, enjoy. It's not *'Fifty Shades of Grey'* but you do learn to accept the pain and actually start to like it. So delight in the joy of pain, just don't cry out in ecstasy and scream, *'more, more, MORE!!'*… especially, when you're at the gym.

When life gets tough, head to the gym and get buff!!
A gymnasium is a great place to alleviate some stress, especially if you're doing some cardio. Whether that's rowing like you're trying to win an Olympic medal, sprinting on the Treadmill pretending you're being chased by the Old Bill, or knocking ten bells out of a punch-bag. You'll release more than just sweat, you'll release your worries, your fears, your troubles. You'll **de-stress!!**

Stop punishing yourself; find something else to hurt instead….

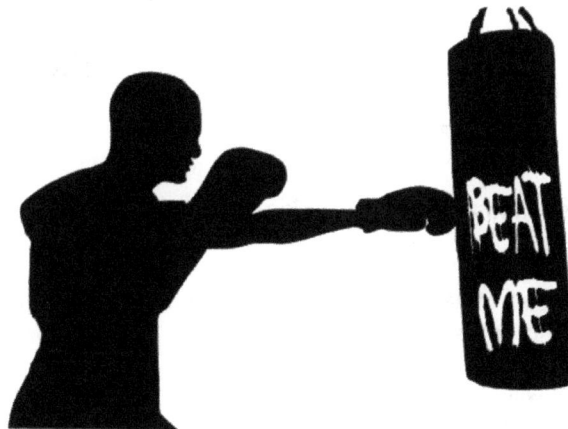

People often worry about loose skin when they start to lose weight. Therefore to reduce this look, you need to complete exercises that utilise your full range of body movement. This will help tone and tighten skin in alliance with your weight loss. Boxing or boxercise is great for *'toning'* and an excellent form of cardio because of the twisting, ducking, diving, bobbing and a-weaving, you can't beat it.

rules

A punch-bag doesn't care if you're upset, happy, unemployed, ugly or fat; it just wants to be punished.

And you don't see many fat boxers either… oops, sorry Ricky Hatton… and Prince Naseem… ok there's a few actually but they're retired.

rules   Nothing is out of reach, when you learn how to stretch.

Whether its hoovering, ironing, washing the car, doing it, hiking, martial arts, dancing, jogging, skipping, yoga, rock-climbing, Pilates or even parkour, they are all great for fitness, burning calories, de-stressing and losing lard. So go unfat yourself.

READER: *What's parkour?*

It's the adult version of climbing trees but you may break a few limbs and get told off for trespassing.

Oh! Let me warn you about Yoga. Be prepared to experience the unexpected flatulence symphony. Don't worry; it happens to the best of us.

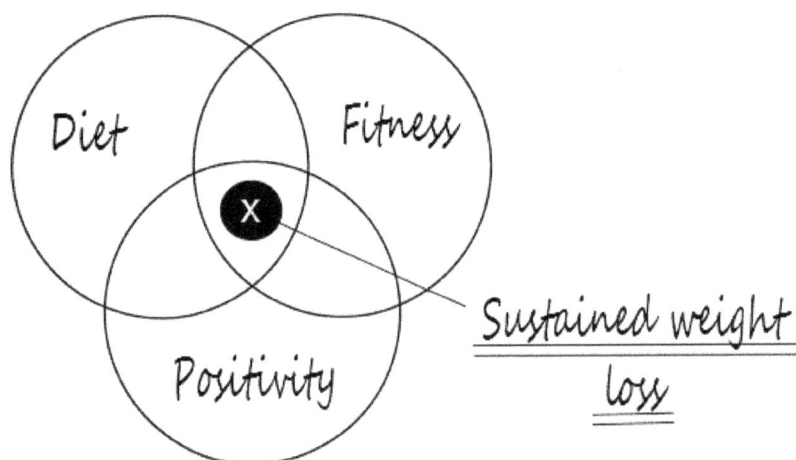

To get the best results out of fitness, find a form of exercise you know you'll enjoy, that you can tolerate and you'll be able to sustain.

If you exercise at home, wear the gear, otherwise you won't get into the right mindset. So don't attempt it in jeans and a t-shirt, you'll just flop about and not take it seriously enough.

Get your friends involved too. They will help inspire, motivate and mock. But above all, they'll make it enjoyable. And exercise, just like life should be **fun!!**

You could even join a cycling, running, martial arts or boxing club which will not only help you get fit but has the added bonus that you might meet some new friends.

Go on activity holidays too. There's plenty of adventure parks where you can hike, play tennis, go swimming, cycle or even take part in water sports.

fitness

food

happiness

happiness

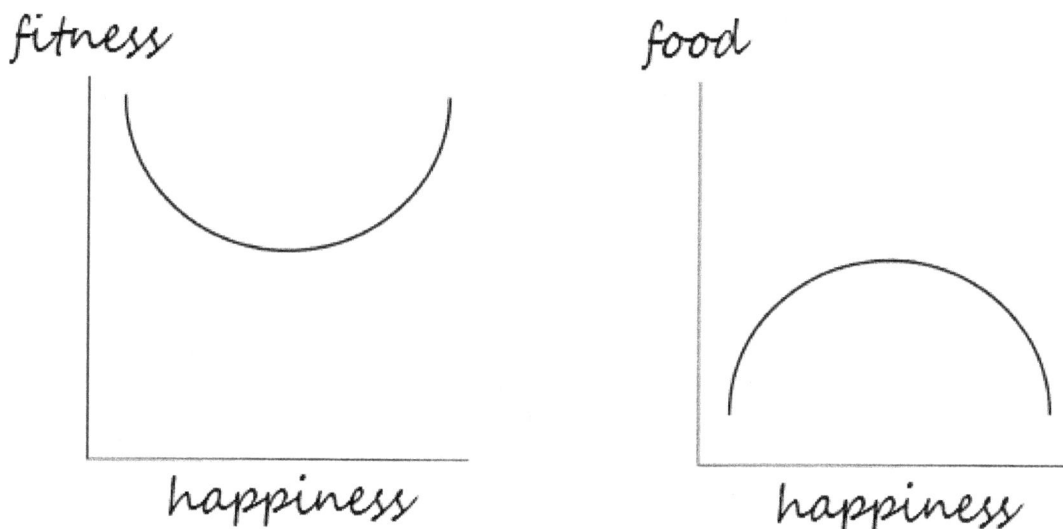

IT'S YOUR CHOICE

Another fun form of exercise is dancing at a concert. Obviously you've gotta buy a ticket for the right band. Granted, Coldplay do have a few nice tunes but nowt that you can get bouncing to in the mosh pit. I remember seeing The Hives at a Uni gig, no not the infestation; I mean the band from Sweden and I danced like a maniac. For about an hour and half.

I say dance, it was more like pogoing in the middle of a crowd, with beer chucked all over me but it was a good laugh. Imagine dancing like a loon at a Stormzy concert or to Run The Jewels, or The Savages (Oh aye!! I'm down with the kids!! But not in an *'Operation Yewtree'* kind of way).

Whatever form of exercise you do, make it **fun**, make it as intense as possible and continually strive for progress, not perfection. Exercise will help you shrink fat and increase your confidence. Basically just be fit and healthy, as if your life depends on it... cos it does.

So, are you ready to get physical?
READER: *Ok!! What's the best form of exercise for long-term weight loss?*
Great question, I'm glad you asked.
Cardio. cardio, cardio... and more cardio.

HEY HO, LET'S GO, HEY HO, CARDIO

READER: *What is cardio?*
The word *'cardio'* is short for *'cardiovascular,'* a term used for the circulatory system, consisting of the heart, lungs and blood vessels. Cardio is the ability of the heart and lungs to deliver an adequate supply of oxygen to the working muscles. The fitter and healthier you are, the more effective the system. Forms of cardio such as running, cycling, swimming and rowing, are all endurance exercises that help to strengthen this network.

These exercises **force** the heart to beat faster, which pumps more blood through your system, allowing each cell to absorb essential nutrients and oxygen, much, much quicker.
Any activity that gets your heart rate to about 50 – 75% capacity can be classified as *'cardio'* and this is known as *'moderate intensity'*.

READER: *Why is cardio so good for me then?*
Cardio will definitely help you lose weight... and increase nipple burn. Those boffins in the science world have calculated that moving your body around burns more calories than just lounging and decaying in front of the television. Who would have thunked it?!
And the faster you bez about, the more calories you burn. And the more calories you burn, the more fat is melted. **Yay!!**

ENERGY

Fuel for the body

Your body has several energy systems that it draws upon to fuel activity and movement. However, certain systems take precedence over others depending on what type of fitness is being performed, and the physical exertion required.

Two of these systems are *'Anaerobic'*, which means they do not use oxygen.

The first system is called the **ATP-CP System** (ATP - *'adenosine triphosphate'* and CP - *'creatine phosphate'*) which is generally used for short, intense bouts of work. Without getting too technical (its ok there won't be a test at the end of the chapter), a molecule in your muscle cell is split to generate energy and creatine phosphate is used to rebuild that molecule so more energy can be produced. This system is especially important for high intensity activity, such as weight training or sprinting, but it only lasts for around ten seconds.

The second anaerobic system is known as the **Lactic Acid System**.

This is the predominant energy source for moderately intense activity that lasts around two minutes. And it uses glucose (a form of sugar) present in your blood or glycogen stored in your muscle cells, for fuel. Sometimes you might find you hit the wall. Not literally, obviously, unless that's how you roll.

Anyway if exercise intensity is high, more lactic acid is produced which challenges the body's ability to clear it and this results in *'Acidosis'*. No, that's not the name of some funky rave club, it's the primary factor that leads to muscle fatigue. And it hurts. When marathon runner's hit this metaphorical wall, it's generally as a result of acidosis but some jelly beans, willpower and facial gurning will pull them through. Trust me, I've hit it and smashed right through it too. **Aarrgghh!!**

Another energy system, and the one that takes centre stage with aerobic activity (cardio), is the **Oxidative System**, so called because yes, it uses oxygen. This system can use protein, carbohydrate, or fat for fuel too, but relies mainly on carbohydrates. What is interesting about this system is that the lower your heart rate, the more it will use fat for fuel, rather than carbohydrate or protein. Which is why the oxidative system, coupled with low intensity cardio is great for *'fat-burning'*.
It is good for your heart; helps to burn calories and will contribute massively to your weight loss goals.

So, if you wanna lose some lard, get your *'low-intensity cardio'* game going.

However, don't **overestimate** how many calories you burned during cardio, which is the downfall of many a failed dieter.
You have to be aware that doing a run, aerobics class, cycle etc, etc is **not** an excuse to eat crap.
READER: *What do you mean?*
Ok! Let's say you've been on the treadmill for half an hour, you did some sit-ups, a few lunges and stretches and then sauna time. You might lose about 400-500 calories at the **very** most.
And that's if you've been running at a moderately high intensity.

If you then decide to get yourself a snack as a reward for your effort, you may end up consuming upwards of 1000 calories.

If you then eat normally for the rest of the day in line with the average RDA, you will **put on** weight, rather than lose it.

All that effort is therefore wasted.
READER: *But I get hungry after a workout and surely I deserve a treat?*
Completely understandable but try a banana, some eggs or porridge, rather than a mocha-chocca-crapachino with a side order of toffee-caramel cheesecake. Fair do's, drink like billy-o (water preferably, not vodka!!) but the less you eat after a workout, the more you'll gain.

And don't give me this *'Oh! But I'll be famished'* routine either, you'll probably be having a meal a few hours afterwards and that's more than adequate to re-energise you. I could go on about the *'fasting'* state but I'll save that for later in the book.

It's often overlooked by Bodybuilders but your heart is a muscle too. Billy-Big-Bobs don't seem to realise this...
READER: *Sorry, what's a Billy-Big-Bob?*
Oh! It's my fancy moniker for the meatheads. The beefcakes!! The ones that are obsessed with protein shakes, skinless chicken, vests, deadlifts and their own reflection. Anyway, they don't seem to understand but the heart is just like any other muscle in your body, and needs exercise through cardio to strengthen and improve its performance. And if it doesn't receive it, it will get weaker like any other muscle in their heavily fake-tanned, shaved bodies.

For those *'Top-Gear'* fans (YAWN!!), imagine that your heart is like the engine of a sports car.
When it's brand new and costs the equivalent of a small house, it's all pristine and full of raw power. Over the years you'll thrash the pants off that motor and the engine will start to malfunction and won't work as efficiently. Therefore it needs extra maintenance, it needs love and attention. The more you put into maintaining that engine, the more you'll get out of the car.

Hey!! No-one wants to be put on the scrapheap, so look after your engines, your pipes and especially your horn. ☺

When you start to do cardio, your body's cells **crave** more oxygen and nutrients therefore your body is forced to adapt to keep up with this new demand. It will strengthen the delivery system bringing it to them: the lungs expand capacity, the heart is able to pump more blood and the blood vessels are reinforced.

If you think of your veins and arteries as a complex road network, to be effective, the blood should flow efficiently. However, when folk consume a diet high in sugar and fat, these *'roads'* get impeded, traffic congestion occurs and on occasions there's roadblocks and closures. These roadblocks are the strokes and heart problems you *'may'* sustain in later life, if you don't get fitter and sort out your diet. Don't trust the Government to maintain the roads, they're bloody useless.

Did you know that conducting cardio actually makes you smarter?
READER: *You'll tell me anything.*
It's true.
On this occasion, size does matter.
People with weaker hearts, have less brain mass than those of the same age whose hearts are stronger. Thus, the weaker your heart, the less blood is pumped around your body. The less blood transported, the less oxygen and nutrients get to your brain. As a result the brain ages quicker, which leads in some cases to Dementia. Therefore I recommend Crosswords, Scrabble, Sudoku and Cardio for a gooderer brain.

Cardio increases your self-confidence and for those few hours after, you'll feel more alive than you ever have in your life. A bun can keep you happy for a few minutes but the buzz from cardio lasts for hours. And a runner's high is still legal... for now.
READER: *Why do you feel so elated then?*
Cardio, in fact any type of exercise causes the brain to release a group of hormones called, *'Endorphins'*. These endorphins have the ability to offset pain and induce euphoric states which mimic the effects of mood enhancing drugs, resulting in positive emotions occurring **during**, and **after** exercise.

Doing cardio can also **ease** and **combat** depression. Take that, Dr *'medication is always the answer'*.
So the more you cardio, the happier you'll be.

Cardio will improve your sleep patterns, heart rate, brain function and help alleviate stress and anxiety. Now you know why so many people do it.

Cardio exercises also increase bone density and strength, which is great for the ladies.
READER: *Why's that then?*
As women get older they are more susceptible to suffering osteoporosis, which is a thinning of the bone tissue and loss of bone density. If you have ever seen an old dear with a stooped over back, chances are you are

looking at a prime example of osteoporosis. Together with strength training, cardio can increase your chances of preventing this from happening.

READER: *So will cardio get rid of the fat round my stomach and legs?*
It will eventually but you can't just *'spot fat'*.
READER: Of course you can its right there round my belly and thighs.
No! What I mean is that fat loss is genetically predisposed, as in fat disappears from different areas of the body, based on your personal genetics.
It's all to do with this little guy again:

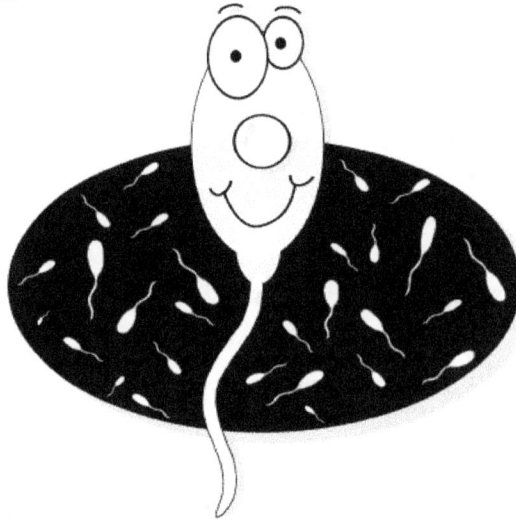

Could be arms first or the face, bum, legs, tummy or even from around your internal organs.

So you can't just focus on exercises specific to problem areas, i.e. crunches for stomach fat, arm circles for bingo wings etc, etc in the hope that fat will disappear from there first. I'm sorry but when it comes to fat loss, the most important element is your diet, diet, diet... **DIET!!** That's why every gym should really have kitchens and classes for nutrition, not just aerobics.

READER: *Wait a minute. You have fat around your internal organs?*
I'm afraid so and it's the fat you can't see that is often the most dangerous.

There are two different types of fatty tissue, *'Visceral Fat'* (sometimes called active fat, although it doesn't do much activity) and *'Subcutaneous Fat'*. Subcutaneous fat is stored directly below your skin and is also known as *'Adipose'*, which ironically sounds like a new sportswear range. Oh! If only it was. Adipose fat can be found draped around your belly, bingo wings, thighs and your Khyber Pass.

Visceral fat is stored around your internal organs, predominantly in your abdominal region and surrounds and protects your liver, pancreas and intestines. Too much visceral fat can restrict the organ functionality, leading to diabetes, erratic blood pressure, high cholesterol levels and also increase the risk of developing heart problems.

High visceral fat storage has also been linked to breast cancer, strokes, Alzheimer's and Dementia.
READER: *So what can I do about it?*
You can make some drastic lifestyle changes that include a moderately healthy diet, some low level fitness and some raucous laughter.
READER: *Which is the best form of cardio for getting rid of the flab then?*

In my opinion of humbleness, the best form of cardio for long-term weight loss, which can be performed by almost anyone, is… actually, try the wordsearch below for some clues.

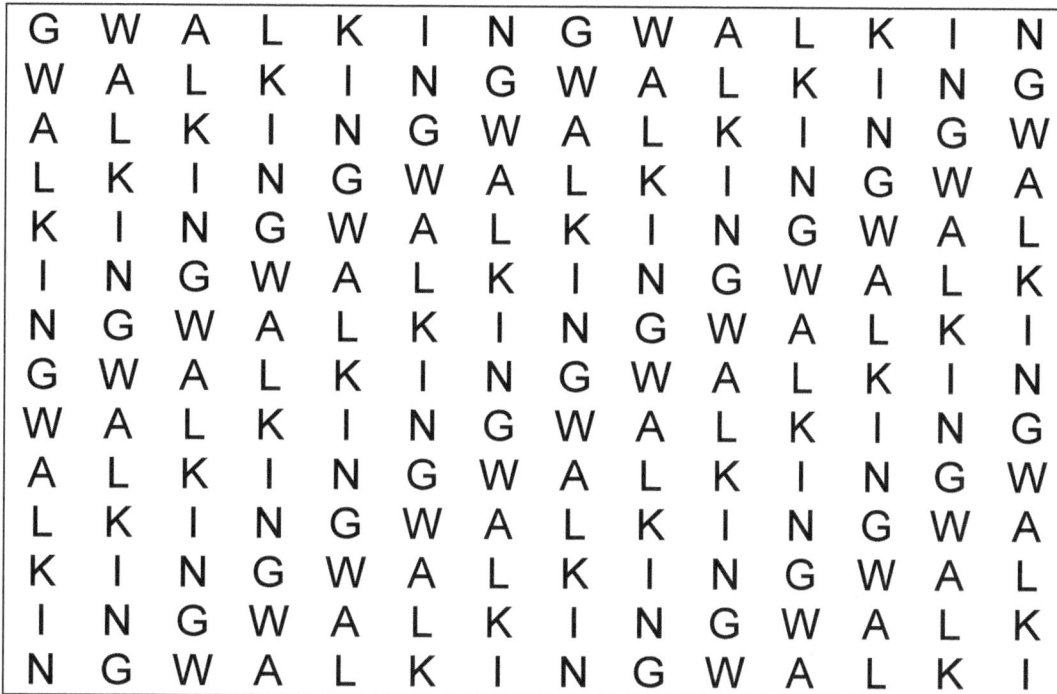

```
G W A L K I N G W A L K I N
W A L K I N G W A L K I N G
A L K I N G W A L K I N G W
L K I N G W A L K I N G W A
K I N G W A L K I N G W A L
I N G W A L K I N G W A L K
N G W A L K I N G W A L K I
G W A L K I N G W A L K I N
W A L K I N G W A L K I N G
A L K I N G W A L K I N G W
L K I N G W A L K I N G W A
K I N G W A L K I N G W A L
I N G W A L K I N G W A L K
N G W A L K I N G W A L K I
```

It's a puzzler alright

WALKING

Shanks's pony

Whether you're trying to lose a few pounds, five stone, eight or fifteen, walking is the **best** method of fitness for your goal.

You've got to walk. Everywhere.

- Walk to work.
- Walk to your Mums.
- Walk to your mates' house.
- Walk to the local shop.
- Walk to school to pick up the kids.
- Walk to the park.
- Walk to work.
- Walk at lunchtime.
- Walk home from work.
- Walk on a weekend.
- Walk, walk, walk, walk, walk... **walk!!**
- Walk some more, and then walk back.

The most efficient, low-impact, low-intensity workout to improve fitness and help you lose weight in the long-term, is walking. It is the cheapest and simplest way to get active, and I won't stop rambling on about it. So, if you can't afford a gym membership don't waste money trying to lose pounds, walk, it's free!!

And before you come up with more excuses as to why you can't walk all of the time, here's a comprehensive step-by-step guide, as to why walking is the best way to get fit.

It's underrated as a form of exercise but if you want to be more active, walking is **ideal** for people of all ages and fitness levels. Walking briskly for fifteen to twenty minutes a day has been shown to reduce the risk of chronic illnesses such as heart disease, type 2 diabetes, asthma, stroke and even some cancers. Admittedly, it does increase the risk of bird poo on the shoulder, and many a car driver will stare at you in bewilderment because you're actually *'walking'* rather than driving an automobile.

You don't need to buy any expensive trainers or equipment because **all shoes** are walking shoes.
<u>READER</u>: *That's so corny!*
Yeah! Like the Podiatrist said to the patient... sorry, my bad.

Walking is brilliant for fresh air and scenic views. Crisp packets floating serenely upon the surface of rivers, birds gnawing at polystyrene cups, fag butts left to rot in the rain, discarded needles and small, black, plastic bags of dog shit strewn across tree branches and bushes along the walkways of this wonderful, strikingly beautiful country. Try and see as much as you can of this green and pleasant land, before they frack the beejesus out of it.

Hiking is an awesome pastime. Rolling hills, cows frolicking in fields, grass cavorting in the wind, flowers blooming, rocks rocking, majestic trees, picture-postcard stone cottages, pints and a roast in the pub afterwards, what's not to like?!

If you dislike running then don't worry, *'walking'* is so much easier to master. All you have to do is put one foot in front of the other and repeat the motion whilst moving forward. Apparently, even bairns can do it, so you shouldn't have much of a problem, ya big whiner.

BRIAN, 67 - *I didn't realise until I got into my 60's how amazing being alive, truly is.*
A couple of very close friends have passed away recently, which has made me really appreciate just being able to breathe. You start to discover the true value of simple things. And walking is simply marvellous, a wonderful experience. The colours, the noises, the buildings, the people... everything is great. Every instance, every event becomes something to savour.
It really is a joy.

HERE ARE THE BASICS:

Select a pair of boots, shoes or trainers which are **comfortable**, provide adequate support and don't cause blisters. Do be careful if you borrow some shoes. I borrowed some from a drug dealer a few weeks back. I'm not sure what he laced them with but I was tripping all day.

Wear loose clothing that allows you to move freely. Choose thin layers, which you can add or remove depending on the conditions.

If you're walking to work, slip on a comfy pair of trainers and change your shoes when you get into the office. Yeah, I don't advocate walking long distances in kitten heels. They cause me some right grief whenever I try it. For long walks, you may want to take some water (or rum), healthy snacks, a spare top, sunscreen, Werther's originals and a sunhat, which you can pack into a small rucksack. Or if you're a Recruitment Consultant, in your expensive LV handbag (that's counterfeit, we all know).

Once you find your feet and you actually start going for regular, longer walks over t'hills, then buy some specialist walking shoes for the more challenging routes, 'cos you gotta protect them tankles. Get yourself a decent waterproof jacket too, so you can tolerate/enjoy the rain.
READER: *Walking in the rain? Are you mad, I'll get soaked.*
Chuffin' 'ell, calm down, you're waterproof you know, you won't melt, you're not made of suede.
There's no such thing as bad weather, it's just incorrect clothing and footwear choice. So **wrap up!!** When you go for your strolls that is.

In cold environments there's an added bonus for those trying to lose weight, stored fat is used to heat the body.
READER: *You mean I burn fat when it's cold?*
Of course you do, you're a mammal right?!
READER: *Am I?! I mean yes, yes I am.*
Well, as a mammal your stored insulation is used as an energy reserve in the colder climes and burned for energy to maintain your core temperature. But it's only ever cold outside, if you're standing still.
READER: *Hang on a minute, if I was cold all of the time, even at home, could I lose weight?*
Theoretically, yes. We're talking complicated science here which is all to do with *'brown fat'* and *'white fat'* but this isn't my area of expertise, so do your own research.
READER: *Charming.*
Ok! Basically, we are so accustomed to being supremely cosy at all times. Electric blankets, radiators, insulated winter jackets, Bovril and onesies. However, this prevents our bodies from functioning as they were designed to, back in the prehistoric days of Ug and Gug.

We are all the descendants of a long line of successful survivors, who had to endure some very unforgiving and extremely harsh times. In those freezing temperatures, Ug and Gug used their stored fat to produce heat, which lead to fat loss. This in turn led to a faster metabolism that naturally produced more energy and kept those survivors, lean and mean. But these people were warriors not molly-coddled, wet behind the ears, couch potatoes. Anyway this book is called *'Wake the Fit Up'* not *'Turn the Thermostat Down'*, so back to walking.

As in any exercise programme, start slowly and try to build your walking regime gradually.
To get the health benefits from walking it needs to be of moderate-intensity. In other words it needs to be faster than a stroll, get your *'brisk'* on. When you start, if you can only walk fast for a couple of minutes that's fine. Don't overdo it on your first few days.

You can break up your activity into bitesize chunks, as long as you're doing your activity at a moderate intensity. Sit yourself down on a bench, or a wall for a rest. There's nowt wrong with having a breather or six. You're not being timed. Go at your own pace. If you want, you can walk slower than a constipated emperor penguin, carrying it's young... over a frozen lake... covered in ball-bearings. As long as you're walking you'll be burning calories. And that's what counts. Towards the end of your walk, gradually slow down your pace to cool down. Finish off with a few gentle stretches, collapse in the garden and then put your feet up for a few hours.

It'll get easier I guarantee it, as long as you make walking a **habit**. So, think of ways to include walking into your daily routine.

And then mix it up a bit.

Add variety to your walks. You don't always have to travel to the countryside to find a rewarding stroll, wherever there's a path there's a walk to be had. Towns and cities offer interesting walks including parks, heritage trails, back alleys, canal and riverside paths, ginnels, commons, woodlands, heaths and nature reserves. Walking in a group is also a great way to start getting into the habit, you'll make new friends and they'll help you stay motivated.

If you've put on some pounds,
And got a little bit chunky,
Make walking your hobby,
Become a pavement junkie.

READER: *Well that's all well and good but I don't think I'll have time to walk.*
Excuses, excuses, **excuses!!**

! ! ! WARNING ! ! ! SPOILER ALERT ! ! ! WARNING ! ! ! SPOILER ALERT ! ! ! WARNING ! ! ! SPOILER ALERT ! ! !

I'm sorry but excuses, don't burn calories. I'll repeat that, **excuses don't burn calories!!**
If you drive to the local shops. I'm not interested in your carbon footprint; it's your fat arseprint that's more of a concern. Walk, you **lazy arse!!**

Ok! If you have to drive to work, that's fine. Just park further away than you normally do and walk the rest of the journey. If you get the bus to work, get off the bus a few stops earlier and walk the rest of the way.

If your kids moan about walking, tell them to grow a pair.
KIDS: *But, but, but, that's impossible, shoes don't grow on trees, so there!!*
Ok! Well, **buy** a decent pair of shoes/trainers for them too and try to make the experience fun.
Play games during the journey. Pretend that you gain points for viewing animals, coloured cars, cyclists without helmets, motorists using their mobiles, muggers, smokers outside hospitals etc, etc.
Make it enjoyable. Think of it as a bonding session.
READER: *I get bored walking though.*
EVERY MUM in the WORLD: *Well if you're bored, you must be boring!!*
Cheers Mums.

Walking gives you time to unwind, to contemplate your *'alleged'* worries, to check out the scenery, to ponder life's many mysteries. And more importantly, you can listen to music or podcasts. After all, that's why God invented the I-Pod.

READER: *I'll get blisters though.*
Blisters are like stretch marks, scars and war wounds. They heal (no pun intended). They show that you took part; you contributed to life. You took some action. You lived.

Walking is ace, walking will definitely get you fitter and if you're about as active as an amoeba on Prozac, walking is the best way for **you** to lose weight. All I ask is don't walk a mile in my shoes... you'll ruin them with your clown feet.

And finally, to summarise.
People that like to go walking don't do shortcuts and **everywhere** is walking distance, if you have the time.

PETER, 37 – *Sometimes Birchy, you can annoy the hell out of me by thinking you're always right. But I tell you what mate, you were right about walking. I used to drive all over the shop as you know and as a consequence I'd end up going to drive-thrus and garages to buy fast-food and snacks.*
You suggested that I start to walk places instead. At first, I bloody hated it, especially in the wind and rain.
After a few weeks mooching about, I got myself a decent pair of walking boots and then started listened to audio-books on the I-Pod whilst I walked. It got to the stage where I used to look forward to an hours walk after tea and at the weekend. I then started searching for more books to listen to on my jaunts. I really enjoyed it and then I noticed that the weight was dropping off. I didn't make that many amendments to my diet but with less junk food and more walking; I'd lost nearly 2 stone in about 8 weeks. I was absolutely stunned. Damn you and your good advice.
*Cheers fella and as a fellow Reds fan, walk on my friend, walk on. **YNWA!!***

JOGGING

Leg it

A lot of old sayings don't resonate these days, but the one that goes something like, *'don't run before you can walk,'* is definitely on the money regarding general fitness. If you're not a big fan of walking, how do you expect to enjoy running? You won't, simple as.

But so many people trying to dechunkify, make a schoolboy error thinking that they'll be marathon runners before they've even mastered walking to the local newsagents. They set off on their merry way, new trainers a-poundin', sweat a-drippin', tongue a-droopin' and before they complete their first mile, all they can think of, is a-quittin'.

Why do this to yourself? Once you've mastered the art of strolling, **then** and only **then** is it time to start jogging.

I once asked a scouse PT what the best exercise was to lose the flab and he replied, *'jog on mate!'*
I don't know if he was trying to abuse me cos he was an Evertonian, or give me brilliant fitness advice but those were wise words.

I love to jog, in fact the only time I really, truly feel alive is when I'm jogging. It's just me against the pavement. And I just love **to kick ass-phalt**.

A run is like an orgasm. It's great whilst it lasts but when it finishes, you can't wait for another one.

We spend our first nine months locked inside the womb, that's why we scream when released, joyous at our new found freedom. The umbilical cord is the first of many chains and luckily that's cut but then we have school, college, Uni, work, mortgages, unhappy marriages, credit card debt, internet providers, social media, neighbours etc, etc.

Running is unadulterated freedom and any opportunity to breathe fresh air before they start to tax oxygen use, should be positively encouraged.

GRAHAM, 34 – *Dude I'm so tired, my feet hurt, it's difficult to breathe, I have sore nipples, my face is beetroot red and I've got bloody big blisters on my toes… same time next week?*

Solo runs are great for self-discovery and like life, no matter how long you have been travelling in the wrong direction, you can always turn around.

But I'm not fit 'cos I run, I run 'cos I'm fit.
READER: *Ok! I get it, you like to run, I'm not sure I'll ever feel the same way.*
You could do, that's entirely up to you of course but knowing how to run and not running, is almost the same as not knowing how to run.
READER: *Whatever?!*
Anyone can achieve the couch to 5k to extreme marathon runner, merely by slightly adding intensity and time to their walks and runs.
READER: *I can barely run a bath and I turn about as quick as UHT milk.*
Look, no matter how fast you go you'll still be going faster than the people stuck in their houses watching the boob-tube. Plus, you don't want to get eaten when the Zombie apocalypse arrives, so you need to be prepared, you need to run.

The following suggestion (not set in stone, adapt as necessary) will help you progress to a decent level:

Week one – 3 times a week
Begin with a brisk five-minute walk. Then alternate between 30-60 seconds of running and 2 minutes of walking, for a total of 20 minutes.

Week two – 3 times a week
Begin with a brisk five-minute walk. Then alternate between 90 seconds of running and 2 minutes of walking, for a total of 25-30 minutes.

Week three – 3 times a week
Begin with a brisk five-minute walk. Then alternate between 2 minutes of running and 30 seconds of walking, for a total of 30-35 minutes.

Week four – 3 times a week
Begin with a brisk five-minute walk. Then alternate between 3 minutes of running and 30 seconds of walking, for a total of 40 minutes.

Each additional week you should try to increase the amount of time you spend running and reduce the walking breaks.

Perhaps add some lamppost sprints into your session.
READER: *What are they?*
During your run, as you pass a lamppost, sprint to the next one. Reduce the intensity for a minute or so and then repeat the exercise. Don't worry about looking a bit odd, who cares what other people think. The only thing that counts is **you**, your fitness and achieving those weight loss goals.
Alternatively, add an extra day to the schedule. It's up to you. But by increasing intensity your body will adapt and the workouts will become easier and easier.

Continue this programme until you end up entering one of those extreme Marathons that take place in the desert, probably in about ten years from now.

Good luck with that.

Running is just ace!! **It's awesome!!** You don't need to pay a fee, it's rarely double booked and the pathways are never full at peak times. It's just you against the pavement, your worries disappear, you forget about your debts, insurance premiums, wallpaper, Brexit etc, etc. You concentrate on your breathing, on relaxing, on living. So c'mon, run both ways and walk coming back.

Running will boost your health, your fitness, your vitality and your endurance. You'll become a **staminal**. And when you get to that moment when your muscles ache, your stomach knots, breathing is shallow, your mind is weak and all you can think about is giving up. That's when it's working. Embrace it. **Enjoy!!**

LOG OFF
AND
JOG ON!

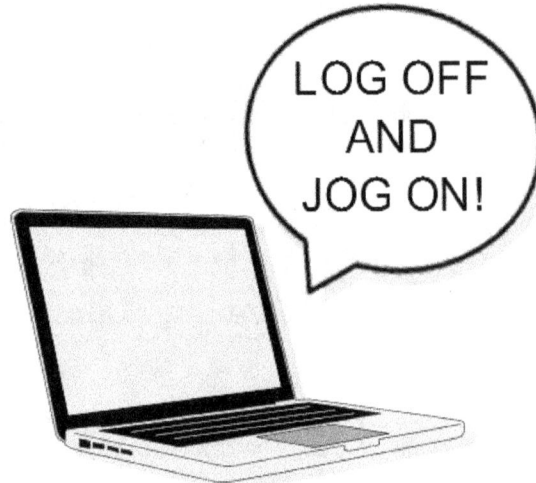

Yes, jogging can be sole destroying but the more you do it, the more you love it. Try asking one of your friends if they want to run with you too, it will help with your motivation. And everyone needs a **solemate**.

Run like there's free cake at the end, or run like you're a shoplifter being chased by the Police.
Don't worry they're so unfit you'll easy outrun them.

Whatever works for you, just run... **It's the law!!**

And if the voices in your head are saying stop, run further until you can't hear them anymore.

If... sorry, **when** you start to enjoy it, buy yourself a decent pair of trainers (£70 max) that offer support and flexibility. Don't overdo it and always intersperse with walks, jogs and even sprints if you can. Plus, don't fret about motorists hurling insults at you. They're morons. You push yourself, they just push pedals.

READER: *What if I'm no good at it?*
Ok! So you might be as elegant as a dog trying to control a balloon, and run like a drunk zombie limping through mud, with your shoelaces tied together but at least you'll be running.
READER: *I'm not sure.*
What have I told ya?! If you're not positive, you won't achieve anything.
READER: *Here we go again...*
Yes I know that I sound like a cracked record but it's true and if you run as much as your mouth does, you'd be in awesome shape.

Both positive and negative people experience fear, but the person with a positive mindset uses the fear to push themselves on, to give it a go. Whereas the negative person just cowers away and hides. You're not unique, we all experience fear, we all worry, we all suffer from pain, but it's what you do with it that matters. It shouldn't matter what time of year you start to run either because the weather is always naff anyway, whether it's winter or summer.
READER: *Is it ok to run when it's hot and sunny?*
Yep definitely, you're not a vampire are you? Don't worry you won't burst into flames if you venture outside in the sun. Just take some water with you and have a few gulps, you'll be fine.

And if it rains, that's no probs either; you get the added bonus of sloshing in puddles... **Yay!!**

Not everyone knows this but I have the secret to successful running.
READER: *Oh yeah?! Here we go again, Mr Know-it-all...*
Well I do, and even though you're having a go, I like you, so I'll give you this invaluable tip.

It's not the width of your shoes, or the length of your stride that makes you a good runner, it's all down to breathing. Controlled breathing reduces the amount of energy expended and utilises oxygen more efficiently, especially up hills.

You see the harder and faster you breathe, the more energy you waste thus the more difficult the run becomes because your muscles don't receive the adequate fuel.

Therefore relax, control and regulate your breathing pattern, and you'll master the art of running in no time.

DANNY, 41 – *I've always enjoyed running but I started to get arthritis in my knee that was very painful and made me feel older than I was. I stopped going for jogs in my thirties and naturally the weight piled back on.*
Yes, I know the scoffing of whole Battenbergs didn't help either but doing no exercise made it worse.
But I took your advice and started to go on walks.
After a few months I stopped getting the pains, so I started going for short jogs. As you mentioned, I made sure I stretched before and after each run, plus I also incorporated squats and lunges into my warm-up routine.
In no time I began losing the lard, I stopped getting the aches and throbbing in my knees and I felt full of energy.
I now complete different park runs at the weekend and even the wife comes along. I think she only does it so she can take selfies at the end but who cares, we both feel vibrant and our health has dramatically improved.
I used to get grouchy because of my knees, now I get twitchy and grumpy when I can't fit a run into my day.
Mate, I'm a runner again and I feel fantastic.

READER: *Will running hurt my knees then?*
Well everyone's different, so what works for one doesn't necessarily work for someone else.

Therefore running *'may'* cause some pain and discomfort in your knees.

My advice to you is exactly the same as what I mentioned to Danny and will help you avoid what is commonly known as, *'runner's knee'*.

Without fail, always stretch **before** and **after** a run.

You could also try to add some lunges and squats during your warm-up routine too.

But most importantly, when you're running don't **stomp** when you land with your feet.
READER: *Huh?!*
During your running motion, if your footfalls are striking hard on the heel, then the entire shock of the impact is traveling directly up your shin to the first flexible part that can dissipate that energy - your knee.

Beginners tend to gravitate toward *'heel-striking'* because that's the running style we're used to from the time we were bairns. By striking at the midfoot instead (balls of your feet), the shock is distributed more evenly and dissipated **before** it gets to your knee. In addition, whenever you land, your feet should always be straight, never at an angle because this places undue pressure on your ankles and knees, which often leads to injury.

But posture alone won't always be the solution. Sometimes, we do have to fork out for a decent pair of trainers that offer adequate support.

READER: *Do you suffer from runner's knee?*
Nah!! I run so fast my feet hardly touch the ground... ☺

As I said, I make sure I perform a stretching routine **before** and **after** my runs and I incorporate squats and lunges into my workouts. I tend to be *'light on my feet'* during a run, and push up with my toes as my foot strikes the ground, so this landing technique reduces the impact and lessens the chance of injury.

Many independent running shops offer guidance on running styles and your gait, plus which trainers would best suit your plates of meat. Some runners actually purchase trainers a size bigger than their normal shoe.
READER: *Bonkers!*
Who are you, *'Dizzee Rascal'*?!

It might be a tad strange but it allows the feet and toes some wiggle room, which reduces your chances of getting blisters. Whatever works for you, I don't really care, as long as you run.

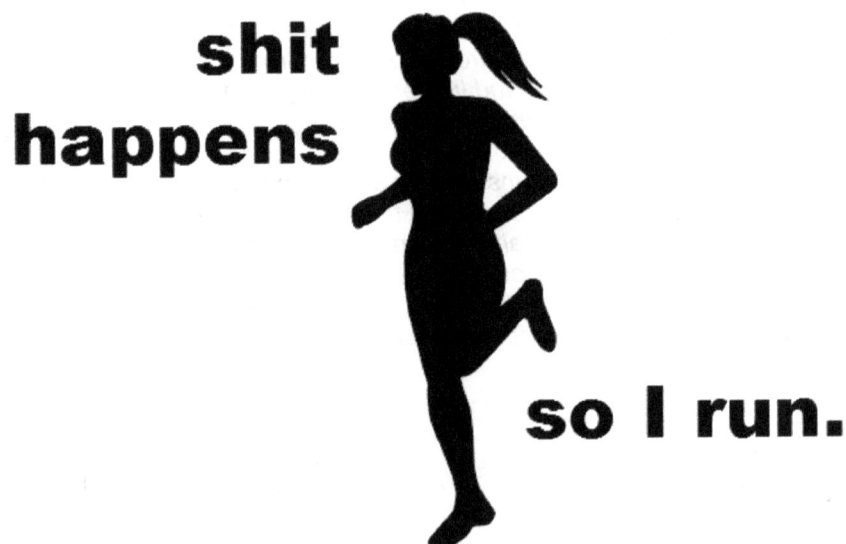

shit happens so I run.

READER: *My friend goes running a lot but sometimes blokes shout and harass her?*
On behalf of the entire male population of the world, let me apologise. But quite frankly, most blokes are **knobs!!**

It could happen that you *'may'* suffer abuse, wolf-whistling and name calling, so I recommend you either run in a pair or a group, and/or wear earphones to help ignore it.

I'm not gonna lie to you, folk shout stuff and generally it's abuse, so if you do start running, it won't just be your feet that need to develop a thicker skin.

Before I forget, let me give you a few running tips regarding safety.

If you're about to run into some mud, slow down, 'cos you could end up sliding and falling on your sweet derriere.

It's a blast sploshing in puddles but be careful when other pedestrians are around, they might not take too kindly being drenched in mud. Although you'll be faster than them, so they won't be able to catch ya to punch ya!!

When running down a hill, take it slowly. The faster you travel down a hill, the more pressure you place on your joints and the more likely you'll sustain an injury. And never stomp!!

When running in the dark, make sure you wear some illuminous clothes. This way, teenagers in gangs will easily notice you, so they can give you dodgy looks and hurl abuse. Motorists might see you too.

As you get more experienced as a runner you start to develop a sixth sense near junctions and drive ways, enabling you to slow down and stop, preventing possible accidents. Before you develop this Spidey-sense, always be careful when approaching potential hazards.

And just like when driving a car, you have a blind spot when running, so get used to looking over your shoulder before crossing roads.

As well as being a fantastic fat burner, running is also a great metaphor for life. You can't run from who you are but you can run towards your fears and seize opportunities whenever they present themselves. Each day, life will send you little windows of opportunity and how you respond dictates your destiny.
So **always** try to go the extra mile... and then jog back.

TREADMILL

The good thing about running is that expensive equipment is not required. Yes you'll have to buy some decent trainers, a few tops, shorts and protective socks but all in all not a costly hobby, especially when you consider the benefits.

Perhaps you want to run but feel you don't have time, well there's an easy option, buy yourself a treadmill for your home. You can get a decent second-hand one for about four hundred quid these days, which is probably the amount some of you spend on a handbag, games console or some Avant-garde furniture for your home.

All I ask is that if you're buying a treadmill, rowing machine or exercise bike for use at home, don't just use it as a clothes hanger. Use it for what is was designed for, losing timber.
READER: *As if I'm going to have one of them in my home.*
Think about it. If you run at level 6 or 7 on a treadmill, you'll burn about 400 kcal in 30mins or so. Which means you can watch your soaps **and** lose weight. All from the comfort of your very own uniquely designed, LEGO, new-build, starter home.

No, not convinced?!

Consider this... *'Life is like a treadmill'*, you may feel like you're going nowhere but the more you put in, the more you get out of it.

10k/MARATHONS

With respect to running, you don't have to be training for the Olympics, setting a new world record or trying to impress that girl in the sandwich shop. You should do it, for yourself. To just, be.

However, once you've got the run-bug, you might decide to enter a 10k, half-marathon or triathlon perhaps, which I whole-heartedly recommend. And if you do it for charity, you'll have to raise funds which increases your motivation 'cos you don't want to let people down.

In 2005 when I did the Great North Run, I raised money for *'Whizz-Kidz'*, a charity that helps disabled children. It really helped inspire me on the run because when I felt low on energy and in pain, thinking about those kids really put into perspective. Who was I to internally moan about a few minutes of anguish, when they had a lifetime of disability to contend and cope with?! This pushed me on and helped drive me forwards, which was definitely required for that last mile. Yeah, once you run down that hill and you're onto the finishing stretch, it's **a bloody killer!!**

When **you** complete the course get in touch (birchygoober@hotmail.com), I'd love to know how you got on. And how good are the crowds? They really get behind you, especially near the end when you need encouragement the most.

So whether it's a 10k, half-marathon or you hanker for the extreme, I suggest that whatever you have to do, do it.
READER: *As if, I'll never do a marathon.*
Of course you can, I believe in you, **you** can do it.

The satisfaction of finishing a marathon is incredible and so rewarding, whether you're breaking records, or you crawl over the finish line after seven and three-quarter hrs. It's called pride and it'll last forever.

Dead last is better than did not finish, which is better than did not start.
READER: *How about, just dead!!*
Nah! You'll be fine. I'm convinced… I'm positive.

It's such an amazing feeling when you cross that finish line, although it's difficult to fully describe so have a go yourself and we'll compare notes.

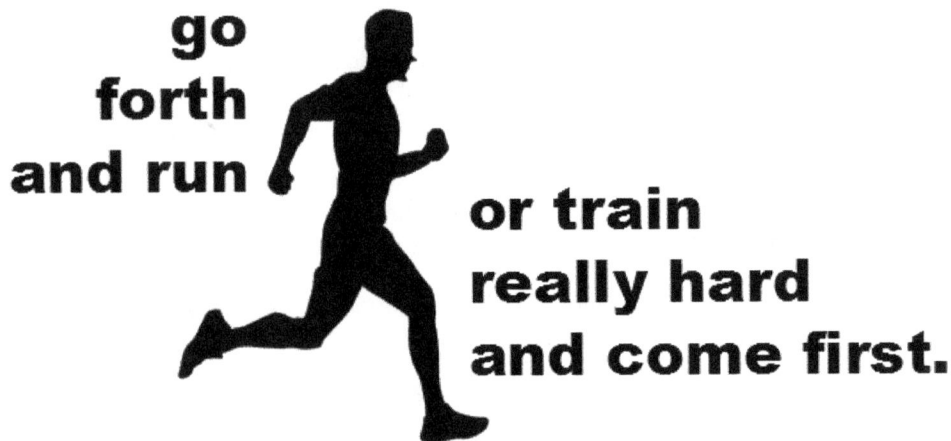

go forth and run **or train really hard and come first.**

You're trying to lose weight right?
READER: *Derr… yeah!!*
On average a runner burns 3500 kcal by completing a marathon (not a Snickers, sorry!).
That equates to 1lb of fat therefore if you complete a marathon a day, in a fortnight you'd lose a stone. However, you would have blisters the size of tennis balls but it's all swings and roundabouts.

Don't be giving me this *'I haven't got time'* malarkey. The only **time** you should be worried about is your PB. Your best, your personal best.

And if you want to get faster, the nerds have established that runners who listened to fast music completed their run quicker than runners who listened to calm music, or ran without toons. So, if you want to take your running up a notch, listen to songs that **get your freak on!!**

If you do decide to start running and it becomes part of your life, you will categorically, 100%, lose all that flab you want rid of.

So get involved, I mean you want to look better naked don't you?
READER: *Well yeah, I suppose.*
You will, you definitely will if you take up running. But if no-one's seeing the new you, become a streaker.
Although if you don't want to get arrested, you'll have to be speedy and quick as a flash.

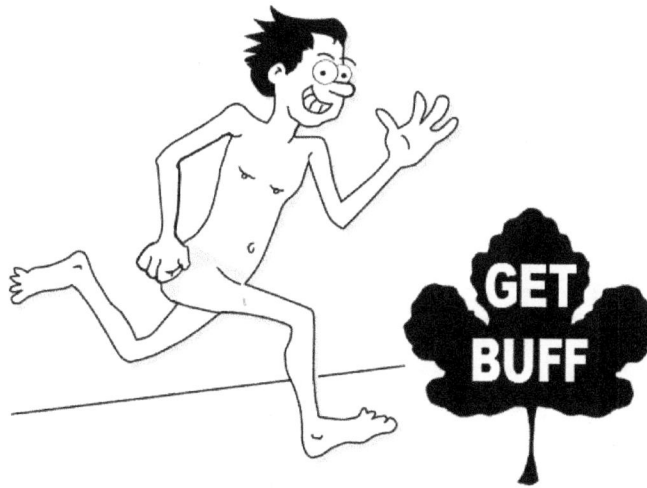

CYCLING

Kilom-eaters

Another great form of cardio is cycling. Aye, you can't go wrong with the ol' push-iron. There seems to be more and more people biking these days, clearly inspired by the drug-taking participants of the many tours. But you don't get nicked for this type of joyriding.

If you've got a bit porky,
Can't fit into your kegs,
Put something powerful,
Between your legs.

Cycling is cheap, fun and everyone loves a ride now and again.

As well as walking, cycling is one of the easiest ways to fit exercise into your daily routine because it's also a form of transport. You can cycle to and from work, to the supermarket for some bits and even to the pub if you so wished... although don't drink and pedal.

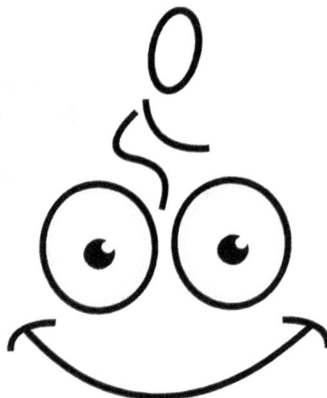

Joy-rider

It's a low-impact form of exercise, so it's easier on your joints than other types of cardio such as running which is high-impact and can cause some wear and tear on the ol' knees.

If you're just getting started, here are some cycling tips for beginners.

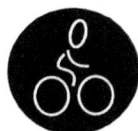

Always take a look behind you before you turn, overtake or stop. And try to use arm signals before you turn right or left, other road users aren't mind readers. Plus, traffic lights and road signs are not just for motor vehicles, **obey them.**

Don't be a maniac and ride on the pavement, unless there's a sign that says you can.

Be extra careful on busy or narrow roads. And when overtaking parked cars, watch out for car doors opening suddenly and allow adequate room to pass safely.

Don't listen to music on your headphones while cycling. It's dangerous!! No, not the Wacko Jacko album, I'm talking safety here.

Never use a mobile phone while cycling, you can check FB for status updates when you complete your journey. If you ignore this advice, I suppose you can use your mobile to call for an ambulance.

If you perform wheelies, bunny hops or skids, make sure there's a decent crowd there to watch first, otherwise that skill is wasted… I'm jesting of course, there's a time and a place for stunt riding and it's not on the highways and byways. It's in music videos and adverts for tampons, as you very well know.

Wearing a cycling helmet can help prevent a head injury if you fall off your bike. Although if you need telling to protect your melon, perhaps it's a brain not worth saving. Be prepared for spectacular 'helmet hair' once you've finished your ride, and take some piccies 'cos they are defo worth sharing.

If you use your bike at night, it is compulsory to have a white front light, a red rear light, a red rear reflector and amber/yellow pedal reflectors - front and back, on each pedal. Be seen, be safe, be lit up like the Blackpool 'luminations.

You may sustain terrible thigh related chafing and have hilarious tan lines but the fun and thrill of the ride is worth it, although blokes, watch your knackers in those tightly packed shorts… it might affect your sperm count.

And finally, always follow the Highway Code; you're not a taxi-driver.

Cycling is challenging, fun, sociable and is the type of fitness that is suitable for everyone of any age or level of fitness, so **no excuses!!**

READER: *I didn't say anything.*

More and more cycle paths are being opened, and biking to lose weight is becoming a more fashionable and enjoyable recreation. What a great way to get out in the fresh air and help achieve your weight loss goals.

Paul Birch

READER: *I don't get the appeal, what's so good about cycling then?*

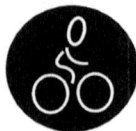

> Just like rumpy-pumpy, the longer you ride, the more fat and calories will be burned.
>
> Cycling strengthens the major muscle groups in the legs (the quadriceps, bottom region, hamstrings and calves) and improves your stamina.
>
> Pedal power is a low impact exercise, so for many people who cannot do high impact sports because of the pressure it puts on their joints, cycling is a great alternative.
>
> Most of us can already ride a bike and it's not complicated, so you're more likely to take it up as a hobby because you don't need any special training.
>
> You can cycle for a long period of time at a low intensity without your leg muscles getting too tired, although you may feel the burn. But the more you cycle, the hotter you'll be.

READER: *Ok! I'm sold, what type of bike should I get?*
There are hundreds of different cycles to choose from – mountain bikes, road racing bikes, touring bikes or even a BMX. It's up to you whatever you want; after all, it's your pins you'll be working.
Get a mountain bike if you're keen on riding in the mud, or a road bike if you fancy yourself as one of them Tour de France type riders (performance enhancing drugs, not included).

A top of the range bike can cost thousands of pounds but when you start out, get a standard one for about a hundred quid or so. Or you can get on the net and try and find a bargain, just make sure it's roadworthy!

READER: *What about them electric bikes?*
You lazy git, that's shocking, **No!!** Kind of defeats the object really, so make sure you get yourself a bike that can only be moved by your pedal power. Actually some electric bikes are pedal-assisted so it's up to you but if you want to lose the timber I don't recommend them.

Once you get your bike, start off slowly and build up. You can keep off the roads too if you want, until you improve your confidence. Try out short journeys initially, like around the block or to the local shops. Also where possible, stick to flat roads and paths until you have worked your way up to a decent level of fitness.

Your weight loss journey will be more enjoyable if you start off gently. Remember, you're not competing on the velodrome; it's not a time trial, so easy does it.

You can then increase the distance and speed the more you get into it, and try cycling to places you would normally go to by car or bus. Within a month or so, riding a few miles will no longer be a problem and you could even consider cycling to work, if it's a manageable distance.

Once you feel that your cycling has improved enough, why not take on a challenge and complete one of the many cycling events which go on throughout the country. Setting yourself a challenging goal will help to give you the motivation needed to train regularly, and stick at it when the going gets tough.

Obviously biking is a great way to view your local scenery. Unlike a jog or a walk, you can travel a much greater distance in a shorter time frame and take in more of the wonderful world around you.
Try varying your cycling routes as much as possible too as this helps to keep pedal power fun and interesting, preventing boredom and a lack of motivation. Which as you know are major obstacles when trying to lose weight.
READER: *Will cycling bulk me up?*
On the contrary, it is much more likely that your thighs, bum and waist will all slim down and tone up, making cycling an ideal exercise for those wanting to lose some flab.

As you progress and start to bike longer distances, your body core, abdominals and back will all get stronger and firmer, and unsurprisingly your pins will start to look defined too.

128

ALEX, 30 - *I took your advice and have been cycling about 3 months now and I cannot believe how much my shape has changed. I'm absolutely amazed. As well as losing weight on the scales, I have lost inches off my bottom, legs, stomach and jelly belly! It is an activity which my husband and I are doing together and I have to admit, I love it. I wish I had taken it up years ago.*

Cycling can help you save money as well.
READER: *How?*
Bicycles are very much an understated form of transport, especially with the increase in congestion on today's roads, not to mention the soaring fuel prices. Riding your bike to work requires no petrol, insurance, MOT or fluffy dice. And say goodbye to trying to find a parking space.
Unlike fossil fuel-guzzling vehicles, bikes omit zero emissions, so they're beneficial for the environment as well.
MOTHER NATURE: *Yay!!!*

Most people who drive to work by car, travel five miles or so, a distance easily achievable after some cycling training. So you can improve health, increase fitness and burn off calories every day without having to allocate time for a babysitter, gym session or aerobics class.

STEVE, 25 – *I began cycling to work last summer, it's only six miles and it's usually quicker than driving. I did it because I felt I wasn't getting enough exercise and I wanted to lose some weight. It was also because driving or taking public transport through the city is so expensive and stressful these days. My journey to work is fun now.*
Some of it involves busy roads where I find myself actually overtaking queues of cars. But I've also discovered some nice quiet cycle routes through the back streets.
I feel so much healthier these days and much, much fitter, plus I've lost the lard.

Whatever the weather, strap your helmet on and see new towns, villages, parks and Cities.
And if you want a dirty weekend, go mountain-biking with your partner... or someone else's.
In fact, don't go for a *'City break'*; go for a *'City brake'* instead.

READER: *I don't fancy the idea of cycling in the rain though. Blimey just think how messy I'd get.*
You big girl's blouse. Mud washes off you know.

Ok! Well, you could always buy an exercise bike and cycle at home instead. This will allow you to watch your fake reality shows **and** burn calories... whilst destroying brain cells.

When you're dropping the kids off at school, why not cycle?

READER: *But that'll take too long, the kids will take ages.*
Excuses, excuses... **excuses!!**
Have you heard of *'Cargo bikes'*?
READER: *No.*
Well check 'em out on t'internet, they're amazing. They're specifically designed to help ferry your children **to** and **from** school. And you can fit up to four of the little blighters in the cabin area.
READER: *Are they safe?*
You betcha.

Your children can be safely seated on plastic moulded seats, with a five point harness and are protected by the spacious impact-resistant cabin. A rear opening window in the cabin allows **you**, the rider, to keep an eye on your sprogs and share the delightful journey with your passengers.

You can even ride at night. The cabin has built in lights and Hi-Viz stickers to make sure you are as visible as can be.

So no excuses, you can exercise and fight the flab whilst doing the school-run.

READER: *Are you selling these?*

Hey!! These babies sell themselves.

There's always a fun way to get fitter and pedalling a bike will help get you there. Cycling is great for losing that lard, so slip your Lycra on and join the revolution.

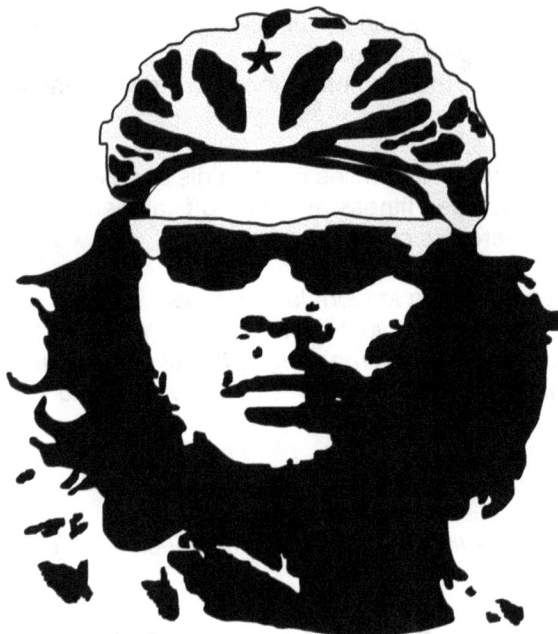

SWIMMING

Aqua-tastic

You want a low impact exercise that will help you lose weight, whilst being weight-less?
READER: *Do I?!*
Then swimming is for you.

Swimming is great for slimming. It's good for people of all ages and all fitness levels but especially useful for people who are corpulent, preggers, have leg issues or lower back problems. So get your goggles on and get thissen splashing, but watch out for the rowdy kids depth-charging, soggy plasters, verrucas and furtive ogling from that bloke in the slow lane.

Exercising in the water at your own pace can be a great way of staying fit, without taking a toll on your joints.

It will tone you up and slim you down.

Swimming is a particularly good form of exercise because:

It uses almost all of the major muscle groups and places a vigorous demand on the heart and lungs. It develops muscle strength and endurance, whilst improving posture and flexibility.

It provides most of the aerobic benefits of running, with many of the benefits of resistance training thrown in.

It doesn't put the strain on connective tissues that jogging, aerobics and some weight training regimens do because the water supports and cushions the body, eliminating the kind of pounding associated with high-intensity training.

It's easy on the joints and muscles, so the water resistance allows you to work out for longer, with little chance of injury.

It will improve your health and may reduce the risk of chronic illnesses such as heart disease, diabetes and stroke.

There's also a relaxing, meditative side to swimming which is difficult to replicate in other forms of cardio. Bathed by soothing water, your mind starts to drift as you focus on your breathing and your movements. This stress-busting aspect is why so many people love the experience of a dip in the pool.

Swimming is also great fun. You don't just have to do length after length after length in the pool. Things like treading water, playing underwater tig and pretending you're a dolphin, burn calories too. Your liddle urchins will love spending some quality time messing about with their Mum in the pool, so it's great for bonding.

So if you have kids, take them down to the pool and have a good ol' giggle, splashing about like you're a mermaid trying to woo Forrest Gump.

You could also join a water aerobics class if lane swimming isn't your thing. These are

held in most pools so check in and ask at your local centre to find out more.

READER: *Ok! I'm sold, how do I start?*

Check out your local pool; most public pools have separate times for different groups - adults only / men only / women only / mother and toddlers.

Try to set aside time at least once a week when you (and the kids) can go swimming.

Remember to warm up and stretch before you swim to avoid possible strains.

Don't forget your legs which are often overlooked when swimming. Stretching them will reduce drag in the water by improving your form and also help prevent cramp.

Get a family member or friend to join you too. Anything that helps motivate you.

Start off by swimming a few lengths of the pool and build up the distances each week.

Change your stroke to add interest and exert yourself in different ways.

To begin with have breaks every few lengths to get your breath back. Each session you can then decrease the duration of these breaks, until you can cut them out entirely and swim nonstop.

READER: *I don't need any fancy equipment do I?*

Costume/budgie smugglers/Wetsuit – There are hundreds available, you decide which you feel most comfortable in.

Goggles – Improves underwater vision and prevents chlorine irritating the eyes.

Ear plugs – Useful if you don't like to get water in your ears, or if you're susceptible to ear infections.

Water Bottle – Remember, you are exercising so need to keep your body hydrated. Keep this at the end of your lane so that you can drink in your breaks. But don't sup water from the pool, unless you fancy an emergency trip to the bogs and possibly your GP.

132

READER: *Swimming at my local pool is safe isn't it?*
Of course it is… apart from the fact you might drown and die… ☺

You'll be fine, there's always a lifeguard around and they won't be spending **all** of their time chatting up girls or sharing make-up tips with the ladies on reception. They'll be watching out for you, so don't worry. Don't be a dawdler though, if you're swimming in a particular lane that is designed for faster swimmers, respect your fellow dippers and give them enough space to go by, especially if they are quicker.

Have fun, relax and enjoy the experience, just make sure you don't get out of your depth.
Ha! Ha! Did you see what I did there?! Oh! I'm so funny.

READER: *It all sounds great but it's not for me.*
Here we go again, excuses, excuses. What is it this time? Not enough time, too old, can't get a cossie to fit?
READER: *I can't swim.*
Fair enough, that's a pretty damn good excuse.

Not to worry, most pools offer adult-only beginner lessons, so have a look at your local leisure centre to see what is available.

READER: *I'm a bit scared of trying.*
Okay doke!! Well I can completely empathise with that 'cos I'm not a very good swimmer at all, in fact when I go to the pool, I resemble a startled brick with asthma… who's just been tasered.

My main issue is *'treading water'*; I'm rubbish at it, which is ironic because in life I do that very thing.

If you can't swim, I strongly recommend you at least **try** to learn. It's a fantastic form of cardio to help you lose weight and who knows, it could even save your life. I had swimming lessons about seven years ago and I have to admit that I used to get so nervous before each one.
READER: *Aha!! It's not just me then?!*
Hey, we're all human.

I'd be fine all day but then about an hour before the lesson I'd start to get anxious and… well put it this way, I had to visit the toilet a fair few times and not for a wee. But as soon as I got into the car and began the drive to the leisure centre I was fine. Until I got into the changing room.

For me, it's the smell. Swimming pool changing rooms have a strange aroma. Chlorine mixed with deodorant, mixed with sweat, mixed with shower gel, mixed with the mild panic of rookies visiting the toilets. A potent concoction indeed.

It was also the impending realisation and dread, that I was about to be putting myself through an activity I don't feel very comfortable participating in at all, and I'm going to be making loads of mistakes. I hate making mistakes. I'm a perfectionist at heart and stupidly feel it's a sign of weakness to blunder.

But then I'd pull myself together and remind myself that no-one's perfect, everyone makes mistakes and to just be positive. I can do it, it's no big deal. So I'd pull on my speedo's and get on with it.

Face my fears.

Once I was in the water with the instructor I'd feel fine. Until I started to feel myself out of breath, or close to the deep end, then the panic would set in.

It's ridiculous really because when you're in the water and completely relaxed, you float to the surface anyway but as a novice you think you're going to drown, so flail about getting out of breath and losing your cool. Oh aye!! You can't be cool as an adult when you have to wear arm bands, or swim with those flotation boards.

But like anything, the more you do it, the easier it becomes. You start to feel calm, your movements are more relaxed and before you know it, you're swimming. Like a swimmer. Smooth as silk as you propel yourself through the water with the poise of a porpoise. It's easy, what was all the fuss about?

I'm not gonna lie to you, I'm still not great at treading water but I faced my fear and now I can swim.
If I can do it, then so can you, so c'mon give it a go.

And once you've mastered the art, you'll realise that swimming is just like life.
<u>READER</u>: *Here we go again, another metaphor about life.*
Hey! I'm Yorkshire's newest Philosopher, folk will be quoting me for years to come and when I die, there'll be a blue plaque placed on the wall of the disused Council house I grew up in.

Anyway, back to swimming and life.

You can spend your days in the shallow end of the pool, or you can test yourself and go out in the ocean. Oh! Before I forget, please don't pee in the pool, it's disrespectful to the other swimmers and it's bloody disgusting. And never, never, **never**… pee **into** the pool, that's just downright repulsive.

THE GYM

Members only

Being a member of a gym isn't like buying a lottery ticket and hoping for the best, it's a commitment to a lifestyle but it will pay out dividends, if you put in some hard graft. But you have to go, to see results.

You're forever swanning off to the gym,
Toning your legs, your arms and your botty,
But I know the real reason you're there every night,
It's 'cos you love to check out the totty!!

The majority of people try to get fit at the gym, so let's take a look at the **pros** and **cons** of joining one. First of all, joining a gym is a costly business. The monthly membership, the personal training sessions, the physio, the massages, the over-priced drinks, the protein bars, the parking, the trendy new sports gear and the beauty therapy that is required 'cos you're trying to catch the eye of that fitty who turns up on a Wednesday.

Aye, it's no wonder that there are more Gyms in this country than Greengrocers. In fact, in 2017 it is estimated that there were about nine million gym members in the UK alone. Yet. **YET!!** Two-thirds of all adults are categorised as *'obese'*. Odd that isn't it?

Nevertheless, it's patently obvious that being a member of a gym doesn't preclude you from putting on the lard, they don't always make you fit and they often make you skint.
READER: *So why bother??*
Good point. Although, it appears to me that people are just not utilising the equipment properly and like a middle-aged Police Officer, they haven't got a clue about fitness (so I've heard… please don't arrest me Mr Officer).

Here's what some of my clients said about their experiences at the gym:

LISA, 47 – *I used to be a gym member and I hated it, you can smell the testosterone as soon as you walk in the door. It's so male orientated and I felt really uncomfortable in that environment, so I quit.*

ROSE, 28 - *I struggled to keep up with exercise classes, they seemed so frenetic and the instructor just assumes everyone is at the same level. So I don't go to them anymore. I'm still a gym member, although I can't remember the last time I went.*

ALEX, 30 – *I've been a gym member for 3 years and still can't seem to lose weight.*

SHARON, 40 – *I go to the gym a few times a week but I don't enjoy it and I'm not really sure what equipment or machines will benefit me the most. It's just become part of my routine now.*

MOHAMMED, 35 – *I actually had a personal training session at the gym but felt like I was just printed out a generic plan that they give to everyone else. It's not helped me at all.*

135

Maybe you're one of those people that detest gyms and have *'Gymaphobia'*?
READER: *Yeah, I think I am.*
If you're honest with yourself I don't think you do really, you're just embarrassed to go or you're not sure what to do, so don't bother trying. This is a common problem with respect to people who just can't seem to lose weight in the long-term.

Gyms are extremely intimidating places, what with all the Lycra clad beauties and pouting meatheads. If you're not very confident, you can be put off for life.

The first thing you should do once you've decided to join is ask for a guided tour. Most gyms will do this and you can ask lots of questions regarding fitness classes, when the busy times are, what services your membership fees include etc, etc.

If they include a PT session within the price, then take advantage of that service and explain to the PT your *'specific'* goals and ask them to provide you with a **tailored plan** and **why** it will benefit you.

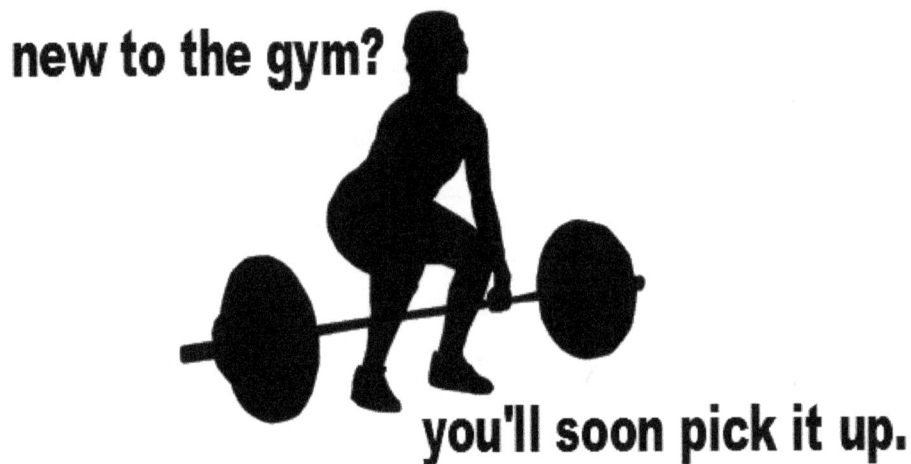

new to the gym? you'll soon pick it up.

Ask questions, lots and lots and lots of questions.

Don't be embarrassed to ask anything, they'll actually enjoy being quizzed so they can show off. Just don't ask them about their tattoos, you'll be there for hours and learn nothing about weight loss.

Once you decide to join a gym or utilise the services of a PT, you'll be asked to fill out a PAR-Q.
READER: *What's one of them?*
It's a medical related *'Physical Activity Readiness – Questionnaire'*, designed to establish if you're healthy enough to actually undertake exercise.

It will ask questions regarding the history of heart conditions in your family, if you've ever suffered from chest pains, bouts of dizziness, high blood pressure etc, etc.

Therefore I recommend that you're 100% honest in your answers. If you're worried that you're not quite fit enough to join a gym (irony overload) then consult your GP and ask for an *'informed consent'* form. Once you're *'fit'* and ready to go you're likely to encounter a few common issues that can hinder your enthusiasm, motivation and chances of improving your fitness level. So let's have a look at 'em and let's get rid of that lard.

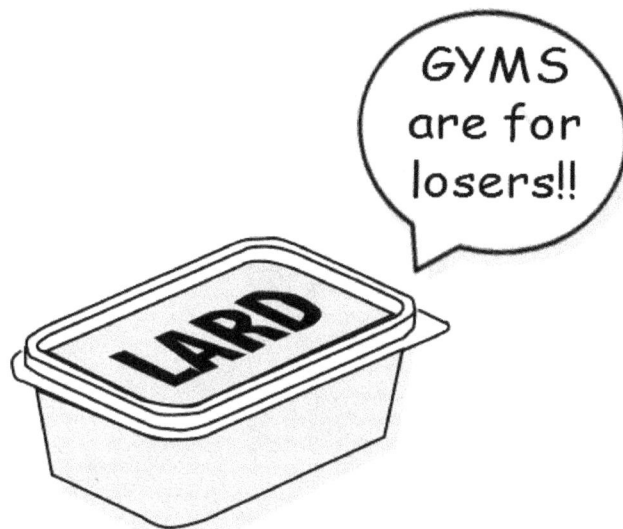

COMMON ISSUES – Generic

Monotony is bad enough in life but especially in a gym routine therefore keep your workouts varied so you don't get bored. Mix it up a bit, variety is the spice of life after all. Try out a new class such as kettlebell, boxercise, spinning or insanity, and attend at different times of the day if you can so you don't keep seeing the same ol' beetroot faces.
READER: *Insanity? That sounds a bit extreme.*
Oh!! Believe me, it is. Personally I love it. If you're gonna have a work out, you want to be sweating cobs. It's based around *'High-Intensity Interval Training'* (HIIT) and it's called *'insanity'*, 'cos it's hard-core man!!

In fact, studies show that 27mins of HIIT, 3 times a week, produces the same anaerobic and aerobic performance gains as 60mins of cardio, 5 times a week. Less is certainly more when it comes to HIIT.

Granted it's a lot harder than normal exercise and you will sweat, boy will you sweat. But it means that you will get more benefit in a shorter period of time due to the lower recovery rates, which **force** your body to work extra.

However, you need to have reached a decent level of fitness before attempting. Otherwise you could sustain injuries, or get disillusioned because you can't keep up.

Who knows though, you might relish it. Give it a go, it might be the making of a new, fitter, thinner and stronger you.

SIMON, 32 – *After your encouragement, I finally psyched myself up to join a gym. It took me a few months to get into the flow and make it part of my weekly routine but I persevered and I genuinely look forward to every visit. Now, life is what happens between gym sessions.*

Don't fear the fancy equipment at the gym; ask an instructor how to use them and which area of the body and **specific** muscles they target. That's what the instructors are there for, not just to chat up the lasses and compare shaved chests with the men in vests.

Whether you're using a treadmill, exercise bike or cross-trainer please don't try to read a book or magazine, or scroll about on your phone. You should be giving it your all, putting in as much effort as you can. If the program isn't demanding enough then **up** the intensity by increasing the level, speed or gradient. Make it, oh I don't know – **challenging!!**

If it's too easy, it's not worth the bother.

CV MACHINES

Common issues

STATIONARY CYCLE

If you have back problems, select a machine that has a back support. Be sure to ask a gym instructor **how** the machine works and be aware not to slouch forward, or rock from side to side because this puts extra pressure on your back (when you're on the cycle that is, not when you're talking to the PT).

Make sure your feet are secure in the foot straps but not too tight that you start to see stars and feel dizzy. Don't lock your knees when pedalling or have the seat too high, otherwise you may sustain stress on the ol' knee joints.

This is a good machine for those on the *'heavy'* side due to the fact that this type of stationary cycle supports body weight more evenly.

ROWER

The rower exercises the lower and upper body, but the rowing action can appear complicated thus some people are actually discouraged from using this equipment.

It's actually very simple once you get into a nice, controlled rhythm. As with all machines located in the gym, if you're not sure how to use them ask an instructor. Don't be shy; they're paid minimum wage to do summat.

Try to keep your shoulders in line with your hips during the rowing movement and most of the power should come from your legs, not the arms. Keep the wrists straight as the bar approaches the body, don't twist your arms and your knees should be in line with your feet. Try not to let the bar hit your kipper or your crotch. Pull it into your midriff.

And be careful that your t-shirt doesn't get caught in the chain, you don't wanna rip that fancy sports top. Although people with back problems seem to ignore the rower, conducted correctly it can promote back and core strength.

Finally, your bottom should stay in the seat, at **all** times. If your rhythm gets messed up, you can be prone to slide off and it's not graceful and everyone in the gym will stare at you and laugh. Secretly remembering the time it happened to them and thanking the Lord someone else did it.

TREADMILL

The treadmill is so easy to use, although your coordination may be slightly off initially, as you start the belt going. Ideally, although I hardly see anyone doing it, you should stand with each foot either side of the belt. Therefore when the machine starts to move, there's less strain on the motor.

Once the belt is going, whilst holding onto the rail, place your feet on the belt but don't set it going too fast or you may slip, fall and slide off the belt in a comedic fashion. It's difficult to regain your cool once that's happened and you might graze your knee too, **Booooo!!**

Always run centrally within the belt, looking straight ahead and close to the front of the machine, which again reduces the possibility of arse-your-on-falling, from occurring.

X-TRAINER

There are several types but the most efficient is the Nordic version which simulates the action of a skier, with both the arms and the legs operating in a sliding motion (good for the abs).

The technique is straightforward enough; it's all down to a smooth controlled rhythm, with both your arms and legs moving at the same pace. A lot of people tend to put too much emphasis on their legs which can cause them to slide off balance. But **you** won't do that, 'cos I've warned you about the risk.

The foot plates can get slippery, so be careful and have a towel handy to wipe the sweat off your brow. When you want to finish, slow down to an almost standstill and then and **only then** should you begin to depart.

All of the CV (Cardio-vascular) machines have built in programmes that allow you to increase intensity, duration and speed, so have a play and test yourself.

And if you're getting bored, pick another form of exercise to do, don't waste your valuable time.

The repetitive actions of CV machines can easily create a muscular imbalance therefore to combat this, make sure you perform some stretches afterwards.

COMMON ISSUES – Generic

Don't get het up about your body fat % and resting heart rate. You don't need a PT with a pair of callipers clasped around your muffin top, to know you've put on some lard. But **you** will need to have patience re any exercise programme, 'cos you'll probably increase muscle definition initially, which *'may'* lead you to believe you're not losing weight or making progress.

That is not the case.

And don't rely on scales to gauge success. You don't need a number to dictate or destroy your happiness. You can assess progress in other ways, by looking in the mirror, by the clothes you wear, your energy levels, your demeanour and by your reflection. Exercise can improve your mood for the day, whereas the number on a scale can ruin it.

If you incorporate all aspects of HELP you won't fixate on measurements anyway, 'cos you'll look and feel fantastic, irrespective of the numbers.

Never, ever, **ever** get the lift or an escalator up to the gym. Kind of defeats the object doesn't it?!

Leave your phone in your locker whilst you conduct your workout, it's ok you'll still be able to breathe.

If you're a woman, heck even if you're a bloke, a good man can make you feel sexy, strong and able to take on the world. Actually a gym can do that too and the added bonus is the toilet seat is always down... in the Ladies anyway.

Changing rooms at gyms are enough to put off any gym-goer. There's nothing in this world more unsightly than a between the cheeks, naked, squat-thrust towel-slide. I don't know about you but the sight of another person's dangly genitals, are a bit of a come down after a high-octane workout. These people are super-determined to get dry, with all the nooks and crannies towelled to within an inch of their lives. And what people use that hairdryer for, are not what the manufacturers had in mind. I understand now why a lot of people get showered and changed at home.

However, if you're motivated and can stomach the genitalia extravaganza, then trips to the gym will **definitely** help you lose weight and increase your levels of fitness but you've gotta have a plan, **Stan!!**

Which means you should base your training schedule around your goals, so let's now look at **specific** fitness objectives.

BESPOKE FITNESS

It works for me

What works for one, doesn't necessarily work for another. One size does not fit all. It's all down to individual preference but if you have a **specific** objective, there will be certain exercises and fitness methods that will **definitely** help you attain those goals, and some that won't.

Therefore you can work out in your living room, in the garden or at the gym, but your goal won't work out, unless you work out properly.

Gaining muscle to lose weight

Although cardio is often cited as the best way to lose the lard, gaining muscle can be just, if not more efficient.
READER: *Seriously?!*
Oh aye!
Put simply, a pound of fat and a pound of muscle weigh the same but your body burns **more** calories to maintain muscle than it does for fat. Therefore more muscle, equates to less fat. And less fat, leads to less weight. **Yay!!**

This means that even when you are out of the gym and in front of a computer, or lazing on the couch, you'll burn more calories if you have been lifting the weights, than if you haven't.
READER: *I thought that the more muscles you have, the more you weigh?*
No that's not necessarily the case.
Muscles are denser than fat, so taking up weight lifting *'may'* make you put on weight, but one pound of fat takes up 18 per cent more space on your body than one pound of muscle, so it will still get you into those skinny jeans.

READER: *Won't weight-training make me big?*
NAH!! Lifting cake builds fat, lifting weights burns it.

READER: *So should I do cardio or weight-training?*
Completely up to you.
You've gotta choose the exercise method which you enjoy the most or else you're onto a losing battle.
Rather than either or, why not **combine** cardio with some light, weight training. Your decision of course but you'll lose the weight quicker because it's more beneficial than focusing on a programme of fitness based solely on cardio.

Resistance training using weights, not only burns a ton of calories when performed intensely but can actually raise your metabolism so that you burn additional calories even after you have finished exercising.
READER: *Why exactly?*
Resistance training stimulates muscle growth, which in turn, means your body uses more energy to recover and rebuild muscle tissue even when you are resting.
READER: *Wow, any other benefits?*
You betcha!!

Are you planning on getting older?
READER: *Erm, I bloody hope so!*
Well, as you now know, bone health deteriorates as we get older but weight lifting can help stem the decline and even reverse it.

Some nerds in the US of A conducted a study and found that four months of resistance training increased hip-bone density and boosted levels of *'Osteocalcin'* (a protein in the blood linked to bone growth) by 20 per cent. Therefore a programme of weight-training can help strengthen your bones **and** improve your posture. Which means you won't develop that hunchback look, and are less likely to *'have a fall'* when you enter your twilight years. You can be quite mean sometimes but I know you have a heart of gold when you want to, so let me also mention that weight-training is good for your ol' ticker. Lifting heavy stuff has been found to have a positive effect on blood pressure, which can help to reduce the risk of a stroke, or a heart attack. You gotta love that.

It could even help you quit smoking. A 2011 study found that smokers of both sexes who completed a twelve week weight-training programme, were twice as likely to successfully quit, compared to those who did not regularly lift weights. Don't ask me why, I don't know but worth a shot for those yellow fingered ones who are desperate to quit.

If you're a bloke, lifting weights can also help to boost your sex life. After about thirty years of age, testosterone levels in chaps begin to drop and low levels can lead to erectile dysfunction and more serious illnesses such as heart disease or diabetes. Lugging heavy loads is a great way of reversing this process, as the body positively responds to weight training by producing more testosterone.

Good things **come**, to those that lift weights.

I'm not recommending that you become a meathead but by incorporating weights into your exercise regime (at the gym or at home), this will help you achieve your goal of losing the lard. And as you start to lose weight you may decide you want to get buffer, so here's some basic guidance and a number of tips that will help you attain some gain.

Oh! By the way, if you're an elite athlete or Billy-Big-Bob then please step away from this book, it's not designed for you. Go back to your skinless chicken, dry tuna, egg whites and protein injections.

There are approximately 650 muscles in our bodies which comprise the majority of our body weight and are responsible for all body movement.

There are three different types of muscle tissue in the human body:
- **CARDIAC MUSCLE** - which is only found in the heart
- **SMOOTH MUSCLE** - which is found in organs and within blood vessels
- **SKELETAL MUSCLE** - which is found all over the body and is primarily responsible for movement

All three of these muscle types have distinctly different anatomical structures and functionality.

We know that muscles get bigger and stronger when put under stress, which is called *'Adaption'*.

This simply means that the muscle is preparing itself in case it's put under the same type of stress again and will **adapt** to this pressure, by either growing bigger or stronger. As the body gets used to this new exertion, the next time you train the muscles they will be capable of handling this level of stress.

Within skeletal muscle, there are three types of muscle fibres:
- TYPE 1
- TYPE 2A
- TYPE 2B

TYPE 1 muscle fibre is often referred to as *'slow-twitch'* or *'red fibre'*, is highly resistant to fatigue and has a high oxidative capacity. Which means this type of muscle fibre is responsible for aerobic exercises such as cycling and running.

Slow twitch fibres have smaller nerves, therefore as their name suggests they twitch much slower, however they have a higher number of mitochondria which increases their oxidative capacity. *'Mitochondria'* are often referred to as the cell's engine, or powerhouse. Marathon runners and endurance cyclists generally have bodies with this type of muscle definition.

TYPE 2A muscle fibre is often referred to as *'fast-twitch'* or *'white fibre'* which is an intermediate fibre, larger in size and much stronger than Type 1 fibres.

Fast twitch fibres have thicker nerves that give them an increased contractile impulse. Footballers and tennis players usually have bodies with this type of muscle definition.

TYPE 2B muscle fibre, which are also fast-twitch **and** white fibre, are capable of producing more force than Type 2A but they're low in oxidative capacity and fatigue very quickly. Sprinters and body-builders, typically have bodies with this type of muscle definition.

We all have our own **unique** distribution of these fibres. Some people can be predominately Type 1, and some Type 2A, however the average Joe or Josephine has an even amount of red and white fibre. But if you want a body like any of the athletes described above, then train and eat as they would.

In fact, on a side note, have you ever seen a sprinter who isn't cut?
READER: *Ooh! No I haven't, I've seen their lunchboxes though…*
Blimey, calm yourself. All I was gonna say is that if you trained like a sprinter, even ate like one, it's highly likely you'd end up fit and muscly. Worth trying if you fancy looking like that.

Lifting big weights for serious muscle gain seems to be the norm but for me, it's so boring and you won't be fit per se, you will be strong and look good in a vest, but have trouble running for a bus.

Therefore all these body-builders that lift and lift and YAWN… lift to get a buff bod, should perhaps give sprint training a go. Much more fun and you'll easily catch the number 23.

So now you know a little bit about your muscles, how you gonna use them??

If you're a woman I recommend that you initially look at a weight-lifting programme that centres around endurance, rather than strength. This means that you will select lower weights but conduct higher reps. Your stamina and strength will improve but you won't bulk up, as you would do if you lifted heavier weights. If you conduct lower reps with heavier weights, this will lead to improved strength but also muscle gain. If that's what you're after then go for it.

KATHY, 29 – *I was reticent at first but coupled with changes to my diet I noticed the fat drop off after a few weeks of conducting a weight-lifting programme.*
I remember when I first spoke to you I said that I was never going to be one of those girls who's a size 8 but straight away you responded by telling me if that's what I wanted, then of course I could do it.
And I did.
I have.
Like a lot of women in my position, I felt like my weight was holding me back in every aspect of my life, especially when it came to doing things with my kids. Activities that other Mums might take for granted like swimming or going to the park, seemed off limits because I felt so self-conscious.
Now I'm an active Mum and I love it. And lifting the bairns has become a lot easier too after deadlifting and kettlebell swinging.
I finally feel like the person I was meant to be, and the Mum that my kids deserve.

MUSCLES

Phwooaarr!!

So do you want big muscles?
READER: *Yes please.*
You want to attract women who are impressed by tight fitting, low neck t-shirts, tattoo sleeves and conformity?
READER: *Defo!!*
Fair enough. The traditional way to obtain the big muskles is to lift. And then lift some more.

Bro!! Do you even lift?
To get the best results you'll need to **shock** the muscles for growth.
Muscles are broken down and then rebuilt stronger, based on the stress you have applied to it.
If you repeat the same exercises again and again, you're liable to get strong but may not improve mass due to 'muscle memory'.
READER: *Muscles have memories?*
Sort of.

Many things contribute to muscular power and even though muscle size is the most obvious, there are other factors that are even more important. Possibly the most critical is the central nervous system (CNS), which is responsible for the transmission of impulses to your muscles. The stress placed on the CNS is directly proportional to the load you are attempting to lift, so the heavier you train, the greater the CNS response.

There's a special section within your muscles called a *'Motor Unit'* that innervates, or activates a number of muscle fibres to allow movement. Fibres contract, generating force in response to stress, so the motor unit signals the fibres to contract, which is where your muscular power comes from.

The amount of hormonal signals required to lift a dumbbell is mind-boggling. Millions upon millions of cellular messages take place in an instant, just so you can lift that incredibly heavy barbell over your noggin to impress that chick in the pink leggings. Therefore the more you repeat an exercise, the less signals are required because the stress is lower, and the effort required to conduct the action is reduced thus the gains are limited. So my main recommendation to all you prospective Billy-Big-Bobs who want the big muskles, is mix it up and increase intensity.

POTENTIAL BILLY-BIG-BOB READER: *How do I increase intensity?*
Easy peasy.
Conduct a low amount of reps with heavier weights. Reduce your recovery times and then try to incorporate pyramids into your sets.

POTENTIAL BILLY-BIG-BOB READER: *Pyramids?*
Yeah, low to high to low again. That means your set should include something like:

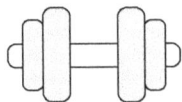

Pyramids

- 5 reps, rest for a minute or so
- 6 reps, rest
- 7 reps, rest
- 8 reps, rest
- Then 7 reps rest
- 6 reps, rest
- And finish with 5 reps, rest.

Repeat with a heavier weight and conduct at least 3 sets.

I'm afraid that gurning and facial contortions are mandatory, whereas farty-pops are optional but entirely possible. But be careful not to pick a weight that's too heavy, you don't want to pass out when the other meatheads are looking.

POTENTIAL BILLY-BIG-BOB READER: *Anything else?*
Well, you could conduct your first set on a higher weight, and then further sets on lower weights because this fools your CNS into sending the same amount of mitochondria and fibres to aid muscle contraction thus increasing mass. You can then train for longer because you're not expending as much energy. With respect to your workout, always target the larger muscle groups first (compound exercises), then you can concentrate on isolation exercises (biceps/triceps etc). This will reduce fatigue and prevent the likelihood of injury.

Deadlifts and barbell squats are both *'Compound'* exercises which utilise more muscles, take more effort and you expend more energy. This extra exertion and intensity will enable significant muscle growth.

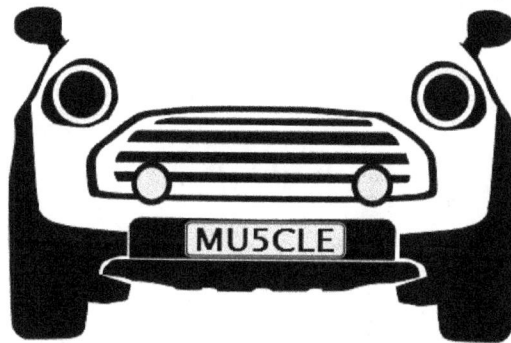

Wrong mindset...don't be a TW4T

You've probably heard some Billy-Big-Bob at the gym saying something like this, *'It's Thursday, so it's leg day!'* My response to them would be, *'Sod off! You boring git!!'*

These people no doubt **have** to conduct *'Isolation'* exercises because they've become such a saddo, and no-one wants to spend time with 'em.

Look, don't be that guy or woman, muscles don't work in isolation they work in tandem with a whole network of muscles. Therefore to increase mass and strength, concentrate on completing **more** compound exercises and **reduce** isolation moves.

You could try supping some coffee about twenty minutes before your workout too.
Apparently, caffeine partially blocks the pain receptors which are contained within muscles, thus you can train for longer.

POTENTIAL BILLY-BIG-BOB READER: *Any tips for bigger biceps?*
Aah!! The holy grail for most Billy-Big-Bobs and hipster poseurs, the *'Biceps'*.
You wanna look good in those tight shirts with the unsubtle logo, I get it.

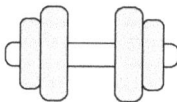

Biceps

If you're conducting a bicep curl, try to make sure that during each rep, the weight takes about two seconds to be raised but five seconds to go down.

This gradual lowering of the weight will put extra strain and stress on the muscle, leading to improved gains.

Your form is extremely important, so I would always make sure you conduct the exercise with a lower weight first to establish the perfect action. This will improve your strength and reduce the risk of injury.

You could even conduct some forearm exercises in your alone time, but remember you have two arms, so rotate, you don't want RSI.

Please also be aware that arms contain *'Triceps'* as well as biceps, so you need to incorporate exercises to target those muscles too.

POTENTIAL BILLY-BIG-BOB READER: *Such as?*

Tricep drops perhaps and the best bodyweight exercise bar none, the press-up. If you work-out six days a week, then alternate between weights and cardio and try to have one day off (Sunday maybe, depends on your work pattern). Or have two days rest if you want, just find a system that works for you. **Hey!!** You gotta have a system.

And, and, **AND** you have legs too. Make sure you work 'em out, they'll improve your overall strength and balance, which will make you stronger. **Yay!!**

Oh! And when you're on the weight-machines at the gym, always add extra weight to the machine before you leave. That way, the next user will think you're just awesome…

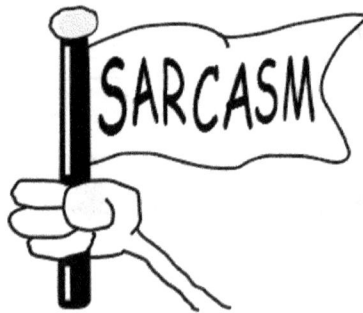

…Yep, that's sarcasm my friend, welcome to my world, come on in and look around. Have a coffee, sit down and take it all in…

But all of the above is useless, if you don't **eat** enough to repair the muscles.

BEEFCAKE

If you want to get bufferer, there's a bit of a paradox going on because even though you'll be trying to lose the timber, you'll need to eat… **a lot!!** Your muscles take a hell of a beating during a workout, so they need to be rebuilt, stronger. That's where food comes in and our good friend, Peter Protein.

The more you exercise them muscles, the more protein is required, although don't forget all the other important nutrients you get from food too (see next chapter).

You should eat an hour or so before your workout, within an hour after and several times throughout the day in order to get bigger and more muscularised.

You can follow the herd and drink protein shakes but beware that too much processed protein, is actually bad for your kidneys. In fact, your body just excretes the excess, unless you're exercising to meet demand.

I've never drunk a protein shake in my life but I do have a valuable tip for you if **you** decide that it's your preferred way to go. Don't mix protein powders with milk because the *'Casein'* contained within doesn't allow the protein to be absorbed into the bloodstream. Therefore mix with water for the best results, or alternatively eat more eggs. It worked for Rocky… *'AADDDRRRIIIAAANNNNNNNNNNNNNNNNN!!'*

Full fat milk contains essential nutrients and protein, so if you struggle to eat enough calories during the day, try to increase your dairy consumption. There's plenty of info on the net about **LOMAD** (Litre of milk a day) and **GOMAD** (Gallon of milk a day), so do some research. Just make sure you buy some Clearasil and lots and lots and lots of toilet paper.

<u>POTENTIAL BILLY-BIG-BOB READER</u>: *Why?*
You'll find out… I certainly did.

Another good tip is to drink a glass of full milk before you go to bed. When your body is recuperating and repairing during your kip, the extra protein will be used to pump up them muskles. Urinating during the night is optional.

In my opinion, stay natural baby!! You don't see many Gorillas taking protein shakes and the like, and they're macker!!

I advise that you add as many of these items to your weekly diet as possible:

<u>FRUIT & VEG</u>	<u>MISC</u>	<u>FISH & MEAT</u>
• Avocadoes*	• Cottage cheese	• Chicken
• Bananas	• Kidney beans	• Liver
• Broccoli	• Lentils	• Mackerel
• Kale	• Natural yoghurt	• Salmon
• Leafy & iron-rich veg	• Nuts	• Steak
• Pears	• Oats	• Tuna
• Spinach		• Turkey

*The plural of *'avocado'*, is in fact, *'avocados'* but it looks ridiculous to me, it sounds like a Greek island, so I'm with Dan Quayle on this one (look it up).

But whatever you do, don't make *'Beefcake'* it sounds disgusting, **eeuurrgghh!!**

And if you eat and exercise how I suggested, you'll be buff and built in no time. However, you will have to get used to one major side effect… Protein farts.

Good luck trying to hide them beauties!!

Paul Birch

KETTLEBELLS

Swing baby, swing!!

When life is getting me down, I reach for the kettle… bell. I absolutely love to work-out with a kettlebell. They're bloody awesome.

You get the benefits of cardio with the added bonus of strength training, all in one hefty package.
Kettlebell training is perfect for those looking to lose the lard and you don't have to be an elite athlete to use them, they're so simple to pick up, even **you** can do it.

Whilst kettlebells have become a go-to piece of gym equipment for many, they can be daunting to any novice not sure what to do with them. Therefore if you don't know how to use them properly, ask your friendly PT to demonstrate the techniques and the benefits of each swing and action.
READER: *I've actually never heard of them, what are they?*
They're basically a cannonball weight with a handle attached and they resemble the traditional *'kettle'* shape, although without the spout.

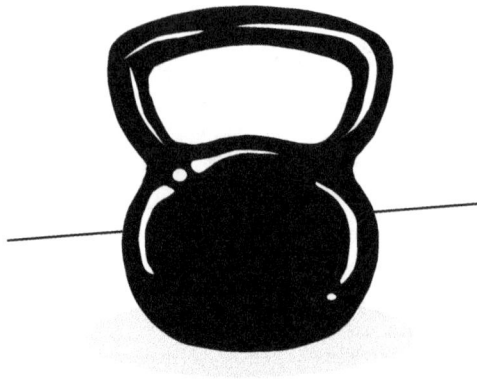

Kettlebells have been used by the Russian Army since way back in the 1800's, but some believe they actually date back to Spartan times, when handles were placed into cinderblocks in order to help move them around and keep the soldiers fit and battle-ready.

SPARTAN SOLDIERS: AWOO!! AWOO!! AWOO!! (Don't understand? Watch the film *'300'*)

Kettlebell or Dumbbell - that is the question?!

You may think a weight is a weight is a weight, but you'd be wrong. What makes kettlebells superior to dumbbells in every way, is that you can do the same things you can with a dumbbell, only better.
The magic of the kettlebell is due to the cannonball shape, and the offset handle which allows you to manipulate the kettlebell in a whole variety of ways.

You can lift a kettlebell in the same manner as a dumbbell but you can also snatch, throw, catch and more importantly, swing them too.

Therefore it's in the name. Either select a kettlebell and be cool, fit and funky or get a DUMB bell and be a fool, a twit and a **flunkie!!**

The dynamic swinging functionality of a kettlebell allows the exerciser to perform countless multi-joint exercises, with **one** or **two** hands and in a range of motions. The body can be worked to the extreme, resulting in greater and speedier fitness gains.

148

While there are many great things about kettlebell training, one of the biggest benefits is that all of the exercises are essentially **total-body** exercises. This means you get full-body strengthening and conditioning, with one single tool. Virtually every fitness goal you want can be accomplished with a kettlebell.

Let's face it, for a lot of people exercise can be a tad boring!! For some, the monotony of the Treadmill, Exercise Bike or X-Trainer is akin to a confused hamster, stuck in a wheel.

If that's how you feel, then kettlebells will definitely help you enjoy the activity.

You want cardio? You want strength? And you want flexibility training? Well buy **one** get **two** free with the kettlebell. It gives you all that and more.

Kettlebells for me,
Kettlebells for you,
Kettlebells a-swinging,
With one hand, or two!!

You're a busy bee and you want to get **in** and **out** of the gym, as quick as poss, right?
READER: *Too right!*
Well, kettlebell training is time-efficient because you can perform a high-intensity workout, in just half an hour. To get the same benefits as this type of high-intensity training, you'd have to conduct cardio on one of those CV machines for double the time. It takes a **lot** of energy to throw and swing the kettlebell weight around, which will not only burn calories but will also stimulate muscle growth.

Although it's high intensity it's also low-impact, making it a safer form of cardio than say, running on pavements. Forces are distributed **evenly** during the kettlebell swing over your hips, thighs, hamstrings, back and shoulders. And you don't suffer from *'kettlebell'* knee, unless you over swing and whack it against your patellar.

It's cardio without killing your joints, so if you're not a fan of jogging, it's the kettlebell for you.

If you're one of those people that alternates training days at the gym, a kettlebell can simplify your trip. You don't have to think about which exercise requires what size weight, or what level to put that resistance machine at. You don't have to figure out which days you do cardio and which days you do strength training because kettlebells combine both elements into any movement. You don't need to worry about upper body and then lower body exercises either. It's all in one.

What could be easier?

One kettlebell, two or three times a week, you only swing when you're winning.

Just **four** basic movements (the swing, clean, press and snatch) and their countless variations, can be used two or three times per week to keep you lean, strong and functional for the rest of your life.

Here's the two-handed kettlebell swing, which is as easy as one, two, Weeeeeeeee!!

1	2	3
Feet shoulder width apart, hold the kettlebell with a two-handed grip, don't hunch, keep your shoulders back and spine straight	Swing the kettlebell backwards between your legs, just past your botty, push down on your heels, press your arse back and then start to swing upwards with your hips	Stand straight, engage your core and swing as high as you can, then return back down to position one. Repeat until red in face and ready to vomit

You have enough to think about with work, children, which cheese to buy and whether you'll reply to that text or not, so let your workout be uncomplicated.

READER: *I'm sold. How much do they cost?*
I know I sound like a Salesman but I'm not personally selling them ☺ although you can get a 20lb/9kg one for about fifteen quid, so they're extremely cheap. That means a massive saving when you compare that price to monthly Gym memberships, personal trainers, parking, milkshakes, over-priced fruit and *'healthy'* saccharin enriched, oat bars.

Just by purchasing a single kettlebell, you can have everything you need to create a healthy, fit and toned body for the rest of your life. They are virtually indestructible and great for holding doors open too. If you're a bit nervous about going to the gym, or it's not feasible to join one for whatever reason, get yourself a kettlebell and work-out at home.

Plus, your entire home gym can be put away in a cupboard, or under the bed.

So if you've tried to get fit before, you'll probably have a room full of fancy machines, swanky gizmo's and DVD's collecting dust, well you can chuck all them away. Or sell 'em to pay for your kettlebells, 'cos the dramatic results will keep you going and as you increase proficiency, you'll end up buying more.

READER: *Are the moves easy to learn?*
Yes, the movements are quite simple and no matter how old or out-of-shape you are, **everyone** can do them, so there's no excuse.
FEMALE READERS: *As a woman, I don't want to bulk up.*
Depending on the weight of the kettlebell you buy, you won't bulk up. Women who regularly use kettlebells get the svelte, lean, firm shape they desire but in a fraction of the time than those lasses who spend hours sweating and preening about in the gym.
MALE READERS: *What about us blokes?*
Yeah you sweat and preen in the gym too…

MALE READERS: *No, what type of body shape could we achieve?*

Oh! Kettlebells will help you build a lean, muscular physique. The training creates broad shoulders, defines abs, builds up arms and pares down the waist. It'll give you that *'toned'* look that everyone desires and goes on about.
READER: *What if the kettlebell gets too light for me?*
Don't worry, you won't outgrow them. As the weight gets too light you could opt for a heavier bell, or even better, you can change the way you work with the one you have. Just holding the kettlebell with a different grip makes each exercise harder and puts extra stress on your muscles.

NICK, 48 - *After you gave me a kettlebell demo at the gym and wouldn't shut up about their benefits, I had to give them a go. Initially I thought I'd get bored using them but that couldn't be further from the truth. You said something about them being **'the thinking person's workout'** and I know what you mean now. You have to be completely focused whilst conducting any exercise. You can't just pick it up and mindlessly swing and chuck it around. You have to concentrate on all elements of the move, which actually makes the time go quicker.*
I love using them, they're perfect for me. I've lost weight, I'm toned, my stamina has improved and for the first time in my life I have noticeable muscle definition.
But the biggest benefit for me is I no longer suffer from pains in my lower back. I used to take time off work, have trouble sleeping and it would just jar sometimes, meaning I had trouble standing. I can't remember the last time I had any pain and I'm putting it down to the kettlebell training.
Cheers mate.

Right, I'm going to punch you in the stomach, so get ready.
READER: *What? Why, what have I done?*
Nowt, And c'mon, I can't really can I? This isn't some 4th wall, matrix type reality. I just want you to enact **how** you would start to pull in your stomach to brace for the impact.
So go on, do it now.
Can you feel it tense up?
READER: *Ooh! Yeah, I can.*
Kettlebells require you to engage and tense the core in almost every lift, so you'll develop exceptional abdominal strength and enhance spinal stability. And you'll be able to take a punch too!!
Kettlebells will help you develop functional strength as well, because the upper and lower parts of the body **must** work as a unit. And by using fundamental movement patterns, this will make everyday activities easier and reduce the chances of injury. You will stand taller, carry packages easier, climb stairs with less effort and have more energy.
READER: *They sound too good to be true?*
I've told you, they're fantastic. I use them every week, without fail. Give 'em a go.
I can guarantee that the fat will drop off and you'll be swinging like the Rat Pack in hammocks.

One word of warning though.
If you use them in your living room, be careful of sweaty hands or else you may suffer a KB shaped hole through your plasma screen or front window.

Kettlebells, kettlebells,
Swinging all the way,
Oh what fun, it is to swing,
Kettlebells every day, HEY!!

BOTTOM

Sweet cheeks

<u>READER</u>: *Does my bum look big in this?*
Yes, yes it does.
<u>READER</u>: *Cheeky bugger.*
C'mon, there's no point deluding yourself. If **you** have a large posterior then it's time to stop chelpin' and do something about it, or you can just accept the fact and get on with your life.

Actually, a big booty is a lot like property.
<u>READER</u>: *How exactly?*
Location, location, location. It's all about perception. For instance, in Central Africa a fuller woman is deemed more attractive than her sisters with the iron-board frame, and these big-bottomed girls are cherished and fawned upon by the males. In the world of hip-hop, Sir Mix-A-Lot loves big butts and that man is telling the truth because he cannot lie.

If you want a hot bot, get down and squat

Just like any goal, you can **wish** for a pert, rounded arse, or you can get off it and try and make it happen yourself. Because you **definitely** won't get the botty you want by just sitting on it. To achieve perfect buns of steel, you've gotta squat, squat and then squat some more.

Few exercises work as many muscles as the squat because it's an excellent multi-purpose activity, useful for toning and tightening your behind, abs, and your pins. A programme of squats will firm up your butt-ocks in no time at all, without placing any undue stress on your back.

Exercises such as running, aerobics and weightlifting often put undue strain on your knees, ankles and back. Whereas squats, being a low impact exercise, do not have this effect. Therefore it is the perfect exercise for those of you who have glass-backs, weak knees or ropey ankles.

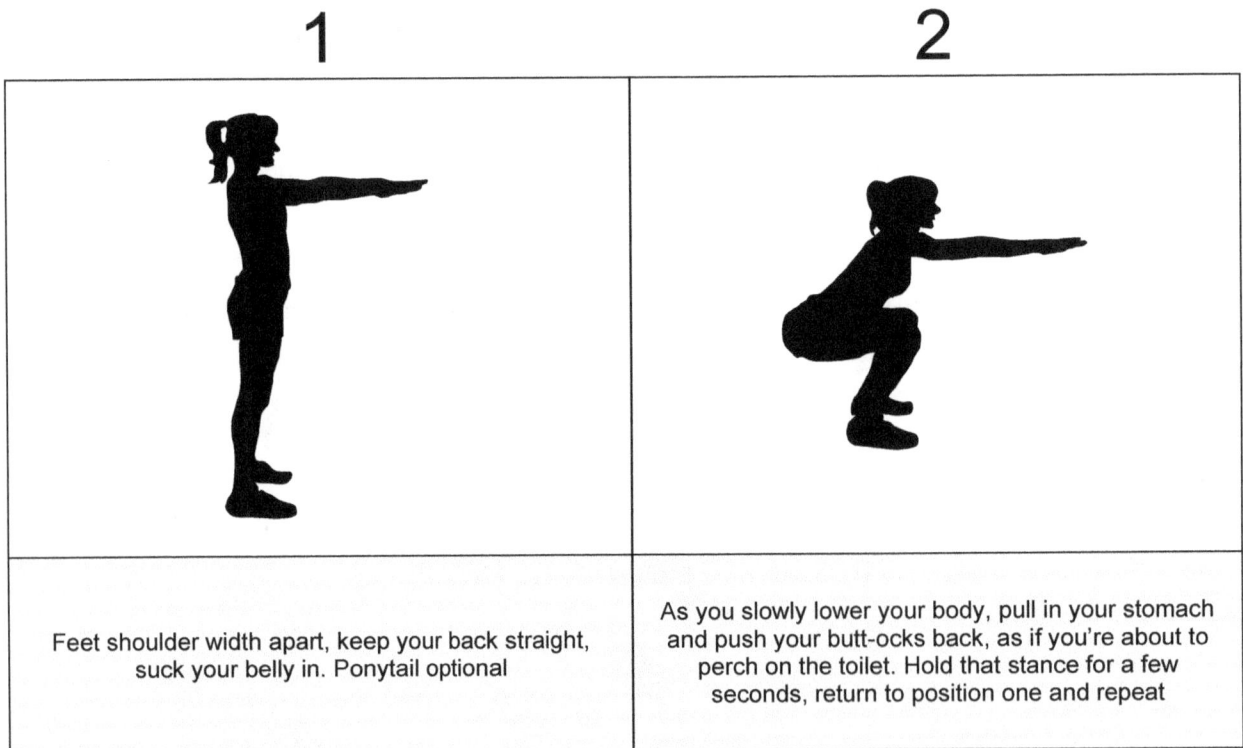

1	2
Feet shoulder width apart, keep your back straight, suck your belly in. Ponytail optional	As you slowly lower your body, pull in your stomach and push your butt-ocks back, as if you're about to perch on the toilet. Hold that stance for a few seconds, return to position one and repeat

SQUATTER'S RIGHTS

When you perform a squat, the act of keeping yourself balanced and upright will give **every** muscle in your leg a workout **and** burn fat, all in one glorious move. Not only do squats help to build your leg muscles (targeting your quadriceps, hamstrings and calves), but they also create this *'Anabolic'* environment, which promotes body-wide muscle building.

An added benefit of increasing your lean muscle mass, is that a higher percentage of calories are burned while you're resting. Since the *'Glutei Maximi'* (or the botty muscles) are the largest muscles in the body, increasing their size has a larger influence on your metabolism than any other muscle.

This extremely effective exercise can be performed pretty much anywhere because you don't need to go to a gym, or use any swanky equipment. You can do squats in the privacy of your own living room whilst watching the box, or waiting for the kettle to boil, or even when you walk your dog.

Squat, 1, 2, 3… Pick up dog poo, 1, 2, 3… Squat, 1, 2, 3 and repeat (especially if dog has diarrhoea).
So you have no excuse, you can do them anywhere.

Squats help you to remove waste from the body.
READER: *You're just making stuff up now!!*
No it's true. The muscular action of the squat exercise improves the flow of fluids in your body, and eases the passing of waste through your bowels. Therefore squats help to keep you regular. Which is a boon for the I.B.S. sufferers out there… and there's a lot of 'em.

Squats are an excellent exercise for cyclists and joggers because they improve muscle flexibility and prevent injuries. The bending and stretching of the knees will strengthen the supporting muscles and allow more oxygen and blood to flow around the joints, thus helping to keep them supple and strong. So, if you wanna smash them PB's, add some squats to your fitness regime.

Have you ever groaned when lifting yourself out of a chair, or bending down to pick something off the floor?
READER: *Ooh! Yeah, I do that sometimes.*
As Snoop Doggy-dog-dog alludes to in one of his raps, you need to:

Drop it like a squat,
Drop it like a squat,
Drop it like a squat!!

Functional exercises are those that help your body to perform real-life activities, as opposed to simply being able to operate pieces of expensive gym equipment, and squats are one of the best functional exercises out there. When you perform them you improve muscle mass, as well as promote mobility and balance. And all of these benefits translate into your body moving more efficiently in the real world too. So you'll have no excuse if you drop litter.

In fact, you could enhance your body whilst enhancing the state of your community, by picking up refuse from your street.

Squat, 1, 2, 3, pick up litter, 1, 2, 3… save environment, 1, 2, 3…
MOTHER NATURE: *Thank you!!*

MOLLY, 29 – *After losing a few stone I wanted to firm up my butt and tone my body. I added a squat and lunge routine to my fitness programme as you suggested and my posture improved no end, which in turn reduced my back pain. I also took your advice and found a 'twerking' aerobics class. Suffice to say, my husband is very pleased with my increased flexibility.*
I've started wearing tight leggings to the gym and even, I can't believe I'm saying this, even hot-pants when going out.
Me, hot-pants… amazing.

WEIGHT FOR IT

Squatting is a form of resistance training because you're lifting your own body weight but to make the exercise more intense, you can hold a weight whilst conducting the move. Using added weight increases the difficulty of the workout, helping you to build additional lean muscle mass which accelerates your metabolism and speeds up weight loss. **Yay!!**

There are a number of variations of the weighted squat, including the *'Back Squat'*, where a barbell is positioned at the base of the neck, atop your trapezius muscles.

The *'Overhead Squat'*, which requires holding the barbell above your head with your arms fully extended. Ooh!! Tough one that, it really targets the core.

The *'Dumbbell Squat'*, where the squatter holds a dumbbell in each hand, straight and at the side of the body, and these are lowered and raised during the squatting action.

Alternatively, a kettle-bell or medicine ball can be held with both hands in front of the body, and the squatter performs an isometric hold throughout the squat.

Weight-free squats that may increase cardiovascular activity include the *'Bodyweight Squat'*, which is performed at a faster pace and at higher repetitions than other variations, and the *'Jump Squat'*, which demands a jump once you rise from the squatting position.

! ! ! WARNING ! ! ! WARNING ! ! ! WARNING ! ! ! WARNING ! ! ! WARNING ! ! ! WARNING ! ! ! WARNING ! ! !

If you are new to the squat, you should start off gradually.

This is especially important if you're using weights because the increased resistance places extra demands on your muscles, especially the lower back. Before each session, take time to warm up your hip joints, knees and ankles to avoid injury.

Be careful to keep your knees in proper alignment as you squat. Ask a PT to demonstrate the correct technique, that's what they are there for, not to belittle you and scream at you and show off their new trainers… but to **help!!**

Life is like a squat, you've got to get down
before you get back up again

LUNGE

Whether you're trying to shape your booty, stimulate muscle growth, develop core strength or increase hip flexibility, the lunge can help you achieve your goal.

1	2
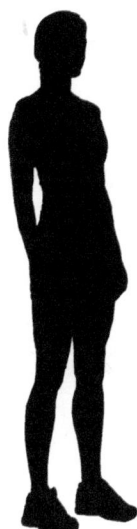	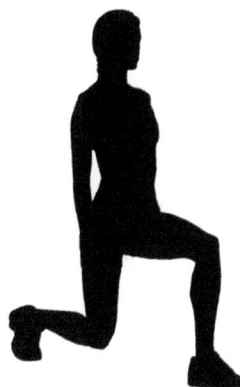
Keep your upper body straight, with your shoulders back and relaxed, chin up and looking straight ahead. Arms to the side, hands resting on your waist. Always engage your core throughout the exercise.	Step forward with one leg, lowering your hips until both knees are bent at about a 90-degree angle. Raise and return to position one, repeat with alternate leg

When conducting a lunge:

- Lower straight down with your pelvis flexed forward and your back straight.
- Ensure that you step your foot far enough forward, so that the middle of your front knee is directly above your ankle during the downward motion.
- Lower your hips until your knees are about 90 degrees bent, and place your weight on the back two-thirds of your front foot during the exercise.
- Lunges are performed on one leg at a time, independent of the other leg. This is known as *'Unilateral'* training. Unilateral training improves your balance and coordination rather than simply developing strength, as with exercises that train both sides at the same time, like squats.

Lunges effectively target your glutes, as well as engaging your hamstrings and quads.

As with squats, strengthening these large muscle groups can speed up your metabolism, which is clearly beneficial if you're trying to lose the lard. When excess fat is reduced from your lower body, lunges can help you shape, tone and firm up your arse and pins.

And just like the squat, conducting lunges can improve your core strength. When performing a lunge, you move your hips up and down whilst tensing your core muscles to keep your body upright and balanced. Having a strong core is essential because it eases daily activities, relieves lower back pain and improves your balance, posture, stability and athletic performance.

Plus you'll look great in a crop top... even you Kev.

Lunges are full body-weight exercises, meaning they make use of the body's bulk and frame as resistance and the beauty is, they can be conducted anywhere that you take your body.

This functional, multi-joint exercise can be modified to meet your fitness level, so if you desire a bit more of a challenge, you can up the intensity of your lunges by adding weights, increasing the number of repetitions, widening your stance or using an inclined surface, such as a bench or chair.

Obviously your diet is a major factor in weight loss and you'll **never a**chieve the perfect botty without making wholesale changes to your diet.

However, by performing an exercise program centred around squats and lunges, combined with a healthy eating plan, you'll maximize your ability to lose weight and tone up the ol' bum-bum.

To get a tight butt, work your ass off,
And get yourself down to the gym,
If you squat and lunge like a demon,
You'll be peachy in no time and trim.

So get a-squatting and a-lunging and leave your old behind, **behind!!**

ABDOMINALS

Cor!!!

The ab-solute goal for most fitness freaks is the six-pack. It seems that no exercise routine is complete without sit-ups, but most gym goers are deluded if they think that completing fifty or sixty sit-ups is going to shift that muffin top.

Doing sit ups to lose excess belly fat, is like repeatedly pushing the elevator button thinking the lift will come quicker. A waste of time and effort.

I'm gonna let you into another secret folks, we've **ALL** got a six-pack but most of us have them hidden under a blanket of flab.

Therefore to reveal them in all their ab-solute splendour, you've got to make fundamental changes to your diet, not your fitness regime.

When it comes to the crunch, have you the stomach for it?

Your core acts as a buffer, linking a network of muscle groups in your upper and lower body.

This complex series of muscles are activated and incorporated, into almost **every** movement of the human body. No matter where the motion starts, it ripples upward and downward through the supporting core and the connecting links of the chain. Whether you're sprinting for a bus, swinging a tennis racket, cuddling your boyfriend, or bending down to pick up a discarded tenner, you'll engage your core in every one of those actions.

The key role of the abdominal region is to support the upper body, primarily to prevent injury to the spinal column. The spine is an amazing design, with each joint allowing about four degrees of movement. If the core muscles are not strong enough, the body may well push the boundaries of this limited range, leading to spinal injury, lower back pain, chelpin' and sick days off work.

Core exercises train the muscles in your pelvis, lower back, hips and abdomen to work in symbiotic harmony. This leads to better balance and stability, whether in the gym, cycling to work or in your daily activities. Therefore a strong, robust core is essential to your health and wellbeing.

When you bend, when you turn and when you twist,
When you lift, reach, sit, you get the gist,
When you run, when you swim and when you drop,
A weak core, won't help, it's just no cop!!

A body is a terrible thing to waist, so to strengthen that weak core you should add the following exercises to your workout:

- Press ups
- Kettle bell swings
- Squats
- Lunges
- Sit ups (much better for your back when conducted on a Swiss ball)
- Toe touches
- Burpees

READER: *What are burpees?*
Oh boy!! Burpees are an intense combination of movements which are fantastic for improving your core, as well as boosting your stamina.
You will love to hate this exercise… it's a **bloody killer!!**

Combined with a programme of lunges and squats, you'll put some junk in your trunk, and some **Phwooarr!!** In your core.

READER: *How do you do them?*
Okay doke! Here's a quick run through:

1   2   3

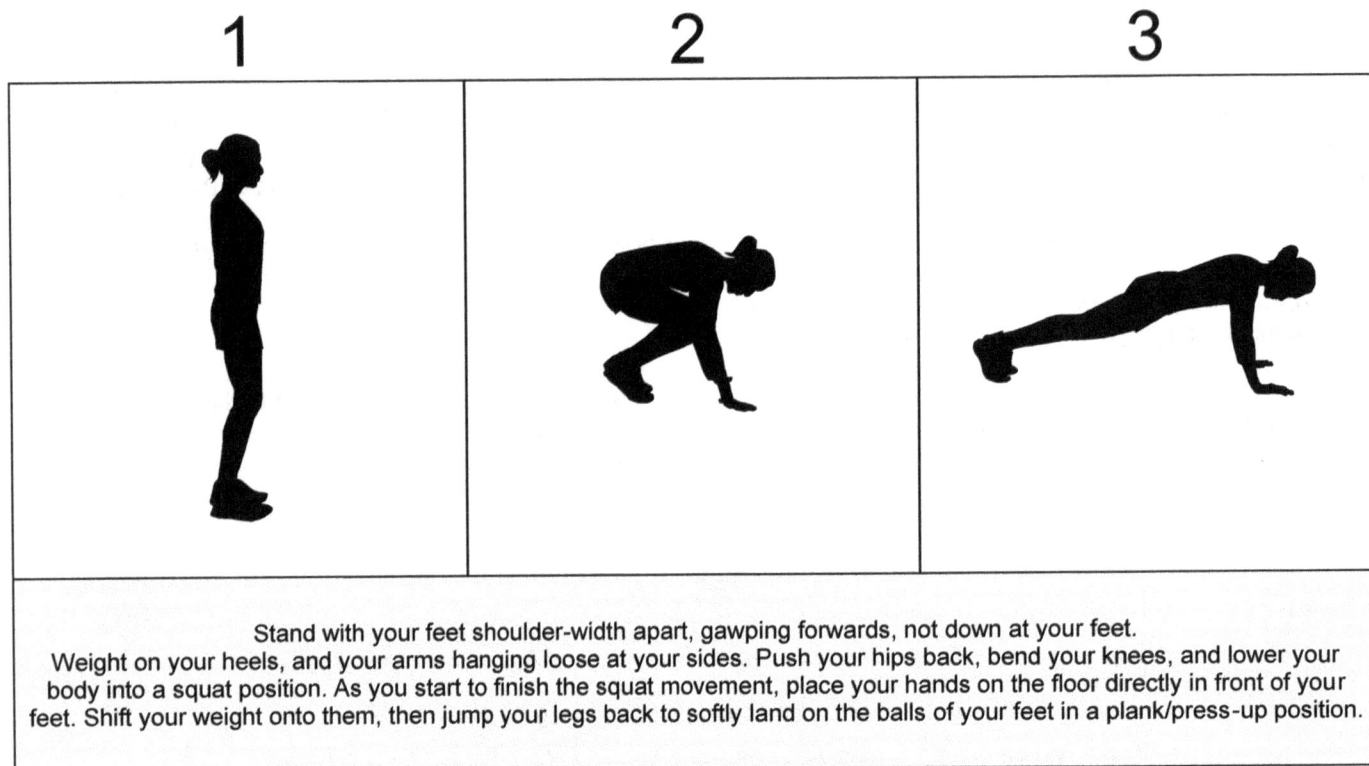

Stand with your feet shoulder-width apart, gawping forwards, not down at your feet.
Weight on your heels, and your arms hanging loose at your sides. Push your hips back, bend your knees, and lower your body into a squat position. As you start to finish the squat movement, place your hands on the floor directly in front of your feet. Shift your weight onto them, then jump your legs back to softly land on the balls of your feet in a plank/press-up position.

4	5	6
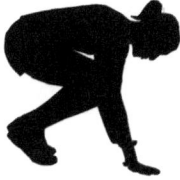		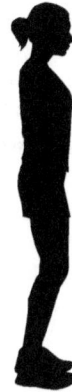

Your body should form a straight line from your head to heels. Be careful not to let your back drop or you booty stick up in the air, and suck your core in. Jump your feet back, so that they land just outside of your hands.
Reach your arms over your melon and jump up into the air as high as you can. Land and immediately lower back into a squat for your next rep. Repeat until you puke your guts out.

It may seem complicated but the movements are quite simple, it's doing them that's tough. Aye, you'll go weak at the knees, after a few burpees.

The faster you conduct the moves, the harder it will be but it's such a great exercise. Try it, they'll be fun… said no-one… **ever!!**

You've heard that saying that goes summat like, '*Do something every day that scares you*', well that could be burpees. They may be horror-ble but they're awesome for your six-pack.

Pilates are also great for the core.
READER: *I've heard of it but what exactly is Pilates?*
I've never done it myself, I'm a Pilates virgin but it is supposed to be fantastic for core strength and overall flexibility.

Tell you what, you do the class and let **ME** know what they're like. You've got my e-mail address, don't be a stranger.

BODYWEIGHT

You can find some snazzy equipment in gyms these days but don't be afraid to go '*Old skool*' by using your body-weight to get fit. I mean **you know** how much you weigh, so try to lift it, hold it, skip it, raise it, shuffle it and jump it around. Bodyweight exercises are a simple and effective way of improving strength, muscular definition and flexibility, without the need for any equipment.

Have you seen male gymnasts? Blimey these guys are stacked, and they train their body to the ultimate limit. Yes they use weights as well but the majority of the time they focus on isometric holds based on their supreme body strength and balance. I'm not saying you've got to dress in those fancy white pants they wear, or that you have to perform incredulous and spellbinding floor routines, but your body can be utilised as a fitness tool. Just don't wear it out.

You could even join an acrobatics class; blimey **they will** help you keep fit, what with all that tumbling and spinning and flipping. Call your local club or gym to check times and costs.
I phoned the local acrobatics club the other day and asked if they could teach me the splits. They asked how flexible I was, I said I can't do Tuesdays or Thursdays.

They hung up the phone.

Whether it's in your kitchen, at the park, in your back garden, or anywhere else you can think of, you can use bodyweight exercises to get in a great work-out any time you can't make it to the gym or a fitness class.
To get the body you want… use it.

Touch your toes, do a lunge, sumo squat,
Shadow box, bench dip, kick your bot,
Raise a calf, star jump, ankle hop,
Once you start, you won't ever wanna stop.
Leg curl, pike crunch, flutter kick,
Crab walk, bear crawl, shuffle quick,
Good for her, great for me and ace for him,
Make your body your own personal gym.

There are countless variations for each bodyweight exercise and they are **all** brilliant for stabilising your core, developing muscle definition and improving your balance. Especially chin ups (on a bar) and press ups, there are hundreds of amazing adaptations which target different muscles from your biceps to your latissimus dorsi.

You could make up your own programme and do a circuit pretending you're in a Rocky style, training montage. Let the other gym goers look, who cares?!

You've gotta put in the effort, otherwise it's a wasted trip and public transport is so expensive these days.
It's very difficult to demonstrate techniques via the medium of a book, therefore check them out on 'You-Tube', or ask an instructor to demonstrate as many bodyweight exercises as possible.

Form is ever so important and reduces your chances of injury, whilst improving strength and flexibility. So once you've mastered the form, it's up to you to try at home, in the gym or on the dancefloor at your local Cinderella's.

when life gets you down...

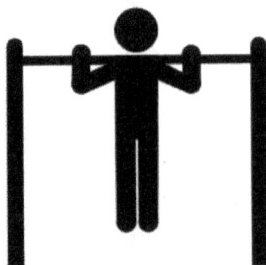

...chin up.

TEAM SPORTS

Are you game?

If the gym or the monotony of running along pavements isn't for you, then perhaps sport can help you enjoy being active. And no, I'm not talking armchair junkies here; I mean joining a team and competing at some amateur level. Team sports will make fitness enjoyable and competitive, with the added bonus of a potential social element too. Working together to achieve a goal, playing to your strengths, the camaraderie, the fun, and you'll get to wear a shiny new kit. It's so rewarding.

You'll train maybe twice a week and have a game at the weekend. Your fitness levels will improve, you'll lose some lard and you'll develop a thick skin 'cos of all the ribbing that takes place. There may be no *'i'* in team but there's one in *'fit'*. Its win/win... unless you lose, or draw but even then it's win/win, 'cos I know **you** and you'll put a positive spin on it.

Can I kick it?

Footy is so simple to play, there's thousands of amateur teams out there who cater for all ages, sexes and abilities. Even **you** can get a game. Well, maybe as a sub.

Mud, half-time oranges, abusive crowds, partisan officials, trophies, outrageous challenges and a few beers in the clubhouse after the final whistle. What's not to like?! And we can all do with scoring now and again. I'll tell you now, playing any sport is better than watching it on the box. And the best thing about it is that there are no commentators or pundits, so you don't have to listen to their inane drivel.

COMMENTATOR: *He's giving 110%*
No he's not, that's bloody impossible. By definition we can only give 100%, 'cos that's the maximum, Mr Cliché-Charlie!!

COMMENTATOR: *He knows where the goal is*
Of course he does, you numpty. He might have an I.Q. lower than his agent's commission fee but he's not an imbecile. The goal is always in the same position on every pitch.

COMMENTATOR: *If that was on target that would've been a goal*
Yeah but it wasn't, so another completely pointless statement.

COMMENTATOR: *It was on his wrong foot*
Hang on, who's foot is he wearing? Absolute clap-trap!!

COMMENTATOR: *Man United, blah, blah, blah, Fergie-time, blah, blah, BLAHHH!!*
Erm, **Hello!!** They're not even playing. For one game, just leave it be you obsessed, biased set of gits... I'm talking to you Mr Tyler and that organisation you work for.

Here's some more advice regarding footy or following a team, especially the *'armchair supporters'*.
I'm extremely passionate when it comes to, *'L – I – V, E – R – P, double O, L, Liverpool FC!!'*
It's very sad.

I'm forever selecting formations, assessing fixtures and *'managing'* the team in my head. Every day.
I told you, very sad indeed. Their results have a massive bearing on my mood; I get quite upset which is ridiculous really, although I'm getting better. Nowadays if we lose (note I said, *'we'*, like I'm actually part of the football team), it only annoys me for an hour or so and then I'm back to my usual happy self.
But a decade ago and more, it used to ruin my entire weekend. Utter madness because I have no positive or negative influence on the outcome of the result, at all. It's out of my control.

And these players have only **one** connection to *'my'* team. Cotton shirts. They still get exorbitant wages, mansions, fast cars and even faster women, regardless of win, lose or draw.

So if you're one of those that base your **entire** state of happiness on your teams results, you've gotta change. Change for your sanity, for your happiness, for your state of mind, for your weight loss.

Your life doesn't change **one iota** after the result. You'll still be fat, thin, ugly, old, single, bald, skint, unhappy or spotty. Win, lose or last-minute draw.

You might be one of those types that wears your lucky pants to support your team, or you only view the games in a certain pub. Well I have some very important news for you... it has no correlation **whatsoever** on the outcome of your fave teams performance. Unless you're the ref of course... but referees don't have any allegiance towards the major football teams...that's what my lawyer told me to say anyway.

Rival fans are humans too... honest!!
Even Man U fans.
Ok, sorry I don't know what I'm saying there... **only joking!!**
No I'm not actually, I draw the line somewhere, sod 'em.

Although I'm not one of these that gets into fisticuffs just because someone else is wearing a different named scarf to me. For God's sake, hooliganism is just mental. I've always thought that if violence is the answer, how dumb is the fuckin' question?!

Anyway, back to the point in hand. If you wanna get fit, have fun and meet new people, then joining a footy team is just the ticket. But if you don't fancy footy, then maybe rugby, or cricket, or netball, or hockey or maybe you're really adventurous and want to try Roller-derby.

Anything that helps you chase the black dog away is fine by me.

So get your skates on, do some investigating and find a kit that fits.

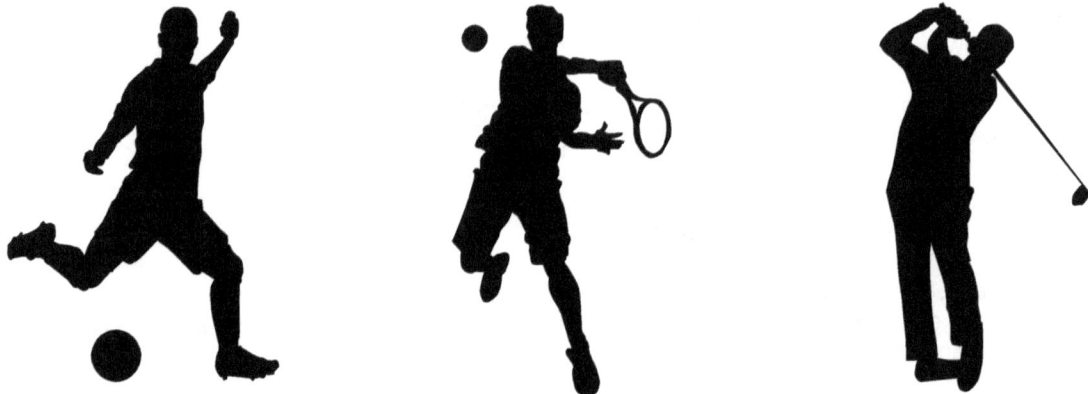

Men in their twenties play footy, in their forties they play tennis, and in their sixties they play golf.

Contrary to popular belief, as men get older, their balls get smaller.

Perhaps team games are not for you but you still fancy competing against others? Then why not try **GALF!!** Or golf, to us non-cockernees.

Birdies and bogies and buggies,
Leather gloves and spiky shoes,
Driving and slicing and putting,
Then the 19th, for some booze!!

I'm not a big fan myself but walking around for three or four hours at a time will be a nice little workout, I just find golfers a bit... boring!!

And why do they have to wear such garish keks? Nah!! Not for me... Fore!!

Why not try tennis instead?
READER: *You cannot be serious?*
Oh! But I am. Very serious. Court violation, point deducted.

Tennis is smashing, you'll love it,
I think you should give it a go,
Serving and volleying and lobbing,
And a racket won't cost much dough!!

Tennis can be played as a competitive sport or as a fun recreational activity with friends and family. It's excellent for maintaining your health, fitness, strength and agility. So, it's gotta be worth a shot, right?!
READER: *Isn't it expensive?*
Not really.
Joining a club is quite reasonably priced these days and if you can't afford an expensive racket, you could always search for a bargain on the net. But it's not all strawberries and cream you know?! It's extremely taxing and some games can go on for hours, so you'll need some balls... but they're quite cheap too.

So you in?

Don't answer that now, but personally I think tennis is great, although no matter how good you get, you'll never be as good as a wall.

OUT!! Game, set and match.

What about rowing?
READER: *I thought that was just for posho students?*
Admittedly it seems that way but rowing is not just reserved for the Oxbridge crowd. There are rowing clubs all over this country, and generally near a river.

It's brilliant for improving stamina, upper body strength and a fantastic fat burner. Whether it's on your own, or part of a crew, rowing is simply spiffing. So, Tally Ho!! **Let's go!!**

Row, row, row your boat,
Gently down the stream,
If you see some commoners,
Don't forget to scream!!

Participating in sporting events is great for mind, body and spirit, and a fun way to help you successfully lose that timber. Fighting for a common goal with your teammates, coaches, managers and supporters, teaches you loyalty and trust. Furthermore, team sports are good for personal responsibility, dedication, leadership, confidence, belief and self-esteem. And your aptitude for piss-taking will improve immeasurably.

These principles can be applied to your own personal life when encountering problems at work, or at home. Above all, participating in sport, especially at a competitive level, will enhance your willpower. And without willpower and self-control, you will have **no chance** in your goal of losing weight successfully.

Look at a tennis match for example. A player might be a set or two down but they fight back because they know the match isn't over, until it's over. Yes they've had a bad start but they are convinced that they can turn it around. They win a few points and game by game, the momentum changes. They begin to realise that the outcome is in their control. Desire and belief starts to grow and this drives them on. That inevitable loss, the possibility of failure soon becomes irrelevant and the only thought is victory. They will not lose.

The exact same principles can be applied to your diet, fitness and state of mind. Yes you've failed in the past, your two sets down but life is a five setter, you can turn this around. But only with drive, dedication, positivity and willpower. C'mon dude, you need to ace it.

When you participate in sport, you realise that any result is possible up until the point that the ref blows that final whistle. You can admit defeat and let your teammates down, or you can work together, pull your socks up and fight to turn the game around.

So what'll be? Early shower or willpower?!

WILLPOWER

Have you got any?

Most folk believe they could improve the quality of their mundane lives, if only they had more of that willpower stuff. With more self-control it would be no bother eating right, exercising regularly or drinking less. There'd be no more procrastinating and it would be a piece of piddle, to achieve all of our goals.

If only it was that simple.

Some more of those American boffins conducted a study a few years ago and established that over half of dieters, felt that their lack of willpower was the most significant barrier to their success. Not the cakes, jumbo-sized soda drinks, mammoth burgers, gargantuan buckets of fried chicken, lack of nutritional knowledge, complete lack of fitness, laziness, or ability to refrain from smothering mounds of cheese on every fuckin' meal y'all, but willpower.

<u>READER</u>: *I'm the same, I've just got no willpower when it comes to food.*
Complete and utter tosh!! It's all in your mind. It's just another convenient excuse. But I'm here to tell you that there's hope, willpower is something that can be taught. It can be developed and improved upon. It can be rebuilt. All it takes is practice, practice, **practice!!**

Willpower is like a muscle and the more you use it, the stronger it gets.

At its essence, willpower is the ability to resist short-term temptations in order to meet long-term goals. Just like money, willpower can be earned.

Think about those internal monologues you have when you're offered a slice of cake, or another beer, or you contemplate getting a takeaway rather than cooking.

You tell yourself *'I can't eat that'*, or *'I shouldn't do that'* but then another voice enters the conversation and says *'Go on, you know you want it'* or *'you'll be good next time, you deserve it'*.

This verbal battle of wills, then gets drowned out by the repetitive drum beat of the sound *'I want it, I must have it, GIVE IT TO ME!!'*

So as you devour that slice of cake, gulp down that beer and put away the pizza menu after phoning your order, you then pretend to yourself that you have no willpower, you're hopeless, you'll never lose weight etc, etc what a load of bollocks, etc.

It doesn't have to be this way.
<u>READER</u>: *What can I do to change?*
Well there's loads you can do.
I'm not saying you can never have cakes again, or pizza or beer but the more you turn down these offers the easier it will be.

If you say to yourself something like, *'I'm trying to lose weight at the moment, so even though I would love a slice of cake, it would have a negative effect on my weight loss goal therefore I will decline the offer'*. Or when you decide to pick up that takeaway pizza menu you could say to yourself, *'Tempting but if I have pizza tonight, it will knock me back because I've been so good this week and I really want to see if I can hit my weekly target. Therefore I'll cook instead and perhaps have a nice biscuit as a treat later'*.

The more you challenge your internal temptress, the easier it will be next time. And the time after that. And the time after that. And so on and so forth and so diddly-on-on.

Who do you want to be? You want to be this new healthier, fitter, happier and thinner you. Right?
RIGHT?!
<u>READER</u>: *Right.*

Well that **you** doesn't do what the old **you** does, so to be this new **you**, **you** must change the old **you**, or fail **you** will do.

Just like Zammo off of Grange Hill, just say *'No!!'*
Do you want a biscuit?
<u>READER</u>: *No!!*
Shall we get a curry tonight instead of cooking?
<u>READER</u>: *No!!*
Shall we give tonight's jog a miss?
<u>READER</u>: *No!!*

You're a bright person, you bought this book so I'm sure you get the idea. The more you say *'no'*, the more it becomes your default setting. Your willpower increases, the weight drops off, you become happier, fitter and after a while you can have the cake, you can have the takeaway and you can miss the odd fitness session. But it won't matter because by that stage you will be living a different life, you will have developed a positive mindset and you won't fall back into your old habits.

You could also make your life easier by not placing these temptations in front of you, in the first place.
<u>READER</u>: *What do you mean?*
If you continue to buy cakes, biscuits, ice cream, crisps and processed crap and then put them in your cupboards, fridge and freezer, then **you** know they're there. And if **you** know they're there, you're more likely to want to have them.

If you don't buy them, then even though you may want these products, **you** can't have them so you have something else instead. Hopefully something healthier or you abstain completely.

You could even choose a voice in your head that you respect...
<u>READER</u>: *What? I'm not schizophrenic!!*
I know you're not and neither are you.

What I mean is that you could place someone you respect and admire as your weight loss Guardian.

It could be Morgan Freeman, it could be your ex, your Mum or a talking grizzly bear.

Whatever. But this individual can pop into your sub-conscious whenever you're faced with a temptation. They can tell you off and remind you that you're trying to lose the timber, so if that temptation is detrimental to that goal, they won't allow you to indulge.
<u>READER</u>: *I don't know, sounds a bit weird.*
Look, whatever works.

Fair do's, what works for some doesn't necessarily work for others but you could give it a go. You could **try!!**

It worked for Isobel. Even though it was a bit weird for me.

ISOBEL, 38 – *Well I did what you said Birchy and found an internal voice and that voice was yours. Every time I felt myself going for the biccies, or thinking about not going for a walk, I'd hear your strange hotchpotch Yorkshire accent saying* **'Do you need that biscuit?'**, **'Will missing that walk help you lose weight?'** *and* **'For fucks sake Isobel, you've been doing so well, don't bloody ruin it'.**
I used to think that my willpower was useless but I soon realised it was just another excuse I told myself to **allow** *me to eat the junk I craved, or get out of doing something I didn't want to do.*
After a while, I'd look at some food and say to myself, **'I don't eat these things anymore'**, *or I'd go for a run and think* **'Hey!! I'm a runner now, this is the new me, this is what I do'.**
I slowly began to change my identity. And initially it was your voice that kept reminding me whenever I felt a little down, or was about to revert to an old habit. But then I killed you. Sorry!!
Not in a murderous rage type way, I mean I swapped your voice for my own. Rather than being chastised by you, I began to empower my thoughts with my new identity. Anyway, I might have had voices in my head but it's worked, I've lost that 3 stone, I'm happier, I feel fantastic and I've got a new bloke. Although I don't mention that you're in my head sometimes.

If the voices in your head are bad for your weight loss goals, destroy them, kill them, tell 'em to **WAKE THE FIT UP!!**

By the by, I genuinely don't swear so much in my day to day goings-on but sometimes it's just a great way to add extra emphasis to a point, whether that's in print or in life.

I mean, I could write *'F**k'* or *'the F word'* instead but in your head you'll instinctively say the *'actual'* word anyway when you're reading, so I might as well type it.

Hey! We're all adults, we all swear occasionally and often cursing can be a cathartic experience.

Anyway, I've heard there's some kids nearby so I'll watch my language.

Paul Birch

MUMS & KIDS

The mother of all excuses

You want the tips?
<u>READER</u>: *I think I'm entitled to them.*

YOU WANT THE TIPS?
<u>READER</u>: *Yes I want the tips.*

YOU CAN'T HANDLE THE TIPS!!

Sorry about that, I went a bit *'A Few Good Men'* on ya there. Okay doke!! Here are some tips for Mums who don't believe they have time to keep fit because they have kiddie-widdie-winkles!!

Walk or cycle with the kids, either **to** or **from** school. Or both ways.

<u>READER</u>: *I don't have time in the morning.*
Get up earlier then. It's just another blinkin' excuse. You don't have to do it every day but give it a pop.
<u>READER</u>: *They'll be too slow, it'll take ages.*
Oh! No! Having to spend time bonding with your bairns, how awful. Look, allocate enough time, make it fun and try it. You know, if you're trying to lose weight n' that. I mean, that is the objective isn't it?!

If you're a Mum that doesn't work during the day then there's plenty of time before you pick up the kids to go to the gym, or do a fitness class at the local Community Centre. Why not try Zumba?

<u>READER</u>: *Ooh! I don't like foreign food.*
Derr!! It's not food, you're obsessed aren't ya?! Zumba is a combination of Latino dance, high-energy music and aerobic routines to help keep you trim, toned and lithe.
Are you ready to live the lithe life?
<u>READER</u>: *Maybe?!*
Zumba is an excellent full body workout, which really burns the calories. Not only do you lose weight but it's also a great opportunity to socialise, as women of all ages partake in the classes. The odd bloke too. De-stress, keep fit and bop away the blubber.

If you've got a child that's still a lazy, selfish git and needs to be wheeled around in a pushchair, don't let that stop you getting fit. You can jog whilst pushing the bairn, or even power-walk. This provides the little sprog with some fresh air and a change of scenery, while you're able to slot in some calorie burning.

In fact, you can actually buy specific prams tailored for this kind of activity which are developed and designed not to topple as you speed along. You could even nibble on a few rusks as a post-workout treat. Now that is a result, 'cos rusks are ace.

Swim - Depending on the age of your ankle-biters you could go after school, at the weekend or during the day. Play underwater games and splash about til' they're crying for the warm embrace of their Daddy. Only joking.

You can do lengths whilst they're pratting about, or you could race each other. Fun, bonding and verruca's. What's not to like?! Check out the activities at your local pool/gym because they might also do water aerobics to exert your body further. Slap that swimming cap over your swede and get your shark face on.

Get up early and let your bloke sort out the kid's brekkie, lunchboxes and tantrums, whilst you go for a quick 20-30min jog or walk each school morning. You'll soon get used to the early mornings and you'll grow to love the quieter streets, birdsongs, the sunrise and the brief elixir of a mardy, moody, mawngy, minor-free morn whilst the other-half pulls his weight. And he needs to, yeah?! Bloody slob, I don't know why you put up with it?! He doesn't deserve you. And does he ever show any appreciation? Does he buggery. Like you, he needs to shape up, or get AHT!!

Play in the garden with the bairns. You could create your own games, allocate points for certain movements and targets. You can't beat 'em legally, so any opportunity to beat your kids has gotta be worth a punt?

Or skipping, jumping, prancing about on the trampoline, playing catch, hide and seek, going as high as you can on the swings, throwing beanbags, whatever gets you messin'. Some bonding time with the nippers, the fresh air will tire them out and you're getting fit. Winner-winner, carb-free dinner!!

As children's TV presenters would say, *'the only limit, is your imagination'*. But don't just do it for you, do it for them too.

It does my head in when kids play computer games indoors, especially sports games like footy. They hit and press a few buttons, score and then celebrate wildly, even though it's glorious outside and they could actually be playing the **real** sport, outdoors in the garden or on a footy pitch. The mind boggles. No wonder there's a kid's obesity crisis... I blame the parents.

Make the play-ground your free gymnasium. If you seriously want to get fit then it shouldn't matter **where** you do it, just that you do it.

So, when you take the kids to the park, get perspiring. You could do tricep dips off a bench, step-ups, chin-ups on the monkey bars, rope climbs, press ups and a whole multitude of bodyweight exercises.

READER: *Sounds a bit weird that last one.*
Really?! You clearly have no desire to lose weight then and are destined to be fat forever.
READER: *That's a bit mean.*
It's not. It's reality. It's the truth. Welcome to the real world.

If you really want to lose weight, you should do **everything possible** in your power to make it happen. Try something different. What have you got to lose? Apart from the lard of course!!

No doubt you take the kids to the park anyway so rather than sitting there scrolling through FB updates, or gassing to the other Mums, get pro-active instead. Who knows, the other Mums might get involved too and before you know it you'll be playing rounders, and setting up a mini league with families from your street.

Enjoy yourself, mess about with the kids, have fun... just **blinkin' play!!**

You could even have a game of tig with the kids and parents.
READER: *What's tig?*
Blimey, didn't you play tig as a kid? Basically one of you is *'it'* and the object of the game is to touch one of the other players, which is known as being *'tigged'*. Once someone has been *'tigged'*, then they are *'it'* and the game continues until you're called in for tea by your Mam.

If you're a working mother and you can't do exercise **before** or **after** your work day, then it's time to use your lunch-hour. There's no excuse as to why you can't walk for at least 45mins every lunch-hour. And when you're at work, never use the lift. Always make sure you use the stairs. If there's an opportunity to either walk **from**, or **to** home during the work day, do it. Essentially it's up to you to utilise the full 24hrs we are blessed with each day to improve your fitness.

Now this next suggestion may seem quirky but what's life without whimsy?! If you're a stay at home Mum, you could squat every fifteen minutes throughout the day.

READER: *All day?*
It's up to you but you could set an alarm at home to go off every five, ten, fifteen minutes or so and when it goes off you complete ten squats. And repeat until you're knackered, or it's time to pick up the kids, or if it's your turn to make the tea. You could mix it up by changing the exercise every day, running on the spot, lunges, kettlebell swings, touching your toes, skipping etc, etc.

The reason this method has been proven to work, is that your body can't switch off. It's not as taxing as completing a forty-five minute workout, and it's extremely effective because you don't feel that you've actually done that much exercise. Before you knock it, try it.

I bet you're one of those kind Mums that ferries your kids around and drops them off at band practice, dance, drama rehearsals, footy, taekwondo, chess club and so on and so forth. Well, rather than driving back home and then driving back to pick 'em up or just sat in the car trying to have a kip for half an hour; use that time productively to go for a walk or a jog. Alternatively, if you speak to the other Mums about your situation and explain you need time to go to the gym or go for a run, they might pick the kids up for you. And then quid pro quo, you do the same for them.

There's always a way, you've just gotta ask. And if you don't ask, you'll never know.

There are no legitimate excuses, as to why you can't do **any** of the above recommendations. The only restrictions are those you impose upon yourself.

DIANE, 42 – *Well Paul, I took your advice and started to jog home from school after I'd dropped the kids off. At first I'd just jog directly back home… slowly. But after a few weeks I'd change the route and add a few more minutes to each run. After about a month I started to lose some timber but what was even better, was I began to really enjoy the runs and a bit of me-time.*

Ok! That's the end of the section on exercise and fitness, so it's time to cool down. Have a few sips of water and then can you please do some static stretching.

READER: *What's static stretching?*

When you stretch for a warm up (dynamic stretching), you're trying to get the blood pumping through your muscles so your body is loose and ready for exercise. Whereas the cool down is performed to bring you back to normality. Static stretches help return the body to a resting state and are more appropriate for the cool down than dynamic stretches. This is because they help relax muscles, realigning the muscle fibres to decrease tension, which can result in injury and DOMS.

READER: *What are DOMS?*

Ah!! Delayed Onset of Muscle Soreness (DOMS), which is the fancy name for muscular aches and pains that are usually felt a day or two after exercise. Static stretching will reduce the risk of DOMS.

Composed of various techniques, static stretching works by gradually lengthening a muscle to an elongated position (to the point of discomfort) and you hold that position for about thirty seconds.

Here are four examples that target the whole network of leg muscles (Calves, hamstrings and quadriceps):

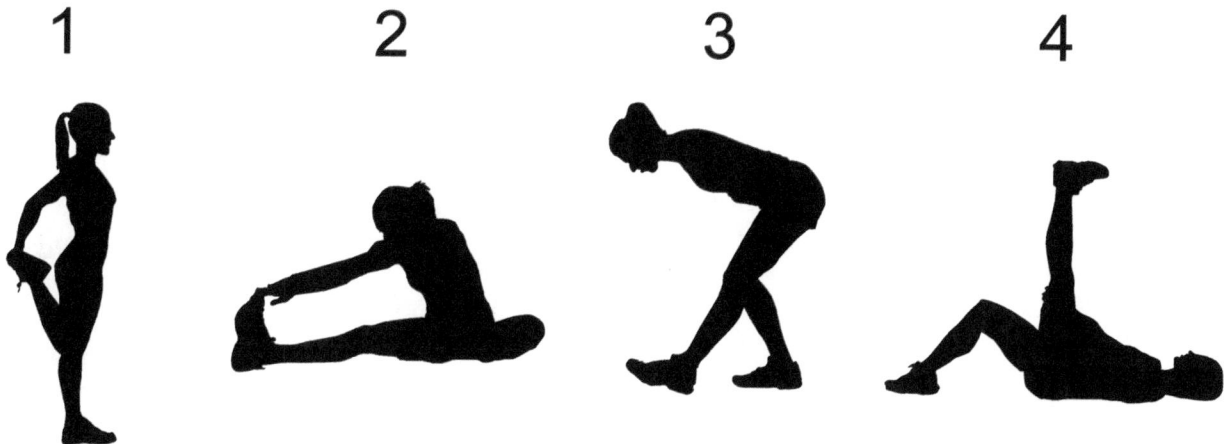

1   2   3   4

Once you start to add a **cool down** stretching programme to your fitness routine, you'll notice that your flexibility and range of movement increases. If you're a keen runner or cyclist this will strengthen joints and muscles, enabling you to train for longer and knock seconds off them PB's.

The post-exercise cool down can also help to prevent dizziness.

Strenuous exercise can cause the blood vessels in your legs to expand, bringing more blood into the legs and feet. When you suddenly stop exercising without taking time to cool down, your heart rate slows quite abruptly and blood can pool in your lower body, causing dizziness and even fainting.

An appropriate cool down will help you to relax after the stresses of the work-out and allow the heart rate to return to its resting rate.

Aah!! Namaste!!

Right then cocker, that's the end of the fitness chapter. I'm sure it wasn't too strenuous.

So, you ready to get your chops round the food section?
<u>READER</u>: *Excellent, I'm starving.*
Well get your elbows off the table, grab a knife and fork and let's tuck in.

Actually, thinking about it, hold on a minute. Before I dish the dirt on food, let's discuss a worldwide epidemic…

OBESITY

It's a wide-spread occurrence

We hear this word so much in the media these days but what does it actually mean?

OBESITY - *the state of being grossly fat or overweight, in a way that is dangerous for health*

There are many ways in which a person's health can be classified based on their weight but the most widely used method is body mass index (BMI).

For most adults, a BMI of:
- 18.5 to 24.9 means you're at a healthy weight
- 25 to 29.9 means you're overweight
- 30 to 39.9 means you're obese
- 40 or above means you're severely obese

In this case, points do not make prizes.

I'm not a big fan of these types of measurement because they can be misleading due to a person's height and muscle mass but I suppose it's a fair enough barometer of whether someone is obese or not.

You might be obese, you might just be a smidge overweight or worryingly, you might be morbidly obese (what a mind-boggling term). However, you don't need to be told by a GP whether you're a bit portly or not, I think you might have an inkling.

But what you probably don't know, and what you need to know, is **how** your weight is seriously affecting your health and wellbeing.

Being overweight or obese is now linked to **thirteen** different types of cancer.

• Bowel	• Liver	• Oesophageal	• Thyroid
• Breast	• Meningioma	• Ovarian	• Womb
• Gall bladder	(Brain tumour)	• Pancreatic	
• Kidney	• Myeloma (bone marrow)	• Stomach	

Hey!! You've gotta die of something right? Why not a devastating, destructive illness, that once diagnosed can dramatically prove fatal within a matter of weeks?!

Apparently, having more fat in the body changes the balance of hormones such as oestrogen, testosterone and insulin, which as a consequence drive tumour growth. Cancer Research UK has estimated that over 18,000 cases of cancer in Britain every year are caused by excess weight, making obesity the biggest **PREVENTABLE** cause of the disease after smoking. And that's just in Britain.

As the amount of people dying from these cancers has increased, the number of fast-food joints has multiplied, people now eat breakfast cereals containing chocolate, there are more takeaway adverts on TV, plate sizes have got bigger, mediums are now large and large is now jumbo, having seconds is par for the course, and all-you-can-eat is now a mantra for the nation.

The situation is getting worse and worse every day, yet a lot of people don't seem to give a shit, or have just accepted their fate and are happy to fill their guts with more and more cheezy, battered, doughy, fried, greasy, congealed, flavourless, processed crap.

But why?

<u>READER</u>: *I don't know.*

I'll tell you why.

Too many folk are weak, molly-coddled and too downright lazy to do something about it. If it takes any effort, they can't be arsed.

Can't…be…bothered…pass me another vanilla slice.

<u>READER</u>: *Yes but there's too much temptation.*

Bollocks!! There's no such thing as temptation, it's greed. Simple as. You **don't have to** shove it in your gob.

If there's no requirement, there should be no need. Food is fuel and once the tank is full you shouldn't attempt to refill it, until it's **empty**.

But no, we've become a nation of sinners with a proclivity for gluttony!!

That's the simple, straightforward reason as to why so many people are obese, they eat too much. It's just plain, unadulterated **greed.** Pretty bloody obvious really.

And if you're tipping the scales, then you eat too much. Case closed.

<u>READER</u>: *Yeah but…*

Nope, sorry but that's the issue and you know it too but you try to blame it on other factors.

You blame stress, you blame work, you blame your relationships, you blame your glands, you blame your genes, you blame Saturn over Venus, you might as well blame it on the boogie 'cos they're all just absurd, meaningless excuses.

But what's even more concerning is that a child with at least one obese parent, is likely to be obese themselves, whilst a child with two obese parents is likely to be morbidly obese.

<u>READER</u>: *Why's that?*

Monkey see, monkey do.

Kids are bloody sponges aren't they? They absorb and replicate the behaviour and mannerisms of their parents, good and bad.

Whether it's swearing, anger, racism, bad diet, or voting UKIP, kids are morons and lead by the folk that are supposed to be role models… not roly-poly models.

It's so disheartening and it genuinely saddens me because folk could do something about it, if only they tried. But too many people choose the easy route and will no doubt continue to lead their sedentary lifestyles, carry on with their poor diets and develop these **preventable** cancers and other such diseases.

There's too many Amanda's out there and I don't want **you** to end up like her. After all, that's why I wrote this book and I will try my utmost to help as many people as I can, get fitter and happier.

The reason I'm trying to be so blunt, is because we're heading towards the chapter on food and I want to prepare you for some plain, forthright and frank opinions.

And I'm afraid I'll be unleashing quite a few truth bombs in this section. Truth torpedoes actually, with some serious nuclear weaponry thrown in. **WDM's - Weapons to destruct mass.**

I'm gonna do my best to help educate, enlighten and entertain you regarding the world of grub but in doing so, this will challenge all of your commonly held beliefs about food, which I'm here to tell ya, are all wrong.
READER: *What even…*
Yep, wrong.
READER: *But what about…*
Wrong.
READER: *And…*
That's wrong too. Wrong, wrong, wrong, wrong, **wrong!!**

Reeto!! I don't know about you but I'm a tad peckish, so I reckon it's time we talked about scran, chow, snap, cuisine, eats, fodder, fuel, slop, provisions, snacks, treats… **FOOD!!**

Let's break some bread…

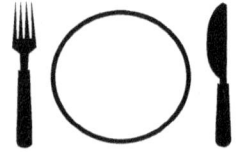

HEALTHY EATING

So here we are, the bit you've all been waiting for, the meat and two veg, the main course but before we start it's customary to say grace... I'll begin.

> *Thank you Lord, for the food on our plate,*
> *I'm bloody Hank Marvin, I just can't wait.*
> ***Amen!!***

Off we go then. Easy one for you to start off with, *'what is food?'*
<u>READER</u>: *Well its stuff that you eat isn't it?!*
Yep, sort of, although it's a bit more complicated than that.
<u>READER</u>: *It always is with you!*
You know me so very well.

Food is any nutritious substance that people eat or drink in order to **sustain life** and without it, eventually your body would break down and you would die.

Essentially, food is a package of potential energy which is released into the body once digested, to be utilised immediately, or stored away for use at a later stage.

Your body is a marvellous and complicated piece of machinery, and the trillions and trillions of tiny cells that make up your beautiful frame need a regular source of energy to perform their basic functions. And they receive this fuel from your scran.

Every millisecond of every day, your amazing body is performing countless tasks and functions that keep you alive and allow you to breathe, pump blood, eat, drink, squeeze cheese, burp, masturbate and moan about the weather.

We all have **five** vital organs that are essential for survival and these are the brain, heart, kidneys, liver and lungs. Without food and water, these organs would malfunction, collapse and you would die.

The central nervous system constantly sends signals via the brain, spinal cord and nerve network to control both voluntary action (like conscious movement) and involuntary actions (like breathing). Without food to provide energy, this system would break down and you would die.

Our bodies are supported by the skeletal system, which consists of 206 bones that are connected by tendons, ligaments and cartilage. The skeleton not only helps us move, but it's also involved in the production of blood cells and the storage of calcium. Without the appropriate minerals obtained from food...
<u>READER</u>: *Don't tell me, would I die?*
Actually, probably not but you'd end up developing osteoporosis, or some other debilitating bone disease, so your athletics career might be over.

I think you get it? Food and water are blinkin' important and without them, me, you and him next door, would all die. Our bodies can't produce **all** of the essential nutrients that we need to function properly, so we have to consume them within our diet.

Therefore ideally, food should offer **value**. We should eat to live, not live to eat.

So if you want to be healthy, the word says it all.
<u>READER</u>: *What do you mean?*

H **EA** L **T** HY

That means a balanced diet that is packed with minerals, nutrients and vitamins... with the odd treat thrown in of course. Although, if you want to be fat, eat foods that make you fat, if you want to be healthy...

<u>READER</u>: *Ok! So what do I eat then?*
Do you want a simple solution to your diet, guaranteed to help you lose weight and never be full again?
<u>READER</u>: *Maybe, although I have a feeling I won't like it.*
Perhaps not but all you really need to live is red meat, fish, fowl, eggs, vegetables, fruit, some nuts and low level exercise.
The ultimate recipe for a long and healthy life. You'll definitely lose weight and that's your aim isn't it? Isn't it?
<u>READER</u>: *But no treats? No chocolate? No pasta? No pizza? No BREADDDDDD??!*
That's right. But ultimately, it depends **how much** you want to be healthy.

Look, if you are what you eat why do you want to be cheap, fast, easy and fake? Why not be fresh, vibrant, healthy and energetic instead?

Anyone can go to the gym for an hour but to control what goes onto your plate, now that's an intensive workout. There's such a plethora of tastes, flavours and textures out there, yet we gorge ourselves on bland, processed, chemically enhanced tat. Artificial crap, containing additives and emulsifiers and fillers and thickening agents...
Ooh tasty!!

Did you know that eating these manufactured, synthetic, processed foods actually restricts the performance of your liver?
<u>READER</u>: *No, I didn't know that.*
Yep, it's true.

The liver is one of the largest organs in the body and an essential element of the digestive process. It performs a multitude of jobs which include detoxification, protein synthesis and converting the nutrients in our diets into useful substances that the body can utilise for growth and repair.

However, when you eat any food that contains additives, artificial sweeteners, emulsifiers and thickening agents, the liver struggles to deal effectively with these toxins, and thus has to work overtime to eliminate them as waste.

But what you're probably not aware of is that another of the livers roles is to actually metabolise and break down fat, but when our liver is operating below its optimal functioning level, it neglects this duty.

Therefore the less harmful foods you eat, the more the liver can concentrate on breaking down stored timber.
So if you're trying to lose weight, you're probably your own worst enemy due to the food you consume.

Admittedly there's so much confusion regarding food promotion, scientific studies, food scandals etc, etc that consumers don't know **what** to believe. But most folk are wilfully ignorant when it comes to nutrition. The majority of people buy food products based on marketing, convenience and the price, not on nutritional value. Which is one of the reasons we have an obesity crisis but don't despair, I'm here to help you.

I'm going to go through the **A to Z of food** explaining the benefits, drawbacks and value of different food types. I understand that radically changing your diet is going to be difficult, so I will be advocating that you opt for the 80/20 method.

READER: *What's that?*

Basically, you alter your diet so that you consume healthy, nutritious foods 80% of the time. The remaining 20% can be split, depending on your personal preferences.

Naturally, I'll give you some more tips to help with this transition but I suggest that ultimately... you just follow your heart.

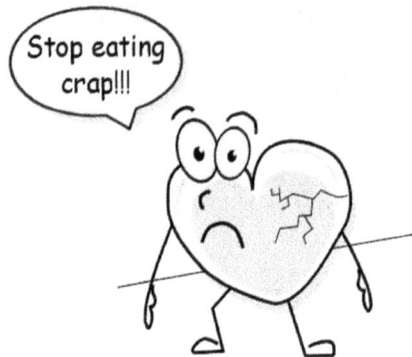

NUTRITION

Food of the Gods

When you consider exactly what makes people healthy and fit, what characteristics define them?
READER: *I don't know, erm, clear skin, a glowing complexion, someone energetic, always active, full of beans with an infectious positive attitude.*
Ok! And what do you think their nutrition is like?
READER: *It'll be good, healthy n' that.*
Nail, on, the head.

Nutrition impacts upon hydration levels, concentration, personality, physical performance, energy levels, immunity, farting and general state of health.

People spend thousands of pounds on moisturisers, vitamins, medication and make up to improve their skin, yet with good nutrition the effects can be replicated at a fraction of the cost.

If you don't get enough of an essential nutrient or vitamin over a period of time, you are known to be *'Malnourished'*. We often think of those poor emaciated children who are starving in Africa as the epitome of malnourishment but many millions in the Western world, exhibit signs of malnutrition too. And the irony is they are often obese.
READER: *What do you mean, I don't really understand?*
Our bodies require certain minerals, nutrients and vitamins in order to perform **specific** bodily functions and without them, our body will start to malfunction and break down. In the most extreme cases that can eventually lead to death.

Certain omissions in our diet lead to specific health issues, and the sedentary are more at risk of sustaining long-term damage than the active.

With a deficiency or an overload of a specific nutrient, a person may show signs of *'Anaemia'*, dermatitis, depression, hair loss, bleeding gums or possible life-threatening symptoms depending on the missing nutrient.
READER: *What's Anaemia?*
Anaemia is a condition where a lack of iron in the body leads to a reduction in the number of red blood cells. Iron is necessary because it's used to produce these red blood cells, which help store and carry oxygen in the blood, as well as ferrying *'Myoglobin'* to muscles.

If you have fewer red blood cells than is normal, your organs and tissues won't get as much oxygen as they usually would, which leads to fatigue, weakness, shortness of breath and a pale skin complexion that a vampire would be proud of. Therefore to combat this condition, a diet rich in iron can alleviate the symptoms.

Cancer, heart disease and strokes can all be linked to your diet, based on an excess of fat and sugary calories, whilst simultaneously avoiding fruit and vegetables.

A high sugar intake can also lead to Diabetes, whereas bone diseases such as osteoporosis are thought to occur due to insufficient calcium and vitamin D consumption.

The body requires **OVER 40** essential minerals and nutrients to function optimally, and these **all** have a tailored role in the maintenance of our body.

READER: *What exactly are minerals?*
Minerals are defined as solid, inorganic, naturally occurring substances which cannot be synthesised by the body therefore they **must** be obtained via the diet.

Each mineral plays a crucial role in the body. For instance, Calcium maintains the rigid structure of bones, Potassium and Sodium control water balance, and Zinc is involved in cell growth and healing.

There are two types of mineral, macro and micro:

- **Macro** – Calcium, Phosphorous, Magnesium, Sulphur, Sodium and Potassium
- **Micro** – Iron, Zinc, Iodine, Copper, Manganese, Fluoride, Chromium, Selenium and Molybdenum

These bad boys are **all** integral components of the immune system and are **essential** in the formation of bones, collagen, nails, skin and teeth; maintaining normal heart rhythm, muscular contractility, digestion, metabolism, neural conductivity and the regulation of hormones.

READER: *Quite important then?*
You betta believe it, buster!!
Therefore your diet should **ideally** contain a healthy balance of dairy, dark green veg, legumes, nuts, seeds, seaweed, fish, red meat, poultry, leafy veg, garlic, broccoli, onions, tomatoes, mushrooms and dates.
Although dates are disgusting.
And currants.
And raisins.
And revolting sultanas, so I wouldn't blame you if you forgot about any of them. **YUCK!!**

Anyway, that's the minerals sorted, now onto the vitamins.

VITAMINS

What are they?

Vitamins are biological compounds that are **crucial** for your bodily growth and are needed for the functioning of your immune, hormonal and nervous system.

Apart from vitamins D and K, they cannot be synthesized by your body in amounts sufficient to meet bodily needs, and therefore must be obtained from the diet, or from some synthetic source.

Unlike dietary minerals which are elements on the periodic table, vitamins are molecules formed from various compounds. Vitamin C (ascorbic acid) for example, is made of Carbon, Oxygen and Hydrogen and is found naturally in fruits and vegetables.

Vitamins are the superheroes of the nutrient world. In fact, I can't believe Marvel haven't made *'Vitaminman'* the movie yet, watch this space I suppose.

They contain numerous antioxidants which protect cells from damage caused by evil and unstable molecules, known as free radicals.
READER: *What the heck are free radicals?*
Get your lab coat on, 'cos I'm gonna lay some science on your ass.

When oxygen is combined with food to produce energy, *'Free Radicals'* are a by-product of the metabolic process which takes place.

These free radicals have a missing electron thus bond to healthy molecules stealing theirs, which as a result, turns the healthy cell into a free radical too. It's like a game of molecular tig.

This process is completely manageable when a variety of antioxidants are abundant in our daily diet but if your vitamin intake is too low, this **could** be detrimental to your health. There are a number of factors that can dramatically increase free radical production and these include smoking, traffic fumes, medication, radiation, alcohol intake and stress.

If free radicals overwhelm the body's ability to neutralise them, they attack and disturb the action of cellular DNA. And cells with damaged DNA stagnate and are prone to developing cancer and growths. This kind of cellular damage accelerates the aging process, directly causing wrinkles and severely taxing the immune system. It can also trigger life threatening diseases such as coronary heart disease, atherosclerosis, Parkinson's, Alzheimer's and degenerative eye problems.

Therefore to defend against these free radicals, stopping them from becoming harmful, *'Antioxidants'* are the weapon of choice because they soak up free radicals like a sponge.

Antioxidants are naturally found in a varied diet of unprocessed grains, and brightly coloured fruit and vegetables. Citrus fruit, berries, nuts and dark green vegetables are your best source of the antioxidants Iron, Selenium and the vitamins A, C and E.
READER: *Do I have to get my vitamins from food; can't I just take a pill?*
Getting minerals and vitamins from a pill, is like listening to a good song with your fingers in your ears. Don't be a **PRAT!!**

You certainly don't get the full benefit and due to the **concentrated** amounts contained in these pills, your body can't cope with the high levels so they are treated as waste, and excreted via faeces and urine.

If you like expensive piddle then go ahead but in my opinion, the only pills you should ever take are **chill pills**.

Here's a brief summary of all the essential vitamins, regarding their functionality, the food source and the type of symptoms that *'may'* occur in the long-term if you don't get enough consumption.

Vitamin A
Retinol

FUNCTION: It's important for normal vision, the immune system, reproduction, healthy skin and protecting the linings of the digestive and urinary tracts. Vitamin A also helps the heart, lungs, kidneys and other organs function properly.
SYMPTOMS OF DEFICIENCY: Vitamin A contains compounds that preserve the membranes around your peepers, and are an element in the proteins that bring light to your corneas therefore limited consumption can lead to impaired vision, especially at night. Also linked to a weakened immune system.
SOURCE: Meat, poultry, fish, dairy products and brightly coloured fruit and vegetables.

Vitamin B1
Thiamine

FUNCTION: Protects the heart and the nervous system from the build-up of toxic substances and is needed to convert carbohydrates and fats into energy.
SYMPTOMS OF DEFICIENCY: Lethargy and fatigue, muscle weakness, nerve damage, poor memory, anorexia, poor memory, sleep disturbance and constipation.
SOURCE: Lean meats particularly pork, cereals, rice, bread, meat, fish, poultry, eggs, bananas and apples.

Vitamin B2
Riboflavin

FUNCTION: Vital for growth, the production of red blood cells, healthy skin, mucous membranes and nerve functionality; helps to release energy from food.
SYMPTOMS OF DEFICIENCY: Skin disorders, dry lips, bloodshot eyes and sore throat, although B2 deficiency is quite rare in the developed world.
SOURCE: Poultry, lean meat, eggs, milk, fish, yoghurt, apples, bread, cereal and spinach.

Vitamin B3
Niacin

FUNCTION: For growth, production of hormones, maintains healthy glowing skin and assists in the digestive process.
SYMPTOMS OF DEFICIENCY: Skin disorders, lethargy, depression and the dreaded squits.
SOURCE: Poultry, fish, lean meat, peanuts, pulses, potatoes, milk, eggs, liver, kidney, fortified breakfast cereals, broccoli, carrots, tomatoes, dates (eeuurrgghh!!), sweet potatoes, whole grains, mushrooms and sweetcorn.

Vitamin B5
Pantothenic acid

FUNCTION: It is needed for the metabolism and synthesis of all foods.
SYMPTOMS OF DEFICIENCY: A deficiency in this case is extremely rare, however symptoms may relate to fatigue.
SOURCE: Eggs, meat, liver, dried fruit, fish, whole grain cereals and pulses.

Vitamin B6
Pyridoxine

FUNCTION: Aids fat metabolism, required for the formation of red blood cells, helps to maintain nerve function, enhances immune system by creating antibodies.
SYMPTOMS OF DEFICIENCY: Skin disorders, mouth sores, depression and anaemia.
SOURCE: Chick peas, peanut butter, spinach, lean meat, bananas, eggs, chicken, liver, fish, beans, nuts, whole grains and cereals.

Vitamin B7
Biotin

FUNCTION: Vital component in the metabolism and synthesis of essential fatty acids, carbohydrates and fats. Keeps hair, skin and nails healthy.
SYMPTOMS OF DEFICIENCY: Very rare but could lead to depression, muscular pain, hair loss, skin rashes and fungal infection.
SOURCE: Biotin is found in almost all types of food. High amounts are present in liver, butter, yeast extracts, eggs, dairy produce, nuts and fortified cereals.

Vitamin B9
Folic acid

FUNCTION: Required for the production of red blood cells, DNA and proteins.
It is particularly important for pregnant women to have enough folic acid in order to prevent major birth defects related to the brain, or spine (neural tube defects, including spina bifida and anencephaly).
SYMPTOMS OF DEFICIENCY: The human body does not store folic acid therefore we need to consume it every day to ensure that we have enough in our system. Deficiency can lead to anaemia and limited absorption of essential nutrients.
SOURCE: Leafy green vegetables, citrus fruits, lentils, wheatgerm, fortified cereals, liver, pork, poultry, broccoli, melon, peas, green beans, asparagus, spinach and mushrooms.

Vitamin B12
Cobalamin

FUNCTION: Synthesis of red and white blood cells, required for the metabolism process and to maintain the nervous system.
SYMPTOMS OF DEFICIENCY: Tiredness and fatigue, tingling and numbness in the hands and feet, anaemia, loss of memory and... thingamabobs.
SOURCE: Eggs, shellfish, poultry, meat, dairy produce, liver and fortified cereals.

Vitamin C
Ascorbic acid

FUNCTION: Vitamin C is required daily for the growth and repair of tissues in all parts of your body. It helps the body make collagen, an important protein used to make skin, cartilage, tendons, ligaments and blood vessels. Vitamin C is needed for healing wounds, and helps to repair and maintain your bones and teeth.
SYMPTOMS OF DEFICIENCY: Scurvy, slower healing of wounds, swollen bleeding gums, fatigue, loss of appetite, dry skin, painful joints, anaemia and a slower metabolism.
SOURCE: Citrus fruits, melon, strawberries, blackcurrants, peppers, tomatoes, broccoli, kiwi fruit, potatoes, dark green leafy vegetables, mango, cauliflower, pineapple, blueberries, raspberries and cranberries.

Vitamin D

FUNCTION: Vitamin D is needed to absorb Calcium, strengthen bones and teeth, and can prevent the onset of osteoporosis.
SYMPTOMS OF DEFICIENCY: Rickets in kids, Osteomalacia in adults, demineralisation of bones and reduced bone density, insomnia, nervousness and muscle weakness.
SOURCE: Dairy produce, oily fish, eggs and fortified cereals. It is also known as the *'Sunshiii-innnne'* vitamin, as 15 minutes of exposure, three times a week will enable the body to manufacture all the vitamin D that it requires.

Vitamin E
Tocopherol

FUNCTION: An important antioxidant that nourishes and protects the cells from harmful substances and free radicals that could lead to cancer. It is also known to prevent cardiovascular and heart disease.
SYMPTOMS OF DEFICIENCY: Deficiencies are not very common but may include some nerve damage.
SOURCE: Nuts, seeds, spinach, green leafy vegetables, asparagus, whole grains, cereals and Sunflower oil.

Vitamin K

FUNCTION: Vitamin K is a fat-soluble vitamin that plays an important role in blood clotting. It is also absolutely essential for the maintenance of bones and can help prevent heart disease.
SYMPTOMS OF DEFICIENCY: Deficiency is rare because vitamin K is manufactured in the body but signs of deficiency can include easy bruising and mucosal bleeding.
SOURCE: Spinach, cauliflower, kale, green leafy vegetables, soya beans, spring onions and pistachio nuts.

So the next time you're feeling in a mood, or a bit tired, or your skin's looking a tad ropey, or your bowels are playing up, or you've got cold sores and you just feel **bleeuurrgghh!!** It's down to your food young un', and the fact you're not getting enough minerals and vitamins.

Now let's take a look at *'Macronutrients'*.
READER: *What the hell are macronutrients?*
Well they may sound like an alien race of mutants but once again are an **essential** food source for you, me and her with the hair.

In order to get the full gamut of nourishment, every diet should contain water, fruit and vegetables, plus a healthy balance of the following macronutrients:

- Carbohydrates
- Fats
- Protein

It is recommended by the Government that our daily diets should consist of over 50% Carbs, over 30% Fat and over 15% Protein but so many studies have taken place over the years that dispute these figures, it's not surprising that so many people get confused. And if the Government says one thing, then it must be wrong, right?!

Fight the power and all that.

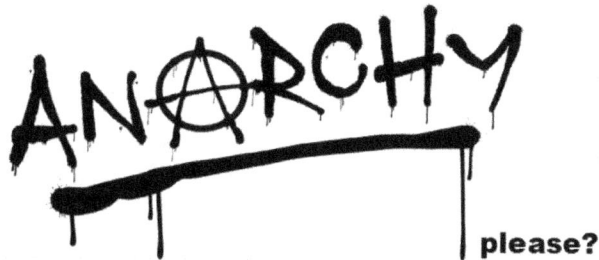

ANARCHY | **please?**

However, what cannot be disputed is that as a nation we consume **far too much** saturated fat, salt and sugar, which is a major contributory factor to the inordinately high levels of obesity.

So how much food should we consume on a typical day?

For men it's around 2500 kilocalories and for women it's about 2000, and this should meet your daily energy requirements. Although this depends on the level of activity, body size and age of the individual, so it's not set in stone.

If you're trying to lose weight, it's an acceptable gauge for those that feel the need to calorie count.
For instance, if you're a chap and you eat less than 2500kcal for that day, you will lose weight. If you eat more than 2500kcal you will gain weight. Simple as dat.

It doesn't matter if you consume all of those calories in one meal, or in tiny meals throughout the day, it will still take the same amount of energy to digest and burn - 2500kcals.

To lose weight, you need a **calorie deficit**, whether that's obtained via your diet, or by physical activity, or both.
READER: *What do you mean?*
Ok! I'll give you an example.
One ordinary day, a woman goes to the gym for an hour and burns off 500kcal. During that same day, she consumes her recommended daily allowance of 2000kcal.
By definition, this woman would have a deficit of **minus 500kcal** for the day and as a consequence, she would lose weight. In the very simplest of terms of course because there's a whole biological minefield to take into account as well, but in principle that's the theory.

READER: *Ok! I get that but what exactly are calories?*
A calorie is simply a weight of measurement for the amount of **potential energy** stored in food.
And if you're interested in this type of thing, one Calorie is equal to 4,184 joules of energy. **Kapow!!**
The calorie measurements you see on food labels are actually *'Kilocalories'* (kcal) and one kcal, is equal to 1,000 calories.

Therefore if we were being completely pedantic, a woman's recommended daily allowance of calories is 2 million not 2,000, and a blokes is 2.5 million not 2500, actually that could explain the obesity problem.

In common parlance, *'Calories'* and *'Kilocalories'* are used interchangeably but to limit the confusion, when I mention *'calories'* in this book, I actually mean one kilocalorie (kcal).
You ok with that? Clear as mucky mud?
READER: *Erm... I think so, yeah!*
Look, I don't make the rules, it's not my fault some boffin in a white coat couldn't come up with a better alternative word for *'Kilocalories'* and decided upon, *'Calories'*.

Anyway, back to nutrition…

Obviously in order to survive you need **energy** and this enables you to breathe, pump blood, move about, perform bodily functions, digest food, compare mobile tariffs and a whole lot more.

And in the main, your body gets this energy from food and water.

The number of calories contained in a food item **differs** based on the type of macronutrient:
- One gram of carbohydrates has 4 kcal of potential energy
- One gram of protein has 4 kcal of potential energy
- One gram of fat has 9 kcal of potential energy.

The calories in both natural and processed food will provide you with the requisite energy your body requires to perform to its optimum capacity but it's the **type** of calories that you consume, that count.

All calories are **not equal**, as many people have been led to believe.

For example, if you ate toast for every meal and that equated to 2000 calories for that day, you'd get the requisite energy your body requires but you wouldn't get the necessary nutrients. And as I keep banging on, your body needs those nutrients.

That toast is likely to contain traces of *'protein'* if it's wholemeal bread, *'saturated fat'* if it's slathered in butter and if it's white bread, a whole host of sugary *'carbs'*. But there'll be a limited amount of essential vitamins and minerals.

Hey!! That reminds me of a fun game.
Say the word *'toast'*, ten times in a row.
READER: *No.*
Oh! Go on…
READER: *Alright then. Toast, toast, toast, toast, toast, toast, toast, toast, toast, TOAST!!*
What do you put in a toaster?
READER: *Bread…*
You're no bloody fun you.

Ok smarty pants, what are carbs?
READER: *Wheaty, starchy, bready type stuff…. Oh! I don't know, what are they?*
I'll tell ya…

CARBOHYDRATES

Brain food

Carbohydrates are the sugars, starches and fibres that can be found in fruits, grains, vegetables and milk products. They are called *'Carbo-hydrates'* because at the chemical level they contain Carbon, Hydrogen and Oxygen.

Carbohydrates are the body's preferred energy source and the only fuel source for the brain and central nervous system. Your body can either utilise carbohydrates right away, or convert them into a storage form called, *'Glycogen'*.

There are two types of carbohydrates (carbs), **simple** and **complex**. The difference between the two forms relates to the chemical structure and how quickly the sugar is digested, and then absorbed into the blood stream. In essence, simple carbs are digested and absorbed quicker and easily than complex carbs, which can lead to spikes in blood sugar levels and sugar highs.

Simple carbs contain no nutrients which is why they are known as, *'empty calories'* and are heavily linked to weight gain (did you see what I did there?!). They include naturally occurring sugars found in fruits, honey and milk, as well as processed sugars such as *'Saccharin'*.

From a chemical perspective, simple carbs contain just one or two sugars, such as fructose which can be found in fruit, and they are known as *'Monosaccharides'*. Carbs with two sugars, such as sucrose (table sugar), lactose (from dairy) and maltose (found in beer and some vegetables) are called *'Disaccharides'*.

Simple carbs are the bad boys of the carb world, hanging out in alleyways, spitting and terrorising old ladies:
- They're high in calories
- They're full of refined sugars, like corn syrup and white sugar
- They're low in fibre because the refining process omits the good fibres and leaves easily digestible sugars
- They're high in sodium
- They're high in saturated fat
- They're also high in cholesterol and trans fats

Quite simply, they have very **limited** nutritional value and in today's extremely knowledgeable society, it's baffling why we eat so much of them. Ah! Yes I know why... they're **bloody delicious!!**

We've evolved to crave energy-dense foods but that doesn't mean we have to gorge on them. By all means eat them but in moderation.

Complex carbs (polysaccharides) have three or more sugars. They are often referred to as *'starchy foods'* and include beans, peas, lentils, potatoes, corn, parsnips, whole-grain breads and cereals.

Good carbohydrate sources are unrefined and fibre-rich, such as oats, wholegrains, quinoa, sweet potatoes, squash and legumes, all of which release their sugars slowly.
They are good little boys who call their Mum when they say they will and **never** forget their partner's birthdays. They smell nice too.
- They're very low in calories
- High in nutrients
- Devoid of refined sugars and refined grains
- High in naturally occurring fibre, which aids digestion and helps lower cholesterol
- Low in sodium
- Low in saturated fat
- Very low in, or devoid of cholesterol and trans fats.

Unfortunately they are seen as **boring** compared to their bad boy brothers, so ignored in favour of sugary, saccharin, sickly sweet pap.

187

Once consumed, all carbs break down into smaller units of sugar and are then absorbed by the small intestine before being transported to the liver. The liver converts all these smaller units of sugar into glucose, which is carried through the bloodstream and utilised as energy when required.

If the glucose is not immediately needed for energy, the body has the capacity to store about 2,000kcal of it in the liver and skeletal muscles, in the form of 'Glycogen'.

Once glycogen stores are full, carbs are converted into 'Lipids' to be stored as fat. Thus the more carbs you eat, the fatter you'll become.

Carbs are an essential food group but scientific studies have shown that the increased consumption of simple carbs, such as those in many processed foods, is linked to heart disease, obesity and diabetes.

READER: I keep hearing about diabetes but I'm not quite sure what it is?
'Diabetes Mellitus' is a chronic disease which is associated with abnormally high levels of glucose in the bloodstream, and ranks among the leading causes of death in adults today.

When food is digested and enters your bloodstream, the pancreas reacts and releases the hormone insulin, which then acts like a key, unlocking cells throughout the body to **allow** glucose to enter the cell and be absorbed and used for energy.

Diabetes occurs once your pancreas struggles to produce enough insulin to keep up with the amount of sugar in your bloodstream, or it stops producing insulin altogether.

There are two main types of diabetes:

Type 1	20% of all cases. The pancreas loses the ability to synthesize the hormone insulin therefore the patient **must** manually inject insulin into the bloodstream in order to allow cells to absorb glucose for energy. Once diagnosed with Type 1 diabetes, you will require regular insulin injections for the rest of your life.
Type 2	There is insulin present in the bloodstream but the body's cells **fail** to respond and absorb glucose effectively therefore medication is required to assist. This is now a common disease suffered by obese adults and more worryingly, children.

Other symptoms that can occur in addition to insulin resistance include:

- The constant need to pee
- Intense thirst and hunger
- Lethargy
- Cuts and bruises that do not heal
- Numbness and tingling in the hands and feet
- Sexual dysfunction in males.

So think about that, the next time you're munching on your third slice of gateau, **Mister!!**

Insulin is the primary regulator of fat storage. When insulin levels are elevated, we stockpile calories as fat. When insulin levels fall, we release fat from fat stores to be burned as fuel. Therefore if you have a diet that is high in carbs and sugar, your pancreas is **forced** to increase insulin levels in order to regulate blood sugar thus you're liable to weight gain because fat metabolism slows.

If you're ever diagnosed with diabetes you'll need to eat healthily, take regular exercise and carry out regular blood tests to ensure your blood glucose levels stay balanced.

But if you want to reduce the risk of you ever being diagnosed with this life-changing disease, I suggest you try to avoid simple carbs.

You could also try eating a diet based on the Glycaemic Index.
READER: *What's that?*
The *'Glycaemic Index'* (G.I.) was devised for diabetic sufferers to help reduce and stabilise their blood sugar levels.

It may interest you to know that a low/moderate consumption of GI foods, can actually aid weight loss.
READER: *How?*
The G.I. ranks foods according to their ability to elevate blood sugar levels, which is known as the *'glycaemic response'.*

50g portions of foods are given a rating out of 100, based on a comparison to 50g portions of table sugar or white bread. The lower the rating, the less the food will affect the levels of glucose in your blood stream. And by combining these carbs with non-sugary foods, this lowers the impact of the GI food on glucose levels, and the overall rating is reduced.
READER: *I'm not sure I understand.*
Ok! If you eat 50g of table sugar or white bread, the sugar in your blood stream will be dramatically elevated thus the GI rating would be 100. If you ate a 50g portion of Rye bread, the sugar in your blood stream would only slightly elevate, therefore in comparison to table sugar/white bread, the G.I. rating for Rye bread would be 41.

Carbs that have a G.I. rating of less than 50 (low) can be consumed more regularly than those that have a G.I. rating of over 65 (high), which should be rarely eaten or at least in moderation.

Please see the below tables for some examples of Low, Medium and High, G.I. rated food:

LOW	Peanuts (14), Soya Beans (18), Lentils (25), Kidney Beans (27), Pasta Fettucine (32), Skimmed Milk (32), Chick Peas (33), Apple (38), Ravioli (39), Rye Bread (41), Spaghetti (41), All Bran (42), Porridge (42), Orange Juice (45), Instant Noodles (46), Fruit Loaf (47), Baked Beans (48), Bulgur Wheat (48), Peas (48) and Carrots (49).
MEDIUM	Sultana Bran (52), Buckwheat (54), Ready Salted Crisps (54), Special K (54), Sweet Potato (54), Mango (55), Butter Popcorn (54), Sweetcorn (55), Sultanas (56), Pitta Bread (57), Basmati Rice (58), Vanilla Ice-cream (61), New Potato (62), Beetroot (64), Raisins (64), Whole milk (64) and Couscous (65).
HIGH	Mars Bar (66), Pineapple (66), Croissant (67), Coke (68), Crumpet (69), Ryvita (69), Wholemeal Bread (69), White Bagel (72), Banana (72), Watermelon (72), Brown Rice (76), Coco Pops (77), Chips (78), Crispbread (81), Rice Crispies (82), Corn Flakes (84), Shortbread (84), Baked Potato (85), White Rice (87) and White Bread (100).

If you decide to opt for a low G.I. carb diet, it *'may'* make you feel tired and irritable initially, so supplement with fruit because the natural sugars within (fructose), will help feed and energise the brain.

FIBRE

A crackin' bit of rough-age

Fibre should be an integral part of a healthy balanced diet because it aids the digestion process, keeps you regular and also decreases the risk of coronary heart disease, diabetes and colon cancer.

Although it won't surprise you to hear that most people in this country don't consume the requisite daily allowance.
READER: *Ok! But what exactly is fibre?*
Fibre is only found in plants and forms the outer walls of grains, seeds, fruit and vegetables.
It's commonly referred to as, *'roughage'* or *'bulk'*.

There are two different types *'Soluble'* and *'Insoluble'* and each type helps your body in different ways, so a normal healthy diet should include varieties of both.

Soluble Fibre dissolves in the water contained throughout the digestive system and helps lower blood cholesterol, as well as controlling blood sugar levels.
If you suffer from constipation, gradually increasing soluble fibre intake can help soften your stools and make *'dropping the kids off at the pool'*, a more pleasurable experience.
CONSTIPATED READERS: *Sold!!*

Foods that contain soluble fibre include:
- Oats, barley and rye
- Apples and bananas
- Root vegetables, such as carrots and potatoes
- Beans and legumes.

Insoluble Fibre helps promote regularity and a healthy digestive system but doesn't dissolve in water. It passes through your gut without being broken down and absorbed into the bloodstream.
It adds bulk to waste in the digestive system, which helps to prevent constipation and haemorrhoids.
HAEMORRHOID SUFFERING READERS: *Yay!! Praise the Lord. Where can I find it?*

Food sources that contain insoluble fibre include:
- Wholemeal bread
- Bran
- Cereals
- Nuts and seeds.

Be warned though, if you start to increase your fibre intake, it's important that you do so gradually because it may lead to incessant trumpety-trump trumps, stomach cramps and leave you feeling bloated.
READER: *Sounds great…*
Hey!! Don't pooh-pooh the fibre, or you may not poo-poo at all.

If you're obese… and I'm not saying you are but if you are, the transit of food through the colon is apparently slower in obese people.

Therefore by eating a fibrous diet of fruit and vegetables and drinking plenty of fluid, this will aid the transit of food through the digestive tract and reduce the possibility of stomach discomfort. So now you know, if you're obese that is… and I'm not saying you are.

Anyway!! Fibre is great for aiding number twos, potentially preventing heart disease, colon cancer and diabetes, as well as reducing your cholesterol levels.
READER: *I've heard that word so many times but what exactly is cholesterol?*
Cholesterol is a waxy, fat-like substance which is made by the liver and produced to make hormones, vitamin D and aid the digestive process.

It's also found in some of the foods you eat therefore you can absorb further quantities through your diet. Cholesterol travels through your bloodstream in small packages called *'Lipoproteins'* and there are two kinds, Low-density Lipoproteins (LDL) and High-density Lipoproteins (HDL).

It's important to maintain healthy levels of both types of these lipoprotein.

LDL cholesterol is often referred to, as *'bad cholesterol'* because high LDL levels can lead to an unhealthy build-up in your arteries, which could ultimately restrict blood flow and lead to heart problems.

HDL acts as the loyal Caretaker, mopping up cholesterol from all parts of your body and carrying it back to your liver to be removed as waste thus lowering your chance of getting heart disease.

Cholesterol is also linked to plaque.
READER: *What, in your mouth?!*
Derr!! No, plaque is not just found on your teeth, it's a nasty substance that gets into your bloodstream and is made up of Cholesterol, Fat and Calcium.

When plaque builds up in the arteries, it leads to a condition called *'Atherosclerosis'*.
Over time, the plaque hardens and narrows your coronary arteries, limiting the flow of oxygen-rich blood to the heart. Eventually, an area of plaque can rupture; causing blood clots to form and if these clots get large enough, it can severely restrict or completely block blood flow, leading to angina or a heart attack.
READER: *I've heard of a heart attack but what's Angina?*
It is not a disease in itself but rather an early indication of coronary heart problems and occurs when an area of the heart muscle, is receiving a decreased supply of oxygenated blood.

Attacks are triggered when the heart is forced to work harder, perhaps during physical exertion or during emotional stress, and has similar symptoms to indigestion.

It may feel like pressure, or tightening in your chest but the pain can also be felt in your shoulders, arms, neck, jaw or back. In some cases the pain can also develop after eating a meal, or during cold weather but it will usually improve if you rest for a few minutes.

If you believe you are suffering from angina, it's a sign that you're at an increased risk of heart attack therefore you should seek medical attention immediately.

Lowering your cholesterol is extremely important, it's necessary, you should do it **now!!**

And when you do, it may slow, reduce, or even stop the build-up of plaque in your arteries, reducing your chances of ever suffering angina, or a heart attack.

That's carbs out of the way,

Now let's talk about a subject that gets more bad press than Putin…

Paul Birch

GLUTEN

Can you tolerate it?

READER: *Oh! I was hoping you'd mention that, should I go gluten free too?*
Gluten is the new kid on the block and it appears to be the font of all food ills. It's like a stray pube on a bathroom tile. **Eeuurrgghh!! Gluten!!**

However, most people don't have a Danny La Rue what gluten is, but they're damn sure it's causing them all manner of ailments. So they decide to cut it out altogether and spend an extortionate amount of dosh on foods that are *'gluten-free'*, even though some of those foods were gluten-free anyway.

Admittedly, it's not **just** an ingenious marketing tool, so what is gluten?

Gluten is a family of proteins that can be found in foods **processed** from some type of grain, such as wheat, barley and rye. When flour is mixed with water, the gluten proteins form a sticky network, which has a glue-like consistency. This adhesive-like property makes the dough elastic, providing a chewy texture and helps it to rise when baked.

READER: *What about corn that's a grain, does it also contain gluten?*
'Yes' and a resounding *'No'*.

Corn on the cob and tinned corn should always be *'gluten-free'*, unless it's been cross-contaminated during the manufacturing process, which should be a rare occurrence.

Although corn is a type of grain, it's from a different branch of the grain family than the gluten grains found in wheat, barley and rye. Corn contains a substance known as *'corn gluten'* but this isn't the nasty gluten that bothers people with celiac or gluten sensitivity. Think of these two gluten strains as cousins, one is an evil get, who takes great pleasure in pulling the legs off ants and the other is friendly, nice to animals and has probably set up a standing order to pay £3 a month to a charity.

Nasty gluten can be found in bread, pasta, bagels, doughnuts, pizza dough, corn flour and you may need to sit down for this… **beer!!**

Although having said that, those canny breweries are now producing *"gluten-free"* beer, so don't worry you can still experience *'gluten-free'* hangovers. And at twice the price.

But the multi-skilled capabilities of gluten don't stop there; it is also a stabilizing agent in ketchup, ice cream and soy sauce; a thickener in yoghurt and an imitation bulker in chicken and beef type products. **Hmmm!! Yummy!!**

READER: *Imitation what?*
Bulker!!
Oh aye!! When you opt for a packaged chicken breast at your friendly supermarket, it might state it weighs 450g or similar, well half of that chick-chick-chick-chick-chicken is actually water and gluten.

Hey!! Those chicken manufacturers have to cut the corners somewhere; they have shareholders, holiday homes, antique wristwatches and yachts to buy.

Most folk can tolerate gluten just fine, thank you very much.

However, as cheaper production methods take place, (austerity cuts aren't just for Schools, Hospitals, Social Care, The Police, Fire Brigades, disability benefits, rail services and Libraries ya know?!) more and more people are suffering ill health due to the declining quality of processed food. It can therefore cause problems for those with certain health conditions such as celiac disease, gluten sensitivity, wheat allergy and irritable bowel syndrome.

READER: *Celiac disease? What's that?*

192

It is an **autoimmune disorder** which causes the sufferer to sustain intestinal damage, as well as decreasing the capacity to absorb nutrients from food.

The body treats gluten as a foreign invader, with the immune system attacking the gluten, as well as the lining of the gut. This damages the gut wall and may cause nutrient deficiencies, severe digestive issues and anaemia. The most common symptoms of celiac disease include digestive discomfort, tissue damage in the small intestines, bloating, diarrhoea, constipation, headache, lethargy, dermatitis, depression, weight loss and clothes pegs at the ready, disgusting smelling **poo-poo-poo-poo!!**

However, be aware of self-diagnosis because these symptoms can also be ascribed to substances other than gluten, or may not be related to nutrition at all.

Therefore many people who **think** they're gluten intolerant, are actively seeking to find a problem in an area that doesn't actually exist. If you think you have an issue, seek medical advice from your G.P. don't take medical advice from magazine articles, day-time telly, your sister or Janice from Sales.

Don't be a gluten for punishment... sorry, had to be done.
READER: *Could it be IBS?*
Blimey, ten years ago no-one had even heard of *'Irritable Bowel Syndrome'* (IBS), now it's a common discussion topic in offices, at Bus stops and Doctor's surgeries up and down the land.

I can't eat that, I've got IBS
Ooh! I feel terrible today, it's my IBS
I can't go to the gym, I've got IBS
I can't stay behind at work, I've got IBS
He broke up with me 'cos of my IBS
I can't complete a sentence without mentioning IBS

Don't get me wrong, it's another common digestive related disorder which causes symptoms like abdominal pain, cramping, bloating, diarrhoea and windy-pops. But just because you feel a little bit bloated after munching on toast, or having your weekly spag bol, this doesn't **necessarily** mean you have to spend the rest of your day saying, *'my IBS is playing up again'*.

IBS is a **serious** chronic condition but it's not the end of the world as you know it, and you can feel fine in no time by carefully managing your diet, making some lifestyle changes and by stopping the whingeing.

But let's say you do have a gluten intolerance, if that's the case you will have to make some changes.
Adopting a *'gluten-free'* diet is not gonna be easy, it could be quite challenging to begin with.

And you'll have to become a label bore.
In fact, you should **ALL** become label-nerds if you wanna lose the lard, 'cos food packaging can be deliberately misleading sometimes.
READER: *What do you mean?*
Food marketing gurus are deceitful buggers and pretend that certain food types have almost magical healing properties; they under-estimate servings and they use scientific terminology for ingredients in order to bamboozle the consumer.

So if was you, I'd take the nutritional content of food packaging with a pinch of salt. Although that pinch, could in fact be a heap.

However, having said that, you're still gonna have to start reading those food labels on **everything** you eat to improve your knowledge. Unless you go veggie of course, then at least you'll definitely know what's in your food. **No?!** Ok! Well you'll soon come to realise that gluten is added to a whole multitude and quite surprising number of foods. Although, I'm not gonna list them all here 'cos there's far too many to mention.

Ideally you should avoid processed muck, cereals and any grains that contain gluten. The more natural the food the better for **you**, your gut and whoever follows you after you've been to the bog.

There are a few grains and seeds that are naturally *'gluten-free'*, including:

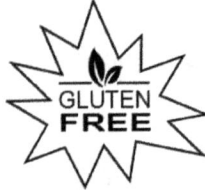

- Rice
- Quinoa
- Flax
- Millet
- Buckwheat
- Arrowroot
- Oats

However, while oats are naturally gluten free, they *'may'* be cross-contaminated in the production plants. Therefore it is safest to only consume oats with a *'gluten-free'* label, and lucky for you they'll be thrice the price.

There are plenty of healthy whole foods that are naturally *'gluten-free'*, honest, cross my heart and hope to die, including:

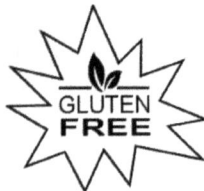

Meat, Fish and Seafood, Eggs, Dairy products, Fruits, Vegetables, Legumes, Nuts, Fats (such as oils and butter), plus Herbs and Spices.

Right this next section is completely *'gluten-free'*, although it does contain a big, juicy, dollop of fat.

FAT

So misunderstood

It may surprise you to learn but fat isn't all bad, in fact, as part of a balanced diet it's another **essential** nutrient and supports a number of important bodily functions. It is only when people consume too much, or too little, that ill health and weight gain follows.

Fat is like *'Star Wars'*.
READER: *What?! What you on about now?*
There is a dark side to fat and a good wholesome side but it's been forced down our throats that fat is just bad, bad, bad, bad, **bad!!** As a consequence, some people become obsessed with eliminating fat entirely from their diet, and as a consequence *'nutrients lack, will essential they'*.

READER: *Why? What's so good about fat?*
Fat gives food its flavour, its alluring aroma, its tenderness and palatability. Without an adequate amount of fat in your diet your body is unable to effectively absorb the fat-soluble vitamins A, D, E and K, which are all necessary for your good health.

Fats help to formulate *'Myelin'*, a fatty material which protects and insulates nerves, enabling them to quickly conduct impulses between the brain and CNS.

Adipose fat stores cushion vital organs, insulate the body and are a structural component of our cells, including the membranes needed for energy, growth and tissue repair.

There are three types of fat:

<u>SATURATED</u> – These are most often found in animal products such as beef, pork and chicken. Saturated fat can also be found in egg yolks, dairy (cream, butter, cheese etc), lard, coconut oil and palm oil

<u>UNSATURATED</u> which includes:
- **Monounsaturated** – these can be found in almond, olive and rapeseed oils, avocado, peanuts and seeds
- **Polyunsaturated** – these can be found in plant foods like nuts and seeds, vegetable oil and cold-blooded fish (mackerel, sardines, salmon, herring – containing antioxidants, vitamins, and Omega 3 & 6 – which although sound like Russian spies, are in fact fatty acids)

<u>TRANSFATS</u> – artificial fats that are found in fast food, fried foods and commercially baked products that use partially hydrogenated oils, such as cookies, cakes, bread, margarine, crisps, doughnuts etc.

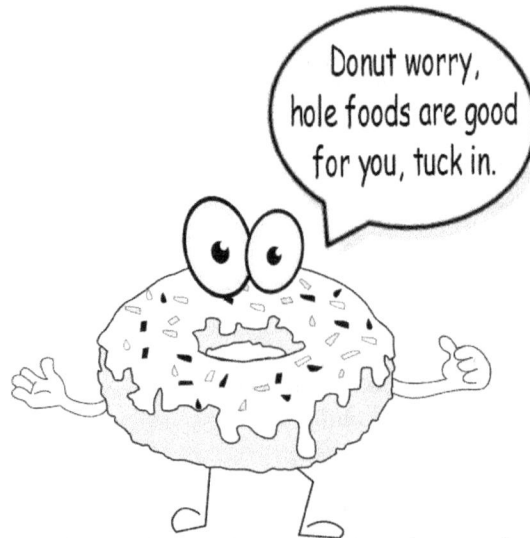

Good fats like those found in fish, nuts, seeds and olive oil, are full of nutrients and will help your hair grow and keep your skin healthy. Bad fat makes you hate looking at mirrors.

If you consume a diet high in transfats, you increase the risk of developing high blood pressure, strokes and diabetes.

These bad fats are not just stored under your skin as adipose tissue but they also start to surround your vital organs too, which is not ideal for your long-term quality of life.

The rest of the fat clogs up your arteries which could restrict blood flow, leading to coronary heart disease and in some cases, may include amputations due to dead blood cells and vessels.
READER: *Not me mate, I'm invincible.*
Oh! Well, don't say I didn't warn you.

If you're one of those people that aren't immortal, my broken record advice to you is simply, enjoy the bad fats in **moderation!!**

And be careful regarding your consumption of products that **claim** to be *'fat-free'*, or have *'no added fat'*.

Many foods **claim** to contain *'no added fat'* but that is a similar boast to saying *'no added alcohol'* to a bottle of whiskey. It doesn't necessarily mean that the product doesn't contain fat; it just means that the manufacturer hasn't added any **more** fat to the product.

'Fat-free' foods do remove the fat content as advertised but this fat is replaced with toxic sugar derivatives to make it palatable (saccharin, aspartame, sucrose, maltose, dextrose, high corn fructose syrup etc) which can destroy neurons in the brain, making us stupiderer and liable to watch *'celebrity'* dating programmes, buy cheese-strings, take out high-interest loans, worry about Soap romances, vote for the Tory party, believe what we read in the tabloids and download Ed Sheeran songs.

But fair do's if you want to eat *'fat-free'* products it's up to you, like everything else it's a choice. It's your choice. And you can choose to be fat and eat more bad fat, to make you even fatter. Or you can choose to be thin, fitter and happier by reducing your fatty-fat-fat consumption. **Good luck!!**

Whey-hey that's the fat section over, now let's discuss **Protein**.

PROTEIN

It makes you biggerer

Proteins are the building blocks of life and fundamental to the structure, functionality and maintenance of our body. Proteins help:

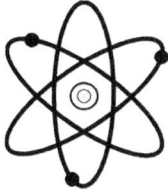

- Control blood sugar levels
- Assist in the digestion process
- Produce haemoglobin to transport oxygen
- Create antibodies to fight infection
- Muscles to contract
- Make vital hormones
- Blood to clot
- Fight bacteria
- Build and repair tissues
- Aid nerve transmission.

Apart from water, protein is the most abundant molecule in our bodies and an essential cellular component of organs, glands, skin, nails, hair, bones, cartilage, tendons and muscle.

Proteins are made up of small compounds called *'Amino Acids'*, of which there are **twenty** different types. But **eight** of these cannot be manufactured by the body and therefore **must** be consumed in the diet. These are known as the *'essential'* amino acids.

READER: *What are amino acids?*
Well, I'd need to get extremely chemical here to describe them and I'm afraid I failed my Chemistry GCSE but basically, amino acids are the chains of molecules that make up protein and include the following elements: Carbon, Hydrogen, Oxygen, Nitrogen and sometimes Sulphur and/or Phosphorus.

What you really need to know, is it's **vital** that your diet includes a variety of protein sources because insufficient consumption can be very harmful to the body and lead to symptoms such as fatigue, atrophy of muscle mass, immune system suppression, oedema and dermatitis. Therefore your diet should include some of these delicious, high protein foods:

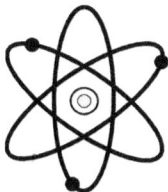

- Beef
- Pork
- Lamb
- Fish
- Poultry
- Eggs
- Milk
- Yoghurt
- Cheese
- Soya

READER: Eeuurrgghh!! Soya?
You ever tried it?
96.8% OF READERS: *Erm… no.*

Well, it's an acquired taste I grant you but full of nutrients.
Give it a go because **tofu** is so good for **you!!**

Incidentally, soya beans are the **only** plant protein considered to be a *'complete protein'* because they contain all eight of the essential proteins:

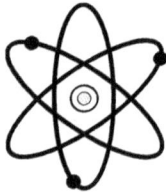

- Isoleucine
- Leucine
- Lysine
- Methionine
- Phenylalanine
- Threonine
- Tryptophan
- Valine

Other plant sources that contain the **majority** of the proteins we need include:

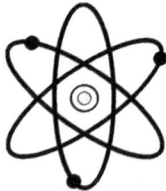

Beans, bulgur wheat, grains, lentils, nuts, oats, peas and seeds

So now you know how important protein is for your body, how much should you eat?
The recommended daily intake of protein should be approximately 56g for the average man and 45g for women, which should equate to about one gram of protein, for every kilogram of body weight.

However, I must warn you (and especially the Billy-Big-Bobs) that if excess protein is consumed, part of it is excreted by the kidneys, and the rest is broken down and added to fat stores.

Excessive protein consumption over a number of years can lead to kidney failure, dehydration and increase the risk of osteoporosis.

Oh! By the by, here's another great thing about protein.

Ghrelin is a hormone that signals to your brain that you're *'hungry'*, and protein compounds decrease ghrelin levels thus helping to reduce your appetite. Therefore a diet that includes a healthy balance of protein, can significantly improve your weight loss goal.
PROFESSORS of ENDOCRINOLOGY: *Yes, there is a link between ghrelin and protein consumption but it isn't a magic bullet, so please advise your readers not to drastically increase their protein intake, in the hope their weight loss troubles will be over.*

Thank you Professors, I'll do that. Hey readers, what they said.

So, that's protein for you, extremely necessary for growth and repair but not a magic bullet.

WATER

H to the O!!

Good old Council pop, where would we be without it? I'll tell you where, in the ground mate, six feet under... **DEADED!!**

Approximately 60% of our bodies contain water and this helps to support the countless metabolic reactions that occur every second, which enables us to *'Ah-ha-ha-ha, stay alive, stay alive!!'*

Water does more than just quench your thirst you know?!

H2OMG

- It controls and regulates body temperature, by the dissipation of heat and evaporation of sweat
- It is part of the synovial fluid that allows movement in joints
- It is a major component of blood plasma
- It helps protect and cushion the spinal cord
- It transports nutrients and gases around the body
- It assists in the excretion of waste products via detoxification
- It is a major component of the digestion process
- It can also make your skin glow, by increasing circulation and creating new cells.

Throughout the day your body loses water through breathing, sweating and digestion, so it's vitally important to rehydrate, by drinking fluids and eating foods that contain water.

READER: *I didn't know that foods contained water?*
Eau Aye!! Natural food sources will often contain water, especially fruit and vegetables.

For example, carrots are 90% water, a strawberry is 91% water, a grapefruit 91%, broccoli is 91%, spinach is 91%, cauliflower is 92%, unsurprisingly a watermelon is 92% water, peppers are 94%, radishes and tomatoes are 95%, and a cucumber is made up of 97% water. Although cucumbers are repulsive, they're just bland, **eeuurrgghh!!**

I'm sure you're aware of this but we can only survive a few days without water, so be aware of the following symptoms, if it ever starts to slip your mind to indulge in some lubrication:

- 5-6% loss of water leads to heat cramps, chills, nausea, clammy skin and rapid pulse
- 6-10% loss leads to reduced sweat and urine production, headaches, dizziness and dry mouth
- Over 10% loss leads to heat stroke, hallucinations, no urine or sweat and then a visit from the ghastly, black-cloaked harbinger of doom. DEATH himself.

The amount of water you need depends on a variety of factors, including the climate you live in, how physically active you are and if you sweat like a pig but the generic recommendation is to sup two and a half litres a day.

Maybe you're one of those peeps who like to show off by spending inordinate amounts of dosh on expensive, sparkling, bottled water, well hey, that's up to you.

We do live in a country where you have freedom of choice. However for those of the frugal nature (saving up for a fantastic holiday, touring the world perhaps) turn the tap on, it's just as good for you and you're paying for it anyway.

naive

Unnatural Spring Water

If you don't like the taste of plain water, add lemon or lime to it. Or get experimenting and create your own concoction by adding blueberries, or chilli pepper, or even a splash of Apple Cider Vinegar.
READER: *What's Apple Cider Vinegar, I've never heard of it?*
Oh!! This stuff is the elixir of eternal youth…
READER: *Is it?*
Is it buggery, there's no such thing. However, apple cider vinegar has been linked to a myriad of health benefits, from curing hiccups, soothing sore throats, lowering cholesterol, stopping the sniffles, suppressing appetite, alleviating dandruff, reducing acne, boosting energy, banishing stinky breath, whitening teeth, lowering blood sugar levels and helping the trains run on time.

Ok! I made the last one up, nothing can do that but it's a powerful liquid nevertheless, which can be drunk or added to meals to give them some **pizzazz!!**

LAURA, 38 - *I used to get awful headaches but then I started to drink at least two litres of water a day. After about a month or so of doing this, my headaches went away, my skin was soft and clear, and I had more energy. Nowadays I notice that when I don't drink enough water for a few days, my body feels like it's running at half the rate it should be. This has been one of the best things I've done for my body.*

READER: *What about hot beverages like tea and coffee are they good for me, they contain water?*
Well they're both diuretics…
READER: *Excuse me?*
Oh! I mean, Eau. They make you pee-pee.

In moderate amounts, caffeine doesn't dehydrate you and it contains water, so yep, they both count towards your allotted two and a half litres of water a day.

Although alcohol is a big no-no regarding hydration because it actually makes you feel dehydrated instead, as well as increasing your curry consumption and lowering your inhibitions so you end up flashing, or snogging your best friend's ex.

Talking of drinks, I'm a bit parched myself and it's gonna be thirsty work this **A to Z game**, so let's start with some liquid refreshment.

Make mine a stiff one.

ALCOHOL

It's your round mate

We all like a drink now and again and I can assure you, I'm no different. Some of the best nights of my life (Hi to Emma, Leonora and Zanelli), worst (beaten up by four blokes because I accidentally spilled one of their pints) and most embarrassing (Pissy-pants Paul), have all occurred after a night on the ale.
READER: *Tell me more.*
Another time perhaps, maybe that can be the subject of my next book.

My mates used to call me *'Jekyll and Hyde'*, 'cos they didn't know which Paul would show up after a few shandies. Would it be the funny, charming, good laugh to be around Paul? Perhaps the cheeky, might take things a bit too far Paul? But too often it would be, *'Oh Shit, what has he done now?'* Paul.

I just didn't know when to stop. I'd get drunk but I always wanted to get a bit more drunkerer.

A single? Make mine a chuffin' quadruple **mate!!**

But that was the old Paul. I've mellowed in my old age. Now I'm happy with a nice tankard full of *'Old Thwackers Bottom'*, a good chat and a nice sit down. And for God's sake, *'turn that racket they call music, down, I can't hear myself think in here'*.

I've realised that it wasn't good for me, so I've knocked those heady drunken, *'who's blood is that on my shirt and who the hell is she in my bed?'* days, on the head.

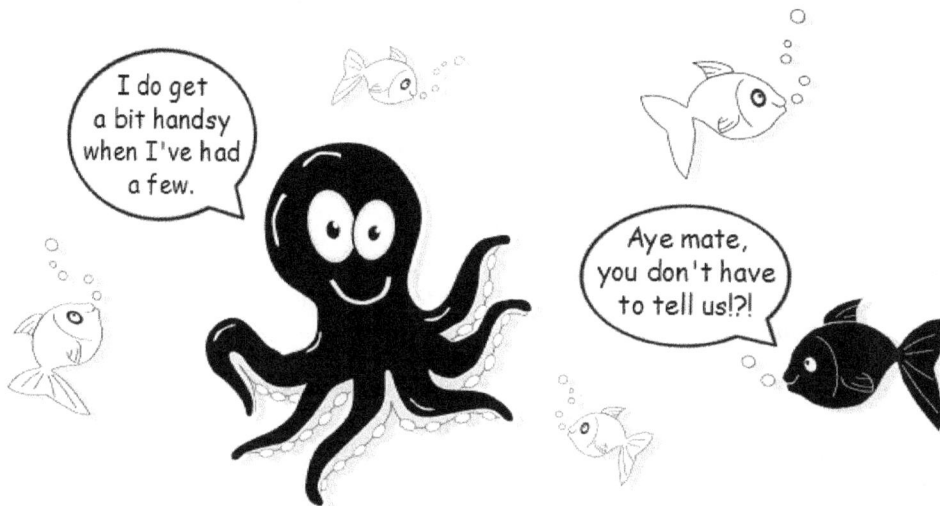

Therefore I'm in no position to tell you to cut down; I'd be a complete hypocrite. Although it's obvious that alcohol should be consumed in moderation, **especially** if you're trying to lose the timber or you use it as a liquid crutch. So if you're pouring it on your corn flakes, I'd think about quitting. It's all fun and games, until you're hooked up to a dialysis machine.

I'm not trying to tell you **how** to live, I'm just making recommendations. However, I can guarantee that the more of my recommendations you take on board, the more likely you are to lose weight and keep it off... for good.
But **you** have to make the decisions. **You** have to take the action. **You** have to reduce the sherbet consumption.
Look, have a few beers, I mean it's not often a great anecdote begins with, *'I remember that time we were drinking green tea...'* but if you are **desperate** to lose the lard, you have to drastically reduce your consumption.
It's just counter-productive. Its four steps forward, three steps back.
Don't ruin your good work.

READER: *But can't I have a glass of wine after a tough day at work?*
Of course you can.
All I'm saying is the more you drink, the harder it will be to lose the flab. There won't be **any** sustained weight loss if you're regularly getting merry, kaylied and mullered!!

READER: *Ok! But why is alcohol so bad for me?*
Well, apart from the fact that getting drunk convinces your brain that you can actually dance, or sing, or it would be a good idea to get off with Darren from Accounts, it is extremely toxic and highly addictive. It's not just the impaired judgement, lack of coordination and incoherent speech; it's the internal damage that makes alcohol so lethal.

Most people are social drinkers and just have a few on a night out, whereas others are *'binge'* drinkers and sup vast amounts of alcohol in a short period of time.

Heavy drinking can cause heart problems including:
- **Cardiomyopathy** – Stretching and drooping of heart muscle
- **Arrhythmia** – Irregular heart beat
- **Stroke**
- **High blood pressure**

It takes a toll on your liver too, which can result in inflammations such as:
- **Steatosis**, or fatty liver
- **Alcoholic hepatitis**
- **Fibrosis**

In worst case scenarios, liver cells die and get replaced with scar tissue, leading to a serious condition called *'Cirrhosis'*, which is irreversible and can result in an early grave, unless a suitable donor can be found in order to **temporarily** prolong your life..

The pancreas isn't safe either. Alcohol causes the pancreas to produce toxic substances that can eventually lead to *'Pancreatitis'*, a dangerous inflammation and swelling of the pancreatic blood vessels, which restricts and prevents proper digestion. It also affects another important organ, which is located in those novelty boxers with that hole by your left knacker, and could result in erectile dysfunction.

Chronic drinking can also weaken your immune system, making your body a much easier target for other diseases such as pneumonia and tuberculosis. And then there's the Big C. Heavy drinking can increase your risk of developing cancer of the mouth, oesophagus, throat, liver or breast.

But for someone who is trying to lose weight, someone like **you**, alcohol is a **bugger!!**

It actually reduces your body's capacity to burn fat as an energy source, by slowing down your metabolism. And the final kicker. Whenever you go out for a night on the pop your liver will convert all that alcohol into *'Acetate'*, which as a result actually **increases** your appetite. Hence the kebab shops of the world rejoice.

I'll be honest with you, I love a beer, I enjoy drinking wine and I'm partial to an Irish coffee or three, so I would hate to live my life without alcohol. Having said that, I live a life where I drink in moderation, for the majority of the time anyway but I'm not trying to lose weight and I'm not an alcoholic.

Yeah, I might have already done irreparable damage to my heart and liver through years of alcohol abuse but luckily I'm not showing any signs of it... **yet!!**

I passed my last health M.O.T. with flying colours but that's me, this book is about helping **you.**

Bottom line - If you're always on the lash, or enjoy daily liquid stress relief, it will take you a long, long, long, long, long, long time to lose the lard. If you reduce your consumption, or cut it out completely, your chances of long-term weight loss will improve dramatically.
Your choice.
READER: *Ok! That's fair enough but I thought that drinking alcohol could also be good for me?*

Yeah that's partially true.
Moderate consumption of alcohol has been linked to health benefits but this varies between individuals, and depends on the quantities consumed, and the type of alcoholic beverage.

Research by some inebriated boffins has concluded that antioxidants in red wine, called *'Polyphenols', 'may'* help protect the lining of blood vessels in your heart. This doesn't mean you should be caning a bottle of Rioja every night but what it does mean, is that the odd glass now and again will have similar health benefits to munching grapes at work, or putting blackberries on your granola.

And I can imagine which one you'd prefer.

But that's ok because M-O-D-E-R-A-T-I-O-N is good for the nation.

Apparently, the hops that are used to flavour beer contain a fancy substance known as, *'Xanthohumol'*, which is a compound that helps to protect the brain from degenerative disorders such as Alzheimer's and Parkinson's.

The darker the beer, the more Xanthohumol it contains, so get yourself some of that Irish stout that has always promoted itself as being good for you. Although don't sup too much, or you might end up forgetting the way home, or waking up the next day wondering why you made a call to your ex at 3 in the morning. And the excretions the day after are something to behold.

If you must drink at home, I have a tip for you to reduce the alcohol content. Add fizzy water to a glass of wine or your lager, then you won't drink as much. Alternatively if you're a spirit drinker, rather than adding a sugary juice, add cranberry instead, especially with Vodka. It's a lot better for you; just don't put it in pints.

Don't do *'dry Jan'* either, abstinence make the heart **desperate** for a beer, and you end up getting absolutely leathered in the first week of Feb to make up for it thus make no gains at all.

The UK Chief Medical Officers' guideline for both men **and** women is that to keep health risks from alcohol to a low level, it is safest not to drink more than fourteen units a week. That means about six glasses of wine, or six pints of low strength beer or perhaps, five pints of cider.

Ideally this should be spread out over the week, not during your Friday lunch hour.

So if you want to lose weight, my advice to **you** is simple, cut down.

Alcohol is for people who can afford to lose a few brain cells, so no offence mate but you've gotta be careful.

A to Z

The food alphabet

READER: *Is this where you tell me what to eat?*
How can I tell you exactly what to eat, I don't know what you **like!!**
No, I'm going to explain the benefits of certain food types and then it's over to you. After all, it's your plate, fill it how you like.

Be aware though, that:
- **Protein + carbs** = muscle gain
- **Protein + fats** = healthy maintenance
- **Protein + veggies** = fat loss
- **And fat + carbs** = muffin tops, love handles and saggy bum cheeks.

All you have to remember is this, *'you can dish it out but can your body take it?'*

ALMONDS

Crunchy goodness

If you're from *'Oop North'*, we call them AL-monds but if you're a soft-shandy-drinking Southerner, you'll most likely pronounce them, AR-monds. Irrespective, these scrum-diddly-umptious nuts are full of nutrients, minerals and vitamins.

The health benefits of almonds are extensive and they are frequently used as an alternative solution to relief from constipation, respiratory disorders, coughs, heart pain and anaemia. They also help in the maintenance of healthy gums, hair and skin. Oh! And if you're a bloke and you have some bedroom related problems, such as stage fright before a big performance, then I have some great news for **you.** They're supposed to be good for impotency, although I couldn't vouch for that, 'cos I'm ok on that score but a mate told me… ☺

Almonds are high in fibre, magnesium, protein and vitamin E. Several studies have linked higher vitamin E intake with lower rates of heart disease, cancer and Alzheimer's disease, so get munching.

Almonds also contain *'Phenylalanine'*, an essential amino acid required for the production of dopamine. Dopamine controls the brains reward centre therefore by increasing foods that release this neurotransmitter, this will improve your mood and help you feel positively super, smashing and **great!!**

Almonds are high in fat though, so be aware of that. I recommend a **Donald J. Trump** handful a day, and you'll be fine. Almond milk is also a refreshing drink, although a tad sweet, so it goes well in coffee for those caffeine drinkers trying to cut down on their sugar consumption.

AL-monds are a superfood and I could fill hundreds of paragraphs in this book pontificating about their brilliance but sod that, you need to learn about these foods off your own back, so **you** do some research too and like me, you'll become an AL-mighty almond advocate.

APPLES

And I'm not talking toffee!!

An apple a day keeps the doctor away, unless you're a hypochondriac.

The original super-fruit, has been pushed aside by the trendy new kids on the branch.

Ok!! They might be a bit boring and not as glamorous as kale, goji berries or Greek whipped yoghurt but they're *'fat-free'* and juicy and crunchy and crisp and cheap. Plus a lil' bit naughty, if you're a lover of the forbidden fruit story. Apples are extremely rich in important antioxidants, flavonoids, and dietary fibre, yet for some reason are overlooked as a snack for summat sweet, chocolatey and full of shite.

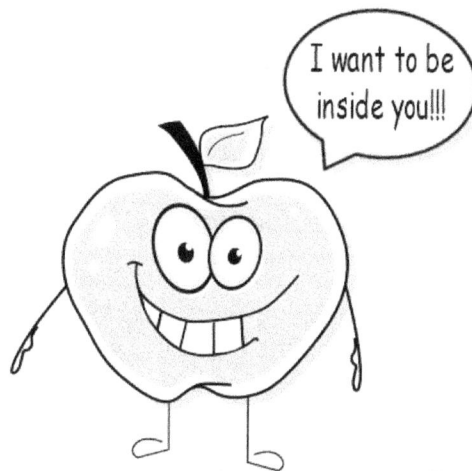

There are more than 7,500 varieties of apples and each one of them is laden with vitamin C and provides countless health boosting benefits.

Boffins from around the globe have conducted thousands of apple related studies, and they have concluded that both the green and the red ones can:

- Reduce tooth decay
- Lower cholesterol
- Improve heart and lung functionality
- Lower interest rates
- Ramp up your immune system
- Prevent gallstones
- Decrease the risk of Alzheimer's, cancer, diabetes, heart disease and Parkinson's

READER: *I thought they were full of sugar?*
Yep! A large apple is about 110kcal and contains about 10g of sugar, which is about the same as a chocolate wafer biscuit.

So, if you're trying to cut down on your sugar consumption, I wouldn't have more than two apples a day.

⬤

Granny Smiths, Braeburn and Cox,
Get one, get a bag, get a box,
If you wanna get the fibre eat the skin,
And the pips should be spat in the bin.

A final word on these fine globules of goodness. Apples contain *'Pectin'*, and when you eat foods high in fat, the pectin binds to some of the fat and helps your body eliminate it through waste, rather than being stored.
So, how do you like them apples?

ASPARAGUS

I'm Asparagus. You're Asparagus. We're all Asparagus.

Low in calories (20kcal per spear) and *'fat-free'*, asparagus also provides a wide variety of antioxidant nutrients including vitamins A, C, E and K, Beta-carotene, and the minerals Zinc, Manganese and Selenium. And it makes your pee smell funny.
READER: *What?*
Asparagus is the only food to contain the chemical *'Asparagusic Acid'*.
When this acidic chemical is digested it breaks down into sulphur-containing compounds which have a strong, unpleasant aroma hence the whiffy wee-wee. But relax, not everyone can smell it and besides, how weird are you if you go about smelling your own piddle?!

Anyway back to asparagus and its unique properties.

You can spend a fortune on anti-ageing creams, or you can eat asparagus every day because it contains the antioxidant *'Glutathione'* which helps protect the skin from sun exposure and pollution.
READER: *What the hell is glue….gloo… glue the phone??*
Glutathione is one of the most important molecules your body requires to help you stay healthy, slow the ageing process, fight cancer, prevent heart disease and combat the risk of Alzheimer's.

Luckily your body produces its own glutathione but toxins from poor diet, pollution, medications, stress, trauma, ageing, infections and radiation all deplete your glutathione stores. This leaves you susceptible to cell disintegration, free radicals, infections and in the worst case, the Big C.

To combat this and help increase glutathione production you can obtain it through your diet by munching on garlic, onions, broccoli, kale, cabbage, cauliflower, watercress and our new mate, asparagus. The more you eat, the better you feel and the healthier you become.

You don't get those benefits with boil in the bag rice, potato waffles, packaged sarnies and ready meals for one.

And as a qualified Personal Trainer, I feel it's my duty to inform you that exercise boosts your internal glutathione production levels too. I told ya, it's bloody good for you this fitness lark. So have a go, you know it makes sense.

Just have a go.

Have a go.

Haveago!!

Avago!!

AVOCADO

Hard, hard, hard, ripe… mush

Here's a fun fact for you. The word *'avocado'* is derived from the Aztec word *'ahuacatl,'* meaning testicle.
READER: *Bollocks!!*
That's right yeah. You'll never look at 'em the same way again.

Ten years ago this fruit was just a pretend hand grenade for kids, now it's synonymous with boosting health and has become a supermarket big-shop, super-dooper staple.

The avocado may have a high fat content but it's also heaving with nutrients and even the fat is the good type of fat, *'Omega 3'* which helps to lower your cholesterol.

The cancer-fighting avocado is a fantastic source of anti-oxidants and high in essential vitamins and minerals. These include Beta-carotene, Lycopene, Pantothenic acid (vitamin B5), vitamin K, fibre, Magnesium, Phosphorus, Iron and Potassium. And if that wasn't good enough it also contains Phenylalanine, the amino acid required for the production of dopamine.

The humble avocado is high in mono and polyunsaturated fats, which can help reduce blood cholesterol levels and decrease the risk of heart disease. It's also another of nature's great beauty products too, due to the high concentrations of vitamin C and E, which help to keep the skin nourished and glowing. And you waste all that cash on skincare products, **madness!!**

They're also good for improving the ol' mince pies because the avocado is an excellent source of the carotenoid *'Lutein'*, which helps to reduce the risk of macular degeneration and cataracts.
READER: *What's a macular?*
The *'Macular'* is the part of the retina that is responsible for your central vision, allowing you to see fine details clearly. Therefore it's not just glasses that help enhance your sight; Mother Nature has provided numerous plants and goodies for your optical needs.

And these rich, creamy gonads of goodness are spectacular, for the macular.

Try 'em, I think you'll love 'em, then like me, you can become an avocado aficionado.
A word of warning though, the stones are not gobstoppers, so for your dental safety please don't crunch or suck on them, put them in the bin.

BACON

Grease me up

I used to think bacon was bad for me, so I stopped thinking.

Aah! The bacon butty, the greatest hangover cure known to man. You can't buy happiness but you can buy bacon and it's pretty much the same thing. I've created a little ditty about our love for the bacon. It's best to sing it in a reggae style. Try it in the manner of someone like Shabba Ranks or Shaggy.

Go on, it'll be fun.

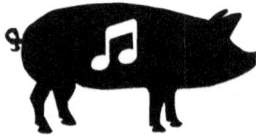

I love BACON, you love BACON,
Everyone is BAKIN', the crispy, greasy, BACON!!

I want BACON, you want BACON,
If it's BACON you're MAKIN', then feed me your BACON!!

We love BACON, they love BACON,
My body's really ACHIN', for smoky, streaky BACON!!

He loves BACON, she loves BACON,
The whole world is WAKIN', to the sizzle of the BACON!!

We want BACON, give us some BACON,
My body's really QUAKIN', for fatty, rindy BACON!!

I love BACON, you love BACON,
The whole world is SHAKIN', to the sound of the BACON!!

Yep, it's safe to say there's a lot of love for the beer-can but what exactly is it? Bacon is a processed meat that comes from the fatty side of a pig's belly. The meat is cured to preserve it and then soaked in a solution of salt, nitrates, spices and sometimes sugar. Two-thirds of each greasy rasher is pure fatty-fat-fat and this breaks down to about 50% monounsaturated, 40% saturated and 10% polyunsaturated fat.

All meat products are nutritious and bacon is no exception. A typical 100g portion of cooked bacon can contain:
- 37g of protein
- The vitamins B1, B2, B3, B5, B6 and B12
- Selenium
- Phosphorus
- And the minerals Iron, Magnesium, Zinc and Potassium.

Therefore in moderation, bacon is good for you. So if you're a bacon lover, then I don't advocate you cut it out of your diet completely, just don't have it every day. It should be a treat.

READER: *Why? I'm confused. You've just said it's good for me.*
In moderation.
And this is because there are major health concerns when it comes to bacon (and other processed meats) because heavy consumption has been associated with cancers, heart disease and respiratory problems.
This is down to how the meats are cooked and the cost-cutting manufacturing processes that take place to produce it therefore the better the quality of meat, the less risk.

If you're going to have some, then I suggest that you always grill the bacon and cut off as much of the disgusting, fatty rind as possible. I could say, limit the ketchup and don't have white bread but then what would be the point?!

However, if your goal is to lose weight and keep fit, then I'm afraid that daily bacon butties are not compatible to that aim.

C'mon, it's bloody obvious really.

READER: *Do you eat them?*
Yeah but probably three times a year max. There's a great butchers near the village where I live and their well-done bacon butties are awesome. If you're gonna have a treat, in my opinion always opt for quality over quantity (I also say that to the ladies, doesn't get me anywhere mind).

As ever, it's your choice re the bacon but remember I'm trying to help **you** add ten years to your life, not take ten from it.

BAKED BEANS

Windy pops, optional

A family favourite for a great number of years, with most pantries containing a least a few tins but how nutritious are these, flatulence inducing, canned haricots in a rich tomato sauce? According to a company that produces a variety of 57 dishes, baked beans are high in fibre, virtually *'fat-free'*, and each serving counts as one of your five a day. They contain no artificial colours, flavours or preservatives, which makes them an ideal snack or accompaniment to any meal. Baked beans are also high in protein and have been found (see what I did there?!), to help lower your cholesterol.

Blimey, they sound like another superfood however there's just one teeny, weeny, **problemo!!**
Most baked beans you buy in a can are **loaded** with salt and sugar.

The average serving has the equivalent of about three teaspoons of sugar and can contain over 50% of your sodium daily allowance, which is scandalous when you bear in mind they are promoted towards kids for their health-boosting qualities. Many manufacturers have now tried to reduce the salt and sugar levels, but they are still too high therefore once again, it's a food source that should be enjoyed in moderation.

You could actually make your own funky healthier beans with this simple recipe.

Warning, *'may'* (definitely will) lead to excessive bottom burps.

Ingredients

- 1 lb. dried Haricot Beans
- 1 large onion, chopped
- 1 chilli, sliced (the hotter, the better)
- A can of chopped tomatoes
- A smidge of tomato puree
- 1/4 tsp cayenne pepper
- 1 tsp black pepper
- 2 tsp sea salt
- A few generous splashes of Henderson's Relish (famous spicy sauce from Sheffield)

Instructions

- Add beans to a plastic container and soak in cold water
- Place in fridge and leave overnight
- When you're ready the next day, pre heat oven to 250 degrees. Drain the beans and then boil in a pan
- Once boiled, drain and then place in a large, oven-proof pot
- Add in the chopped onions, chilli, tinned tomatoes, tomato puree, cayenne pepper, black pepper, sea salt, and Henderson's
- Stir and cover pot with lid
- Place in the oven for about 2 hours, or until the beans are nearly soft
- Toast some thick, wholemeal bread and dish out the beans. Enjoy!!

- Get the kids to wash up
- A few hours later, fart and revel in the sweet aroma of healthy nutrition

Alternatively if you're one of the CBA gang, open a tin of cannellini beans, slap 'em in a saucepan, add vinegar, black and cayenne pepper, sea salt and half a tin of toms.

Heat for a few mins, stir until they reach the desired consistency, then serve on a bed of toasted, buttered bread. Cheap, convenient and saccharin free. **Sweet!!**

BANANAS

So appealing

The world is absolutely bananas for bananas. These phallic, curvy, yellow fruits (**edit:** *It's actually a herb, but yeah good one Billy-Botanists, as if 99.9% of the planet are gonna start calling 'nanas, herbs*) are one of the most widely consumed foods on the planet.

And for good reason.

They're high in antioxidants; contain the minerals Potassium, Pectin and Magnesium, plus the vitamins A, C and B6.

There are a multitude of health benefits associated with this **fruit!!**

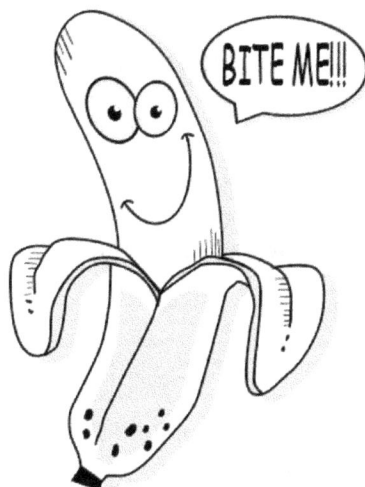

Bananas help to combat depression, aid digestion, make you smarterer, cure hangovers, relieve morning sickness and protect against anaemia, kidney cancer, high blood pressure, diabetes, osteoporosis and macular degeneration.

Bananas are just, **ace!!**

Bananas are great, bananas are cool,

Don't slip on the skin, 'cos you'll look like a fool,

Bananas for brekkie and bananas for lunch,

If you're feeling peckish, break one from the bunch!!

So whenever you feel like a snack, opt for a 'nana rather than a bag of crisps or a choccy bar because they're full of nutrients, low in calories, virtually *'fat-free'* and full of protein. But be aware, that size, does in fact matter...apparently ☺

1 - Are you chuffin' kidding me?
2 - I can't even hold it properly
3 - I have never been so unsatisfied in my life
4 - Well, I've had bigger
5 - Good but not quite enough
6 - Yeah, about right
7 - Nice one, can't complain
8 - Ooh! Perfect
9 - Aah! A bit much
10 - It's hurtin' my insides
11 - It's too big, I can't take it anymore
12 - OMFG!!!

BISCUITS

Get dunking

Everyone loves biscuits, now…
READER: *Let me stop you there. You're gonna rattle on about moderation again aren't ya?*
No… well, perhaps… alright, yes I am but and if it's a big butt, there's a legitimate reason to discuss moderation.
If you're actively seeking to lose weight, then an overzealous consumption of biscuits is not gonna help 'cos they're full of fat, calories and sugar.
Pretty obvious really, do I need to go on?
READER: *You probably will though…*
Look, I'm only trying to help. Hear me out.

I'm not a massive fan of biscuits myself but I do love fig rolls. I don't know what's in 'em and I don't want to know, maybe crack. Whatever it is, they're bloody lovely.
Let's say I'm having a cuppa…
READER: *I'm having a cuppa.*
Cheeky get!! Although I like what you did there, good stuff.

Anyway, I'll have a brew and take three fig rolls out of a new packet, then place the rest of the pack back in a cupboard. After I've wolfed them down, I think, *'sod it'* I'll just have two more. A few minutes later, I'll take my empty cup to the sink and then as I'm passing the cupboard I tell myself, *'another few fig rolls won't hurt'*, so I get two more. Oh look, the packet only has three left, well I might as well scoff them too, no point just leaving a few in a pack. So, in the space of about ten to fifteen minutes, I've eaten an **entire** pack of fig rolls.

Clearly if I did that every day, I'd be a right porker, plus I'd have no teeth left but I don't.

I probably buy two packs of fig rolls in a year, so in the grand scheme of things my biccy consumption doesn't affect my weight too much. And I always feel guilty for ruining my good work, so invariably head for a jog, either the same day or day after to counter-act the fig roll bonanza.

That's what you do when you embrace fitness and it works 'cos I ain't fat, I'm fit.

Malted Milk, Hobnob,
Shove a couple in your gob,
Custard Creams, Rich Tea,
Pass me one, no make that three,
Garibaldi, Ginger Nuts,
Yum-yum-yum, greedy guts,
Jaffa Cakes, Bourbon,
Packet's empty,
All gone!!

Therefore if your goal is to lose weight and keep it off but you have a similar process of caning the biscuits, the best thing to do is just not buy them in the first place. Alternatively, use them as a reward (I know you're not a dog but in this context it works) for your good work. You could go for a twenty minute walk or jog **per biscuit**, or use them as a treat for when you've returned **back** from a walk, jog, cycle or gym session.

You don't have to be a trained nutritionist, to know that excessive consumption of biscuits is going to ruin and hinder your chances of weight loss success. But you are allowed treats in your life; you're not a robot (yet). So find a way to incorporate them in your life but in **moderation!!**

I'll explain more about the perils of sweet stuff in the sugar section later in the book but...

If you wanna lose weight and get real thin,
reduce your trips to the biscuit tin

BREAD

If you're looking to lose weight, you've gotta use your loaf

For over 12,000 years bread has been a staple of the human diet, so is it bad for us or not? It's a rhetorical question because the answer is yes... and no. It depends. Not always. Ermmm... who the hell knows?!

Ok! What we do know, is that sliced bread *'may'* not have been the best thing after all because it led to cheaper production methods and reduced quality.

Back in the day when it was Farmer Giles's wife baking the bread, it was just flour , salt, yeast and water but nowadays it's full of preservatives, additives, gluten, oils, more salt and for some reason, sugar.

This means that most of the bread we buy from the supermarket might taste delicious but it has little substance and provides limited, or even zero nutrients for the body.

Therefore if you continue to buy crappy supermarket sliced bread, you will **struggle** to lose the pounds, unless you reduce your consumption significantly, or at the very least, try to bake your own healthy bread.

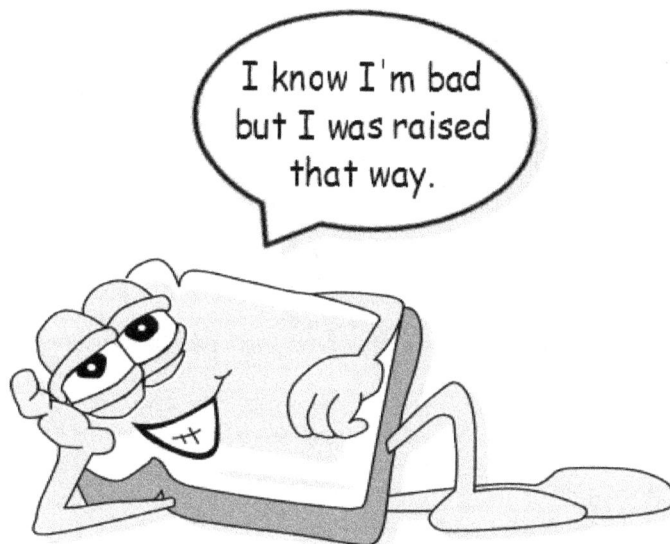

I know I'm bad but I was raised that way.

READER: *Well, there must be some healthy bread out there?*
Yeah, of course there is and the best type is *'whole'* grain bread, which contains very few ingredients but when it comes to the quality of bread, I'm afraid white, is just **shite!!**
In fact, it sullies the good name of shite.
READER: *Why?*
It's all to do with the grain.
And the quantity of the grain determines the **quality** of the flour and in turn, the nutritional benefit of the bread.

The whole-grain of wheat consists of three elements, the BRAN (the outer layers), the GERM (the innermost area) and the ENDOSPERM (the starchy part in between). The endosperm has very little nutritional benefit, whereas the bran and the germ sections are packed tight with all the good stuff, like fibre and the nutrients vitamin B, vitamin E, calcium, iron, magnesium and zinc. During the manufacturing process to make the flour for white bread, the grain is refined and ground up to such a degree, that it strips away both the bran and the germ thus removing those essential nutrients and along with it, all the goodness contained in the grain. All that remains is the endosperm, which is now the main ingredient of the flour.

The resulting flour is insipid, bland, and tasteless with a slightly yellowish colour. So, to give it that pure, whiter than white hue, it is then bleached using chlorine and other fancy chemical agents.

To make it more palatable and to replicate some of the missing nutrients which were lost in the milling process, the flour is enriched with all manner of preservatives, additives, gluten, oils, salt and where would we be without it, **sugar!!**

Once baked, this enriched white flour turns the bread into that springy, light, fluffy texture we know and love and as a consequence, its shelf life is extended. It's not very healthy but admittedly it stays fresher for longer, and tastes great toasted and slathered in **marge!!**

After you've stuffed a few slices down your gullet, the starch contained in this white bread gets broken down rapidly in the digestive tract, leading to a spike in blood sugar and insulin levels. And as we know from our old pal insulin, when blood sugar surges, it tends to go down just as quickly and when it drops suddenly, we become hungry again. Making white bread, a pain in the arse for those looking to lose the lard.

So there you have it, that's white bread in all of its synthetic glory.
If you want to continue eating a food that leads to hunger pangs, contains bleaching agents, miniscule amounts of artificial supplements and has about as much nutritional value as a few teaspoons of table sugar, then go ahead, keep consuming that bread.
READER: *What about brown bread then?*
Granted, it does have a reputation for being the healthier choice but unfortunately many loaves of brown bread, are just white breads in disguise. They contain the same processed, over-refined flour as white bread, but with the addition of caramel and even more preservatives to give it that darker appearance. If you're looking for healthy nutrition in your slices of bread, if it ain't whole-grain, then you're being misled. Be warned though, bread manufacturers are a canny bunch. They can promote **any** type of bread as being made with *'whole-grain wheat'* (such as white bread) but it can still have the bran and germ missing.

When buying bread, the first thing you should do is read the ingredients. The more preservatives, additives and emulsifiers it has, the **poorer** quality of bread it will be. The more the fibre, the **better** quality of bread it will be.

Your best bet is to opt for those loaves that contain loads of seeds, the ones that have a nutty, rich taste, with a dense, heavy texture.
READER: *Hmmm! Sounds... delicious...*
Yeah they do take some getting used to, but those types of bread are vastly superior to their salty, sugary, chemically enhanced mates on the bread shelf. Personally I love 'em and I can vouch for their toasting quality. Alternatively you could try Multigrain bread.
READER: *Never heard of it, go on, enlighten me.*
Well, it's bread that's made from... multiple grains.
READER: *Erm... derr!!*
Ok! Ok! There's more to it than that.

Multigrain bread contains different types of grains and seeds but don't be fooled, this doesn't mean that all multigrain breads are rich in good 'ol nutrients.

Check the ingredients.

If the flour is milled from grains that are 100 per cent whole grain, or 100 per cent whole wheat, then put it in your basket but if it's made from white or enriched white flour, let it rot on the shelf. Although it'll take a while, what with all them preservatives shoved in it. The good brands contain sunflower seeds, raw flax seeds, rolled oats and barley, which gives the bread a firm, nutty texture. **Delizioso!!**

You could also try Rye Bread, which is extremely high in fibre, so it'll keep you regular and tastes great with peanut butter. Like most of the healthy breads, it's heavy man!! But they keep you fuller for longer, reducing your desire to run to the biscuit tin. There's also Spelled Bred... no, sorry that's, '*Spelt Bread'*. A distant cousin of wheat, it's high in fibre and full of minerals and vitamins that **don't** get destroyed in the baking process. It has a comparable consistency to wheat bread, so would offer a similar taste to what you've been used to.

READER: *What about crumpets, surely they're ok for me?*
I'm sorry. I'm the harbinger of bad news, yet again.
Crumpets may seem harmless but these fluffy round snacks can contain as much salt, as three bags of crisps. To be fair they are low in fat, but do contain sugar because they're made from the same enriched flour as white bread, bagels, croissants and the like. Aye! There's nowt in them worthy of the name '*nutritious'*.

Look, it's quite simple.

The majority of manufactured, packaged bread is **not** good for you due to the additives and chemicals, and sugars and preservatives, and whatnot else that is added in the refining and baking process. So if you want to lose weight. I mean really, really, **REALLY** want to lose weight, you will cut down drastically on these products, or even omit them completely from your diet. However, if you decide to carry on eating them, you'll have to either bake them yourself, so you can control what nutrients they contain, or buy products with as few ingredients as possible.

I know I'm a preachy get but I genuinely want to help you, so do us a favour and cut your bread intake down.

Ok! It's early morning and you've put your new healthy, nutty, seedy, whole-grain bread in the toaster because you're ready to start the day with some nutritious brekkie. Well, hold your horses; it's time for me to ruin that for you **too!!**

BREAKFAST

Breaking the fast

The most important meal of the day? Or a scam to increase the profits of the cereal conglomerates?
The greedy flaky gits!!

You've had a night tossing and turning, you've had numerous nonsensical dreams and then you awake from the slumber. You're ratty, miserable and in a right two and eight, so you need something to drag you out of this fug. Maybe you're a crumpet lover, or perhaps you go traditional with a plate of greasy slop, or it's a bowl of muesli, topped with organic goat's milk. Whatever your choice, the common consensus is that brekkie provides the body and brain with the **necessary** fuel it requires to thrive, after an overnight fast. And as well as providing you with energy, breakfast is linked to loads of health benefits, including weight control and improved cognitive performance.

It is also thought that by eating a healthy breakfast this will lower cholesterol, increase happiness and reduce stress.

Eating breakfast is important for everyone, but is especially so for kiddie-winkles and annoying spotty teens. Allegedly, bairns that eat breakfast perform better in the classroom and on the playing field, with better concentration levels, problem-solving skills and hand-eye coordination.

Many studies (financed by Cereal companies perchance?), relating to both adults and children, have shown that breakfast eaters tend to weigh less than breakfast skippers. **WOW!!**

But how can this be?
Put simply, if you eat a healthy breakfast this will negate the need to snack throughout the day and you will select healthier food choices at other meal-times.

However, if you skip brekkie, to compensate you're more likely to gorge on sugary treats, eat a massive lunch and therefore put on more timber.

The brekkie boffins also state that eating breakfast habitually will reduce the risk of sustaining high blood pressure, heart disease and diabetes.

So there you have it, conclusive proof that breakfast is indeed, the most important meal of the day.

Personally, I think that's bowl-ocks but that's just me.

Wake up sleepy head,
The morning's here, hooray!!
Head down to the kitchen,
To start this brand new day,
Toast bread, scramble eggs,
Milk and cereal too,
You can't go wrong with brekkie,
It's just so good for you!!

Actually, hang on a minute; hold onto your spoons because we have a different viewpoint.

The case against breakfast
How can you possibly feel refreshed and able to take on the world, if you haven't had a bowl of sugary flakes bathed in skimmed milk, wholemeal bread slathered in jam, or if you're a teenager, a bag of crisps and a chocolate bar? It's more than likely that you're a brekkie disciple and to be fair, who can blame you after over sixty years of pro-breakfast propaganda but do you start to feel a bit, Oh! How you say? *'Fuckin' ravenous'* by about 11ish? Well, this is completely normal, especially if you opt for a meal based on refined or simple carbs, such as cereal or toast, with a glass of sweetened OJ on the side.

What? How can this be? I hear you ask.

In the words of Jesse Pinkman from Breaking Bad... **Science, bitch!!**

It's all down to *'Cortisol'* and *'Insulin'* levels apparently, so let's go back to those white-coated nerds.

As soon as you start to eat in the morning, this sets off a variety of biological whirrings which kick start your metabolism, and this is where cortisol enters the scene.

Cortisol is a steroid hormone which regulates a wide range of processes throughout the body, including metabolism and the immune response. It also has a very important role in helping the body respond and deal with stress. And when we wake from our blissful, recuperative sleep induced state, this has a profound effect on our body. It's extremely stressful.

To countenance this traumatic event, the body releases cortisol to alleviate and calm the body's internal system. Like offering a cup of sweet, milky tea, to an old lady in shock. And **relax!!**

Once you sit down to munch on your shredded-frosted-enriched-wheaty-flakes, your cortisol levels have reached peak level.
To coincide with this cortisol spike and the consumption of *'food'* for the first time of the day, your pancreas starts to release a rapid burst of insulin due to the rise of glucose in your blood stream.
READER: *Why?!*
The cells in your body need sugar (glucose) for energy. However, sugar cannot be absorbed into most of your cells directly.
After you eat food and your blood sugar level rises, the pancreas responds by secreting the hormone insulin, which then acts like a **key**, unlocking the cells to allow sugar from your bloodstream to enter the cell and be absorbed, and immediately used for energy.

With breakfast being the first meal of the day, blood sugar rises quicker than normal and then falls quite rapidly within the next few hours. As a consequence, the brain starts to crave more sugar and we have this unrelenting urge to eat.
This is when you decide it'll be a good idea to nip to the newsagents for a packet of crisps, or the vending machine for a chocolate bar.
READER: *So what should I eat then to stop this?*
You won't stop it because your body will always react in this way as soon as you start to eat, but you can reduce the speed at which the blood sugar levels drop thus relieving the desire to crave chocolate, like a starved vampire craves blood.

To help you feel fuller for longer and sustain you until lunch time, you should opt for a breakfast that is high in fibre and protein but low in sugar. This will help slow down the digestion process and prevent dramatic spikes in your blood sugar and insulin levels.
READER: *What do you recommend?*
Eggs are great and granola is good but not the sugary induced packet stuff you find in most supermarkets though. Try to make your own by adding nuts, berries or seeds. You could also add natural yoghurt to your dish too. Not diet versions that are full of sugar substitutes but completely sugar free and don't worry about the fat content, it's minimal and not bad for you in any way, shape or form.
You should try and get your oats too. Although, preferably not the convenient, tear here, add milk to line and shove 'em in the microwave types, which contain **loads** of added sugar and very little oats.

No, a boring pack of traditional, 100% oats with no added ingredients are the best ones and you can buy a pack for less than a Scottish pound note. Shove 'em in a pan and gently warm for a few minutes, you know, if you can be arsed that is. Whether you top with sesame seeds or blueberries, or sprinkle some cinnamon, or chuck in a few almonds, or add a dollop of nothing-added-at-all-honest-Guv natural yogurt, or stir in honey, or mix in some dried fruits, or add a splash of maple syrup, or dust with grated coconut, or slice in fresh fruit; oats are endlessly versatile, extremely good for you and will help stave off those snack cravings.

Alternatively, you could eat your previous night's leftovers, a jacket spud, a steak, spag bol, anything your mind desires. Don't just opt for boring cereal or toast, use your imagination.

Remember, food should offer value, at **every** meal time.

READER: *Should you eat breakfast if you're trying to lose weight?*
If you don't eat breakfast, will **you** be famished by 11 o'clock and desperate for a packet of crisps and a chocolate bar, or can **you** manage until lunch?
The prevailing public wisdom suggests that yes, you should eat breakfast.
But the current state of scientific evidence exalting the benefits of fasting means that unfortunately, the simple answer is – *'I don't know'*.

READER: *Thanks.*
Look, it depends on the individual.

I don't eat breakfast and haven't for nearly thirty years. I have had no adverse effects from a health perspective and I don't feel ravenous in the morning. I'm fine to wait until lunch, even after that sometimes, but that depends on whether I'm going to be conducting any exercise or not.

I'll discuss *'fasting'* further on in this chapter but there's no hard and fast rule regarding brekkie.
I've read numerous studies that advocate **not** eating breakfast and others that are firmly in the *'go to work on an egg'* camp. So basically, it's down to individual choice. If you're hungry, eat. If you're not hungry, then don't.
In fact, that should be your mantra for **every** mealtime during the day. Just because you've reached a certain time, don't just eat 'cos you're expected to. If you're not hungry, don't eat.

Oh! Before I forget, I have to mention cereals that contain chocolate.

As we all know, chocolate is very rarely eaten by us Westerners, so if we can jam-pack it into every meal then that is extremely beneficial to our health.

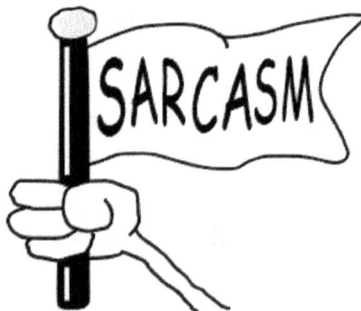

Chocolate breakfast cereals are sacrilege and any parent that gives their child these cereals for their breakfast, should be done for child abuse.
READER: *Bit extreme don't you think?*
Ok! Fined then.
Food should offer value. I'll repeat that sentence again. **FOOD SHOULD OFFER <u>VALUE</u>**.

What **value** is your little cherub getting, if you offer them a bowl of flaky chocolate?

None. It just means more trips to the dentist and the likelihood that they won't be winning any medals at the School Sports Day.

Oh! I wonder why we have an obesity crisis?!

What's next, caramel infused toast and honeycomb, nougat pops? Surely as a nation we can abstain from sugary, chocolatey pap, for one meal a day?!

No? Just me?

Right, onto the next letter. I'll have a *'C'* please Bob.

CAKE

You wanna piece o' me?

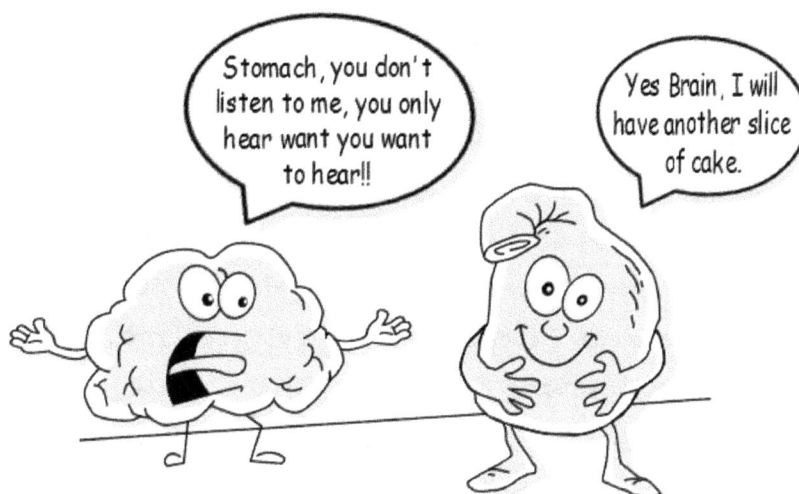

Here's a great tip to help you lose weight, shut yer **cakehole!!**

We all love cake don't we? I mean it's a British tradition, a slice and a brew. How positively **marvellous!!** However, what is now becoming a tradition is we still treat cake as a dessert but also as a snack. And as seconds. And as breakfast. Elevenses. Twelveses. Thirds. Pre-lunch snack. Mid-afternoon no-one's looking; I'll just sneak another slice, snack. And *'Oh! I'm popping into the kitchen, well it can't be a wasted journey, so I'll have a piece of cake whilst I'm here'* snack, etc, etc et-mouth-is-full-of-crumbly-icy-spongey-cakey-sugary-chocolatey-jammy-marzipanny-cetera.

I'm not saying you can **never** have cake again but c'mon, let's knock the consumption down a notch or five thousand.

How is it a treat, when we have it all the time?

You **know** why it's not good for you but if you're trying to lose weight, nibbling on cake is a short term high but a long-term downer, 'cos the only person you're battling is **you!!**

So stop it!! Cut down.

That's all I'm gonna say on the subject because it's bleedin' obvious innit?!

Paul Birch

CHEESE

Grate for any meal

There's hard, there's soft, there's smoked, there's sweet,
There's some that smell, as bad as your feet,
Tangy and crumbly and mouldy and ripe,
You've gotta try 'em all, to find your type.
Some are red and some are yella,
And some are white, like Mozzarella,
Brie and Cheddar and Gruyere too,
Wensleydale and Shropshire Blue.
I love cheese so much, I hate to share,
My Edam, Stilton and Camembert,
Feta, Gouda, Mascarpone,
Red Leicester, on me macaroni.
I'm crackers for cheese, I'm sure you'll agree,
Even though I know, it's bad for me,
So I've cut right down and that is that,
Damn you cheese, why you full of fat?!

READER: *I thought cheese was good for me, full of calcium and the like?!*
Yep, cheese is a great source of calcium as well as protein and zinc, plus it also contains high amounts of vitamins A, B2 and B12. Scoffing cheese is brill for the gnashers, by helping to protect them from cavities.

Butt, butt, butt, butt, butt, whether it's made from cow's milk, goat's milk, sheep's milk, stoat's milk or even that of a buffalo, cheese is bloody fattening.

It's high in calories, loaded with salt and the fat it contains is saturated, which is not good for the 'ol tickerbox.

Therefore once again, an extremely simple message to you if you're trying to lose the lard, cut down!!
On cheese… and lard.

Moderation and all that jazz.

Eat it occasionally, not every day.

And if you have to pile it on your pasta, make sure it's just a smidge, not a whole brick-sized block. Otherwise you're ruining all your good work.

Watch out for products like packaged cheese sarnies too because the fat content in them is ridiculous. I once bought a pack from a service station. It was a well-known pastie company that had diversified into the sandwich game. Anyway, this particular sandwich consisted of three types of cheese, a bit of mayo, onions, mustard and sugary white bread and it came to a whopping 1800 calories for the lot. Madness, I ate it though, I'm not a monster and I was so hungry I could've eaten a scabby oss.

Just be careful, check the ingredients on the packaging, and try and eat cheese products that are as low in fat as possible.

I'm board of cheese now, onto another staple of the British diet, chips.

CHIPS

Fork me, they're good

Who'd of thunked it but chips are, wait for it… **fattening!!**

I know, unbelievable. If only we'd known. Apparently, frying chips in lardy, beef dripping causes the starchy chipped potatoes to be drenched in fat. I for one am shocked, someone should inform the Prime Minister.

Also, some white-coat wearing boffins have had the audacity to link chippy-chippy-chip-chips, with causing cancer. I know! Where do they get the balls?! They'll be telling us next that diets high in saturated fat lead to obesity. Two plus two equals four and all that.

Yeah, the nerds have established that when starchy foods are fried (including bread, cereal, crisps and pre-cooked chips); they contain a toxic substance called *'Acrylamide'*. In the preparation of frozen chips, they are initially boiled in water and then treated in sugar solution (consisting of glucose or fructose), before part-frying them and then freezing.

The lab coat gang have identified that the combination of being cooked at high temperatures and then frozen, creates this chemical toxin. Acrylamide has been found to cause cancer in mice but sod them, they're scary little buggers so they deserve it but us, we're nice people, we pay our taxes and help old ladies with their bags. Not fair.

But it's okay, calm yourself, 'cos it turns out that the link to cancer relates to a very high consumption of these foods, so it's back to Mickey Moderation again folks. Or maybe it's nonsense and the Scientists have miscalculated but if you're trying to lose weight, it stands to reason that if you regularly consume chips you're likely to continue piling on the timber. Choices, choices, choices. Chips or toned hips? Fries or fat thighs?

ROBERT, 45 - *I was 17st 11lbs at my heaviest and my confidence was really low. I felt ugly, tired and depressed and it was ruining my relationship with the kids 'cos I couldn't do anything energetic with 'em. I couldn't play footy with them in the garden, or mess about with them at the park and that really upset me.*
So what did I do? I ate. I pigged out on chips. The way home from work passed a Fish & Chip shop, so I'd pop in even though I was due to have my dinner when I got home. It was just plain, unadulterated greed.
After our chats it seemed like a switch just turned in my brain and I said 'no more'. Simple as that. I just stopped. Coupled with the walks, cutting down on bread, pasta and rice, I'm down to 14 and a half. I look like a new bloke and I can finally play footy with the bairns.
I'm just not eating like a pig anymore, it seems so simple but that's all that I'm doing basically.

If you're trying to lose weight, I'm gonna say it again, cut down on the chippy-chippy chip-chips, or even better omit them from your diet and only, I said **only**, have them as a treat. That's what trips to the seaside are for anyway, fish and chips with mushy peas, an ice cream for afters and being attacked by a psychotic seagull. Aah!!

The British seaside, **spondiddlyumptious!!**

So now I've urinated on your fried spuds, let's see how many more of your favourite foods I can ruin.

CHOCOLATE

I'd give it up but I'm not a quitter

If you had a choice,
Between bonking and chocolate,
There'd only be one winner,
But if you gave up one,
And did more of the other,
You'd certainly be a lot thinner!!

One of my clients wanted to lose four stone and when we first met to discuss a fitness and nutrition plan, she asked me this question:

ANGELA, 37: *Will it still be ok for me to eat chocolate? I mean I can't imagine life without it.*
BIRCHY: There's nothing wrong with eating chocolate now and again but if your blood type is caramel, then you've gotta cut down.
ANGELA: *Noooooooooooooooooooooooooooooooooooooooooo!!*

Chocolate is calorific…
READER: *You're telling me, it's fantastic….*
Well, yes it is but what I meant is that there are **loads** of calories, packed into **very** small amounts.
This means you don't instantly feel full after devouring a bar therefore you eat more. Hence the timber and the requirement, nay need, to get active.

Ok! Here's the good stuff about chocolate:

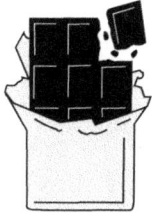

1 - It's bloody gorgeous.

2 - Chocolate contains cocoa, which in itself provides *'Phytochemicals'* which act as antioxidants and the darker the chocolate, the higher the phytochemical content. Bars that contain over 70% of cocoa are the ones to select because they will also contain Iron, Magnesium, Zinc and Selenium. But and once again, if it's a big butt, you should only eat it in moderation due to the extremely high calorie content. That means (and I'm looking at you... yes, **you!!**) have a few chunks and that's it... **THAT'S IT!!**

3 - Eating chocolate is a pleasurable experience.
<u>READER</u> *(munching on a chocolate bar)*: No shit, Sherlock!!

Ok! I know that I'm stating the bleedin' obvious but there is a specific reason as to **why?!**

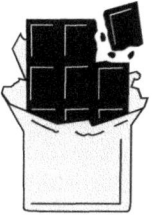

4 - Dark chocolate contains the chemical compound *'Phenylethylamine'*, which encourages your brain to increase endorphin levels thus eating dark chocolate will have a positive effect on your mood **and** improve cognitive health.
However, this is why people get so addicted to chocolate and crave its sweet, smooth, melt in the mouth goodness.

Reeto!! Here's the bad stuff about chocolate:

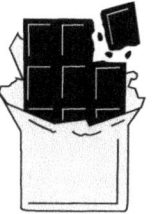

1 – It is **very high** in calories, full of saturated fat and contains loads and loads and loads and loads of sugar and as a consequence, has been linked to extreme levels of obesity.

2 - Due to its addictive qualities, chocolate is extremely hard to give up, in much the same way as heroin. Well, it is another drug after all.

3 - Chocolate is bad for your teeth and worst of all, it's bad for your gut... and your chins!!

You know all of this of course but you also have to remember that:

- Chocolate bars are not a substitute for a meal
- Chocolate bars are not boredom fillers
- Chocolate bars are not post exercise snacks
- Chocolate bars are not breakfast
- Chocolate bars are not 1 of your 5 a day
- Chocolate bars are not relationship replacements.

Chocolate bars will not miraculously solve all your problems. Yes the taste of chocolate is exemplary but the effects are just temporary. Admittedly it is a sweet, pleasurable fix. But a momentary fix nonetheless. Chocolate is **a treat** and should be treated that way, it is not the answer. Positivity, laughter, fitness and healthy nutrition... now that's the answer.

Eating chocolate every day is not gonna help you lose weight, so...

READER: *Don't say moderation again, or I will go all Liam Neeson on your arse. I will look for you, I will find you and I will kill you.*
Alright! Alright, calm down!!
There's nowt wrong with having a chocolate bar occasionally but don't have them every day, eat them in moder... have some self-control.

I think I'm going mad you know. I can't remember what comes after 'S' in the alphabet.
READER: *It's easy, 'T'.*
No thanks, make mine a coffee...
READER: *Yer off yer head you.*
Probably. I've worked in offices for years and years so that statement has got me out of making a brew on countless occasions. It's a tough world out there. Now put that kettle on and make me a *'Stone Roses coffee'*.
READER: *What???*
That's a coffee with cinnamon, *'Sally Cinnamon'*.

COFFEE

Make mine an Irish

Whilst we have a brew, I'm gonna ask you a couple of questions.
How many calories are in a cup of coffee?
READER: *Erm, I don't know, 100?*
Nope, zip. Zilch. Nada. Nowt. But that's only if it doesn't contain milk, or cream or rum.

How many calories in a small *'Caramel Frappe Latte'* from your friendly, train station barista?
READER: *Oh! Well, that probably contains about 100?*
350 calories my friend and that's just a *'Small'*, sorry, a *'Tall'*. And the majority of those calories come from sugar. Those saccharin flavoured brews are full to the brim with the sweet stuff. So, if you have one on the way to work, one at lunch and one after work, that's half of your allotted calories for the **day**, just in coffee. Which is quite frankly, frappe-latte-wappy if you ask me.

A recent study found that some of the drinks sold by these trendy *'chain'* coffee shops include staggering amounts of sugar, up to twenty-five teaspoons in fact. In just one serving. **ONE!?!**

That's **three** times your recommended daily allowance... in one serving.

ONE!?!

And more than one-third of the drinks tested were found to contain the same amount of sugar as a can of Coke.

It's the same for your *'Hot Chocolate'*, your *'Chai Latte'*, your *'Cappuccino's'*, and you'll find the amount of sugar in your *'Mocha'*, is blinkin' chocka!! On average, between six and twenty-five teaspoons of the white stuff. That is disgusting and the mass consumption of these drinks is contributing massively to the obesity problem. Thus another warning from me, and no I'm not gonna suggest moderation, I'm gonna suggest complete omittance. Cut them out entirely.

Although, if you must have a coffee in the morning, invest in a *'Thermos'* and make your own. Or purchase one from the *'chain'* but buy it black and just add milk, or if you're feeling adventurous, cream. Anyway, talking of sugary drinks that offer no nutritional benefit to the drinker, it's time to talk about the biggie, the *'Daddy'* of the cola world.

DIET COKE

Now I can eat anything

Personally, my attitude to coke is this, if there's no JD in it, don't bother.

I've never been a big fan of fizzy drinks in general, which is probably because when I was a kid me Mum couldn't afford to buy 'em, so it was Council pop, or squash, or do without. So in a way, my Mum's frugality helped me to a life free from the saccharin, liquid, caramel-coloured cack!! Cheers Ma!!

Although I don't get the appeal, I can completely understand why peeps get so addicted to it, and it's probably down to the fact that on average, one litre of coke can contain the equivalent of twenty spoonfuls of sugar.

Fizzy pop manufacturers are aware that they've been getting some bad press regarding the white stuff, so they have started to market their *'sugar-free'* alternatives instead. Not only are they promoted as *'sugar-free'*, they are also given the moniker *'Diet'*, which infers health therefore sales have gone through the roof.

But what exactly do these products contain and are they as healthy as promoted?
Well it won't surprise you to read that the above is another rhetorical question and the answer, is chemically enhanced shite and a resounding, teeth rotting, **No!!**

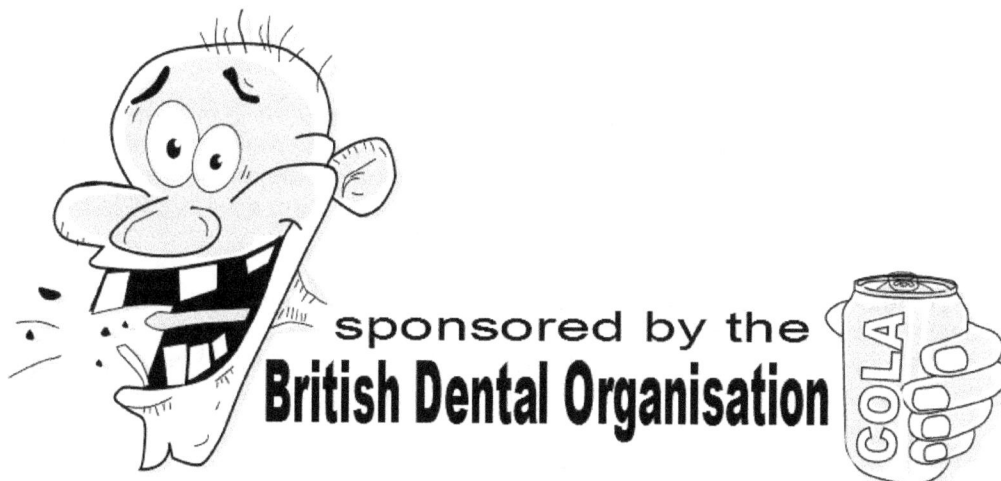

sponsored by the **British Dental Organisation**

These are the ingredients of a well-known caramel coloured diet drink, which is advertised from Trowbridge to Timbuktu:

> Carbonated Water, Colour (Caramel E150d),
> Sweeteners (Aspartame, Acesulfame K),
> Natural Flavourings including Caffeine,
> Phosphoric Acid and Citric Acid.
> Contains a source of Phenylalanine

READER: *Aha!! No sugar, see it's good for me and it contains water.*
Yes, in the same way that the Thames contains water, and would you sup a glass of water from the Thames?
READER: *Of course not, that's full of pollutants.*
I rest my case M'Lud!!
But I'm sure you're gonna go down fighting, so I'll go through each ingredient one by one.

CARBONATED WATER:

My first question would be, *'what the hell'* is in this carbonated water? And then, *'how'* has it become carbonated? But let's assume that those good drinks manufacturers have produced a crackin' source of carbonated water, with limited amounts of sodium and sweeteners to achieve the affect. Maybe it's from the Peckham Spring? All in all, we'll concede that this *'version'* of water is ok, it's good for us. Next...

COLOUR (Caramel E150d):

What the blinkin' 'ummer is Caramel E150d?
This is a food colouring, which is made by the controlled heat treatment of sugar. But that cannot be because diet cokes are *'sugar-free'* even though by default, Caramel E150d is derived from sugar. Erm, curioser and curioser. In fact, a spokesman from a company called *'Coca-Cola Co.'* states that *'Caramel colour is made by a process involving the heating of corn, or cane sugar and other carbs to achieve the desired colour'* – sounds like sugar, comes from sugar, tastes like sugar, **'cos it is sugar!!**

And just for your info, some more white-coat bedecked boffins have conducted tests and found that long-term exposure to a contaminant found in caramel colouring, called *'4-Methylimidazole'*, has led mice to develop lung cancer. And they also concluded that caramel colouring is **possibly** carcinogenic to humans, even though it is found in a host of products like beer, brown bread, chocolate, cough drops, vinegars, custards, doughnuts, gravy, soy sauces etc-who'd have thought it-etc?!

These boffins also found a link to high blood pressure, immune system deficiencies and stomach allergies in humans but what do they know?!
Next...

SWEETENERS - Aspartame, Acesulfame K:

The bittersweet argument over the safety of the artificial sweetener *'Aspartame'* has been going on for decades. There have been thousands and thousands of studies conducted worldwide regarding Aspartame and as a consequence, many of the findings have identified links to brain tumours, cancer, depression and seizures. Check 'em out on the t'internet 'cos I'm not gonna bore you to tears with them here because they are so contentious (not to mention, scary as fuck) but they are a fascinating read.

Tests are still being conducted by Food Standards Agencies (FSA) around the world, with many countries **banning** the substance and I for one, avoid any product that contains it. Yet it is the most consumed artificial sweetener on the planet, and the go-to ingredient for any diet-product that claims to be *'sugar-free'*. Up to you regarding your own consumption and exposure but it's a no from me.

Before I started to write this book, I had never heard of *'Acesulfame K'*, so I had to get my research head on and investigate.

Oh my, it's up to 200 times sweeter than table sugar, and this artificial sweetener can be found in protein bars and shakes, ice cream, cereals, yoghurts, crumpets, doughnuts, sweeties, chuddy and fizzy pop.

Once consumed, it works by stimulating the sweet-taste receptors on the tongue to replicate the taste of sugar but like it's good mate *'Aspartame'*, this chemical granule has a sour reputation and has also been linked to cancer. Again, it needs to be researched to be believed and it staggers me that so many FSA's **allow** these products to be used in every-day products.

Not for me sweet-cheeks, oh and if you're pregnant, then do me a favour and check out this stuff on the web before you carry on consuming any product containing *'Acesulfame K'*.
READER: *Why?*
Because I've read that it can negatively affect the early development of babies during pregnancy and I'd hate for that to happen. I told you, I care, I genuinely care, that's why I'm trying to help **you** and all the others reading this book.
Next...

NATURAL FLAVOURINGS including Caffeine:

Natural flavourings are derived from the essential oils, or extracts of spices, fruits, vegetables and herbs. Lovely, lovely goodness. Although, hundreds of chemicals can be legitimately used to mimic the taste of these natural flavours, so who the chuff knows whether they're actually *'natural'* or not?! However, there is no mistaking that diet cokes contain caffeine and generally 10mg more than regular coke.

We all love a bit of *'caffeine'* to help us get through the day but what exactly is it? Caffeine occurs naturally in the leaves, seeds and fruit of more than 60 plant species and is used as a stimulant to alleviate fatigue, improve concentration and enhance focus. Caffeine can be prepared by extraction from natural sources, or synthesized from *'Uric acid'*.

Once consumed, caffeine is quickly absorbed from the gut into the bloodstream and although it can affect the functionality of various organs, it has a profound impact upon the brain.

Caffeine works by blocking the effects of *'Adenosine'*, which is a neurotransmitter that helps you feel relaxed and sleepy weepy. But by blocking these signals, this temporarily stimulates the brain and promotes a state of arousal, alertness and focus. Thus caffeine has become the most commonly used drug in the world. And just like alcohol, sugar, shopping, Facebook, internet porn and chocolate, it's highly addictive and the withdrawal symptoms are so bad that many people would rather carry on consuming, than give up for good.

Yep, coke withdrawals are not just for politicians, stock-brokers and Z-list pop stars ya know!!
Anyway, next...

PHOSPHORIC ACID:

Whenever I read or hear the word *'acid'*, I instinctively think it can't be good but those FSA guys wouldn't allow us to quaff dangerous toxins would they?! Would they?!

So what is it?

Phosphoric acid is a colourless, odourless crystalline liquid that is used to give fizzy pop a tangy flavour. It also acts as a preservative and helps to prevent the growth of mould and bacteria, which can multiply easily in a sugary, syrupy solution (not that diet cokes contain sugar of course... ya know, being sugar-free and all).

Another interesting fact is that Phosphoric acid is a common ingredient in many fertilisers, liquid soaps, polishes, dyes and rust removal products. And we all love to neck those down don't we?! Of course we don't but is it harmful to swallow Phosphoric acid?

Over to the science geeks again.
Countless studies have taken place over the years to establish if imbibing Phosphoric acid is dangerous to your health or not, and the conclusions have identified that:

- It has been linked to an increased risk of chronic kidney disease
- It has been found to lower bone density
- It can decrease the amount of calcium in your body and has been found to erode tooth enamel
- It can also impair your body's ability to utilise and absorb other minerals, such as iron, zinc, and magnesium

Apart from that, it's positively fantastic and flavoursome.
Next...

CITRIC ACID:

Aah! Another acid but I'm sure it's fine.

Do you remember eating fruit?
READER: *Cheeky!!*
Well anyway, every time you munch on an orange or add lemon or lime to your G & T, you consume citric acid because that's where it's naturally found. Your body also manufactures its own internal supply because citric acid is essential for producing the energy that keeps you active and healthy.

Commercially produced citric acid is added to food, drinks and pharmaceutical products but this type is not sourced from nature because that would be too expensive, instead it's artificially synthesised. The citric acid produced for use in coke, works as a preservative and also boosts the flavour, adding a slightly sour and tangy taste. The same manufactured citric acid is used to clean your tub, remove lime scale from a kettle, polish your best cutlery and added to dishwasher detergent to keep your dishes and plates, spick and span.

Citric acid, should you spit or swallow?

Generally speaking, this is one acid that's not too bad to drink, although there have been links to teeth erosion and digestive complaints. The eyes, skin and respiratory organs can also suffer scratchy, itchy sensations from overconsumption but it's not like you drink loads and loads of coke is it?!

Is it?!

Next…

CONTAINS A SOURCE of Phenylalanine:

Aspartame is a low-calorie sweetener made primarily of two amino acids: *'Aspartic acid'* and *'Phenylalanine'*. Pheny-neny-neny-la-la *'I'm not listening'* la-la-nine or whatever it's blinkin' called, occurs naturally in many protein-rich foods such as milk, bananas, cheese, eggs, fish, milk, meat and nuts.

Phenylalanine is an essential amino acid (a building block for protein), which can't be made by the body and therefore needs to be consumed through your diet but it's not a dangerous, or toxic substance. However, 1 in 10,000 people suffer from a genetic disorder called *'Phenylketonuria'* (PKU), which messes with your liver and makes it impossible to correctly digest and metabolise phenylalanine.

People suffering from PKU need to constantly monitor their protein intake, and have to regulate their diet accordingly. Excessive levels of phenylalanine can lead to seizures, amnesia, anxiety, depression and possible brain damage. Therefore if you have been diagnosed with PKU, or you suffer from epilepsy, or you're pregnant, or you take anti-depressants, or you have high blood pressure, you should avoid diet coke like the plague, in fact, any artificially sweetened fizzy pap, sorry, pop.

So there you have it, that's the ingredients of a particular diet-coke sorted. It offers no nourishment whatsoever, it won't quench your thirst because coke is actually dehydrating but it will deliver a short addictive high… similar to the way cocaine works, although considerably cheaper. Apparently. So people have told me.

I know I've had a go at this drink but I actually used to work for a drinks manufacturer.
READER: *Yeah? What did you do?*
I used to crush cans so they could be recycled but I gave it up because it was soda pressing!!

There you have it, *'diet coke'* in all its glory.

If you want to continue guzzling this cocktail of chemicals in a can, then so be it.

But as sure as eggs are eggs, diet coke is chuffin' bad for you, it will rot your teeth and weaken your bones, although you won't see that in the next advert.

Talking of eggs…

EGGS

If they're not chocolate, I'm not interested

What's the crack with eggs?
Are they good, are they bad? Can you go to work on one? Let's find out...

I like my eggs scrambled and I like 'em salty,

I like egg fried rice, with chicken Balti,

I like my eggs poached and I like 'em runny,

I like chocolate ones, from the Easter Bunny.

I like egg mayonnaise, mixed up with salmon,

I like 'em sunny side up, on top of gammon,

I like an egg salad and I like 'em with cress,

I just love my eggs, yes I must confess!!

Are eggs good for you?
A resounding, categorical, great big **YES!!**

Eggs are loaded with an amazing range of high-quality proteins, vitamins, minerals and good fats. They're low in calories (about 80kcal for a medium sized egg), easy to cook, cheap as chips and should be added to your basket whenever you do a big shop.

These oval, nutrient-packed spheroids contain Calcium, Iodine, Iron, Potassium, Zinc and vitamins A, B2, B5, B12, D and E.

Oh! And Selenium too, which is a super anti-oxidant and vital for the protection of your immune system. In fact, that bloke that used to be in *'Take That'* sung a song about the wonders of *'Selenium'* in 1998, if I recall.
READER: *That was, 'Millennium'*.
Fair do's but the next time you hear that song, you'll sing the word *'Selenium'* to yourself instead of *'Millennium'*, I guarantee. In fact, you're doing it now... ☺

When it comes to eggs, be aware that almost all of the nutrients are contained in the yolk, with the white stuff containing mostly protein. Therefore eggs are great for Billy-Big-Bobs, 'cos they can help you grow biggerer and strongerer.

Eggs are also great for the peepers because they contain two antioxidants called *'Lutein'* and *'Zeaxanthin'*, which help to protect your mince pies. Found in the yolk, Lutein and Zeaxanthin can significantly reduce the risk of macular degeneration and cataracts, which are among the leading causes of vision impairment.

If you decide to include eggs in your diet (and you really should) then make sure to eat omega-3 enriched, or Organic eggs because of their superior flavour and nutritional value.

Are eggs bad for you?
Well, you could catch salmonella from an infected egg, although the chances are about 200 million to one.
Bearing in mind that your chances of winning the lottery are about 14 million to one, I'd say that you should be ok.

READER *(in best Jim Carrey voice)*: *So you're telling me there's a chance?*
Yes there is a chance, in the same way there is a slim chance you could catch salmonella eating contaminated meat, poultry, green veg or fruit. Don't worry about it, you'll be fine. Just make sure that the eggs are kept refrigerated, you wash your hands before handling them, they're well cooked and you don't eat them if they pass their use-by-date. But you could say the same about any food, so don't be a scruffy Herbert and you'll be sorted.

Another reason eggs have been vilified for years is because eggs do contain a high amount of cholesterol (found in the yolk).
The irony is that many studies have shown that eggs, actually **improve** your cholesterol profile.
READER: *Why's that then?*
You see, eggs tend to raise HDL cholesterol (the good) and they regulate and reduce the LDL cholesterol (the bad) thus lowering your risk of heart disease.

READER: *Eggs are full of fat though aren't they?*
Not at all, only 4g per egg, with 1.5g being saturated fat. It's what you have with your eggs that contributes to the lard. For example, if it's part of a fry up, then the whole plate is gonna be full of saturated fat.

But if you're making scrambled eggs or an omelette, that dish will contain very little fat, especially if you only add a smidge of butter and milk. I like to add onions, watercress and mushrooms to my scrambled eggs but if you decide to add a colossal wedge of cheese to yours, then yep, that's a meal destined to send you to the Cardiac Unit at your local Hospital.

Can you go to work on an egg?
I'm sorry but no. It's not a form of transportation and if you sit on one, you'll break it.

So that's eggs. You just can't beat an egg.

Apparently, *'The Iron Lady'* used to eat about twenty-eight eggs a week, so it didn't do her any harm.

Although she did steal our milk, ruin the industrial heartlands of the North and was a child of Satan, so swings and roundabouts.

FAST FOOD

Take it away

If you love food so much, why do you eat junk?

I'm not a massive fan of fast food...
READER: *There's a shock. Now please insert that flagamathingymabob for me.*
In the words of the most quoted line from the fantastic film, *'The Princess Bride'*... **'as you wish'**:

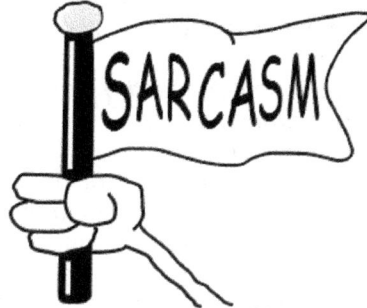

Well, it's probably down to the fact that I used to work in a fast food *'restaurant'* when I was studying at College therefore I have seen **how** the food is dealt with, and stored and cooked and how can I say this, erm... enhanced.
READER: *Enhanced, what do you mean?*
Let's just say that hygiene doesn't always go hand in hand with these establishments and some of the staff are disgusting, repulsive individuals, who delight in redistributing their biological waste.
READER: *Oh!!*
Aye! Although, I'm not saying they're all like that but some of them special sauces, contain very secret recipes, not for the faint hearted.
READER: Ok! Thanks. Move on please.

My main gripe with fast food joints is that the quality of the food is very poor, the food is high in calories, high in saturated fat, high in sugar and offers **very limited** nutritional value.

So if you eat a lot of junk food, stop wearing clothes. You should wear a bin bag instead, 'cos that's where rubbish goes.

It's called **FAsT** food for a reason

It's bleedin' obvious that if you're trying to lose weight and get fitter, you should drastically cut out eating anything from a takeaway, drive-thru, pizza shop or burger joint.
READER: *But, but, but...*
If you carry on, it's big butt, big butt, **BIG BUTT!!**

I can assure you that you won't miss takeaways and pizzas after a few weeks because cravings adapt and go away, but you will need patience and a large serving of willpower.

Don't worry, it can be done.

TERRY, 41 - *Being a tall bloke, I've always had a big appetite. Fry-ups for brekkie, doorstep bacon sarnies for lunch, pizzas and curries and takeaways and whatnot for tea.*

When I reached my 40th I had a big party and naturally folk took pictures and then uploaded them to Facebook. When I saw them I was repulsed and shocked by how big I'd become. I didn't have a neck anymore, I had moobs and my gut hung and flopped over my trousers. I had to do something about it, which is why I contacted you.

I've levelled at about 14st after being over 17st 7lb at the start of the year. Obviously walking every day has helped immensely but the biggest change came with my diet. I won't lie to you but I did cheat and have the odd bacon butty and pizza but overall I did as you recommended. I started to eat scrambled eggs or porridge for breakfast, which was a simple alteration to my old diet and I began experimenting by adding different ingredients to both. That was okay. Not a problem.

For dinner I'd make a packed lunch. At first the blokes at work took the mick 'cos I no longer had a bacon sarnie but after a while some of 'em started bringing in lunches too. It seems ridiculous to admit now but I was embarrassed at first getting my 'Tupperware' out but these days we even discuss different fillings and how to add leftovers to our lunch. It's been a real eye-opener, plus it's saved me a fortune not having to fork out for expensive sarnies.

The toughest change came with the evening meal. Knowing that when I got home I'd have to cook was soul destroying initially and that's why I'd relent and phone for a takeaway but after a few weeks it became easier. I'd plan my meals in advance for the week, and I'd spend my days at work looking forward to tea and some special meal I'd devised. And again, I saved loads of dosh not ordering pizzas and curries and burgers. The weight started to drop off significantly after a month or so and I knew it was worth it. And as I started to save more money, as well as losing the timber, I didn't want to ruin my good work, so I'd stop buying junk food.

When I walk past a pizza restaurant or curry house, I do start to get a bit of a craving but I just think of those pictures. Don't get me wrong, I still eat the odd burger, or curry now and again but that's with the new girlfriend and we try to get the healthiest versions possible.

I'm not a big beer drinker, so I don't get leathered and fancy a kebab or owt, which is great for me but I'm just pleased I have a chin again. And the moobs have gone too. Cheers for all the advice over the year mate.

Another thing that really pisses me off re the food industry is *'meal deals'*, especially those that are targeted towards children. Shops offering a low quality sandwich, a pack of salty crisps and a bottle of sugary pop. Fair do's it's a deal but it has **zero** nutritional value. Then take kids meals, in pubs for instance. *'Chips, beans and garlic bread'*, or *'chips, peas and sausages'*, or *'chips, peas and pizza'*, or *'chips, beans and nuggets'*. Absolute cack on a plate, yet we buy 'em and then wonder why kids grow up fat and addicted to crappy junk food.

Answer me this. Why don't we feed babies junk food?
READER: *Well, they need nutrients to aid growth and health.*
Exactly! So why do **you** eat crap just 'cos you're older? Or feed kiddies processed, cheap, low quality food, just 'cos they've outgrown the booties?

Do you ever feel run down and lethargic, or have stomach issues and headaches?
READER: *Yes, sometimes.*
Well it's 'cos you're eating shite.
As I keep prattling on, food should offer **value** and although fast-food is cheap, it has no positive nutritional value at all.

Look, I'm writing this book to help **you** and to educate **you**, then it's up to **you** to work it out. So here's some more snippets of info for you to peruse, then decide for yourself whether it's worth eating this junk when you're trying to lose weight.

If you really must venture into these establishments, rather than buying the 'extra-large' or 'jumbo', or 'let's make up another word to reflect how fuckin' mega this size is', get the small. At least you'll limit the amount of crap that goes in your gullet.

Be aware that the calories in a **burger** can range between 200-1200kcal and this is down to the fatty sauces, fatty sugary bread and saturated fat of the meat patties. Best option, go plain, this will restrict your calorie intake.

If you opt for a 'meal deal' and get fries **AND** a milkshake, or fizzy drink with your burger, you can end up consuming your **entire** daily calories and more, in this one 'meal'.

MILKSHAKES can contain between 400-800kcals and are full to the plastic lid with sugar, artificial flavouring, citric acid, guar gum, salt, saturated fat, high-fructose corn syrup and artificial sweeteners. Oh! And some milk. Be careful with that straw, brain freeze is not the only risk when sucking on those bad boys.

CHICKEN NUGGETS can contain over 800kcals and when a particular TV advert states that they're made from 100% chicken breast, what they neglect to tell you is that they still contain fat, ground bone and gristle. They're also full of sugar, salt, preservatives, oils and other chemicals.
Bear in mind that I could say a pork pie contains 100% pork, whilst omitting the other rather scary ingredients that are pummelled and mashed together to make up the 'meat'.
In fact, sod it. Here are the ingredients to a well-known brand of chicken nuggets. If you want a clue as to which brand, well I'm not going to McTell you.

Chicken nugget meat contains white boneless chicken, Water, Modified food starch and Salt
Seasoned with: Autolyzed yeast, Salt, Wheat starch, Natural flavour (botanical source), Safflower oil, Dextrose, Citric acid and Sodium phosphates
Battered and breaded with: Water, Bleached wheat flour, Niacin, Reduced iron, Thiamine mononitrate, Riboflavin, Folic acid, Yellow corn flour, Modified food starch and Salt
Leavening agents: Baking soda, Sodium acid pyrophosphate, Sodium aluminium phosphate, Calcium lactate, Mono-calcium phosphate, Spices, Wheat starch, Dextrose and Corn starch
Prepared in Vegetable Oil containing: Canola oil, Corn oil, Soybean oil, Hydrogenated soybean oil, with TBHQ and Citric Acid to preserve freshness of the oil and Dimethylpolysiloxane to reduce oil splatter when cooking

Now, I shudder to think what half of that stuff is but there is one ingredient that I **had** to research, and that is TBHQ.

What the blinkin' buggery is TBHQ?
TBHQ (E319 in the UK and Europe), which stands for 'Tertiary Butyl-Hydroquinone', is a synthetic antioxidant that is used to extend the shelf life and flavour of oily and fatty foods. It is commonly used in foods such as crackers, ice cream, microwave popcorn, noodles, butter and chicken nuggets of course but it is also found in non-food products such as cosmetics, paints, perfume, pesticides and varnish.
TBHQ actually contains elements of butane, which is a toxic chemical and a component of lighter fluid.
READER: *That doesn't sound good.*
No, no it doesn't. However, there are very tiny amounts added to chicken nuggets and even though it's banned in many countries, Europe and the USA have stated that the concentration of TBHQ allowed in foods is safe to consume.
So we can all put our minds at rest.

Yes, if you consume a 5g dose of TBHQ you will die. **Die I tells ya!!**
But who's gonna eat that much?! And prolonged exposure to TBHQ can cause dry skin, nausea, vomiting, headaches, dizziness, delirium, green or brownish urine, elevated liver enzymes, muscle twitching and tinnitus. But hey, all food's a gamble isn't it?

Scientific studies have also linked the consumption of TBHQ to hyperactivity in children, as well as asthma, dermatitis and food allergies for adults. But it's safe in small doses, so you know, go for it, don't worry. Enjoy!!

And we feed these chemical, processed, nuggets of nastiness to our kids **every** single day.
World's gone mad.

Chicken and **fish burgers** are generally higher in saturated fat than beef burgers, which is because they are deep-fried and are a concoction of meats, mixed and ground and pounded together to form what is then called *'chicken'* or *'fish'*. Be aware that they are often marketed as *'crispy'* which just means that they are high in calories, full of sugar and salt, and have been deep fried in fat.

Salad bars contain **huge** amounts of fat, salt and sugar in their cheesy, creamy mayo and dressings. Don't be fooled, sometimes you'd be better off with the burger. Alleged bacon bits, sodium infused croutons, floppy lettuce, fake cheese, rancid onions, sneeze covered tomatoes, warm, rank, over-preserved olives and sliced potatoes swimming in mayo to hide the discoloured, bruised, rotting mould. **Gross!!**

If you want a healthy, nutrition-packed salad, either go to a highly respected, well reviewed, salad emporium (with a sneeze-guard) or make your own.

RUBY MURRAY
Whether it's Indian or Thai or Jamaican or Vietnamese, curries contain a cornucopia of spices, nutritious vegetables, protein enriched meats and mesmerising flavours and tastes. Invariably, the six pints of lager you consume at the same time will mask these savours, but a curry can be quite healthy or extremely fattening, depending on what sauces you have and how much you eat.

A typical meal will also be accompanied with a naan bread or poppadoms, and wolfed down with copious amounts of rice. Effectively you have a very calorie-dense meal (well over 2000kcal in most cases), full of fat and sugar and salt, so any health benefits are negated. Dishes containing coconut milk and ghee, are generally the most fattening, so be prepared to start trying the other, equally as delicious, lower-calorie sauces instead.

We all love a curry now and again, so my advice is simple, don't go mental with the naan bread, remember they're for sharing. Only have a teeny-weeny bit of rice and knock yourself out re the meat and vegetable dishes. Oh! Get yer sophisticated head on too and plump for red wine, rather than lager. If you're trying to lose weight, then having curries every week is gonna hinder your progress, so limit them or that gut just will not go.

CHINESE FOOD
If you want your fortune cookie to read, *'You will wake the fit up, be happy, healthy and fit'* rather than, *'It's a shame you died early of a heart attack, due to a diet high in saturated fat, salt and sugar'* then you've gotta be careful when ordering from your fave Chinese takeaway.

The traditional Chinese diet mainly consists of vegetarian dishes, with meat products making up only a small proportion. This extremely healthy diet consists of stir-fried veg, steamed rice, soy products, fresh ginger, garlic and tofu. Traditional Chinese dishes are generally steamed, poached, broiled, roasted or lightly stir-fried in spices and peanut oil.

Yet what do we commonly order? Heavily battered, deep-fried, oily, meaty stuff coated in salty and sugar-laden sauce, which is oozing with fat, cholesterol and extremely high in calories. With chips. And rice. And noodles. And crackers. And a few beers.

Therefore you gotta play it smart. Chinese food can be **very** healthy if you select the right dishes.
Do some research, expand your choices and order carefully so that your meal contains a source of lean protein, is full of vegetables and contains an assortment of essential nutrients.

Just try a bit of variety, monotony is bad enough in life, so it's just as bad in your takeaway order.
READER: *Like what?*
Well, try a number 6, a number 38, a number 26...
READER: *I meant specifically, ya cheeky git!!*
Oh! Ok! Well, egg rolls are over 300kcal, contain about 30g of fat and are deep fried, so instead opt for a spring roll which has a third of the calories and there's only about 4g of fat. You could even ask them to be steamed rather than fried, although be prepared for a volley of Chinese abuse.

Prawn crackers are high in salt but are actually low in calories and fat, so try those instead of the fatty, deep-fried Wontons.

Having a soup for starters can fill you up quicker, which means you won't scoff as many chips.

Choose shrimp or chicken breast, rather than pork or beef because they are lower in cholesterol and aren't as fatty or gristly.

Steam your dumplings.
READER: *I'm sorry, what now?*
Rather than deep-fried dumplings, ask for the steamed variety and try to have as many stir-fried vegetables as you can stomach with your meal. Make veggies your side dish, rather than rice which is high in carbs, sugar and salt.

Teriyaki, mustard, hoisin and oyster sauces are lower in salt than soy sauce, and watch out for the dastardly *'Monosodium Glutamate'* (MSG).
READER: *Why, what's so bad about that?*
MSG is an additive that is added to a whole host of Chinese foods to enhance the savoury flavour.
It's also found in a lot of packaged food such as canned soup, crackers, crisps, gravy, processed meats, salad dressings, ready-meals, yoghurt and quite scarily, even in baby food.

MSG is made up of Sodium (salt) and Glutamate, and occurs naturally in a large range of foods including tomatoes, parmesan cheese, dried mushrooms, soy sauce, fruits, vegetables and breast milk.
But some people do have an allergic sensitivity to this addictive, toxic additive and can suffer from numerous adverse effects, such as visual impairment, headaches, fatigue, disorientation, insomnia, fainting, diarrhoea, depression, rapid heartbeat and asthma.

If you're happy to put up with that to satisfy your savoury cravings then fair play but in my opinion, you can shove your MSG up your R-S-OLE.

Hey!! Would you look at that, I wrote about Chinese takeaways and didn't even mention cats.
READER: *What do you mean?*
Oh! Nowt.
Nothing to see here Officer...

Blimey, I'm feeling a bit nauseated just typing this stuff about junk food, make the wonder they hand it to you in a brown paper bag.
READER: *What do you mean?*
Well, it gives you somewhere to be sick after you've eaten. **Ba dum tssshhh!!**

And now for something completely different, a food source that will definitely help you lose weight, as well as improving your health.

And there's no catch.

! ! WARNING! ! WARNING ! ! The next section of the book may contain bones ! ! WARNING ! ! WARNING ! !

FISH

If you can think of a fish pun, let minnow

You can grill it, you can poach it, you can fry it,
I really recommend that you try it,
Have it for lunch, or even for your tea,
Haddock and cod and anchovy,
There's more to fish than batter and chips,
Fish cakes, fish soup and even fish dips,
Kippers on toast and kedgeree,
Salmon-en-croute or a hot curry,
Shove it in a pie, or add it to a stew,
Fish is so healthy; it's so good for you!!

It's gone on long enough and I feel we're friends now, so I have to tell you something really embarrassing. I've got crabs.
READER: *Oh! Erm…*
Yeah, I have crabs… and tuna, and mackerel, and sardines, and prawns, and trout, all stocked fresh in the fridge and canned in the cupboard.
Oh! Yes!! I'm sorted for seafood.

READER: *Crabs aren't fish though!!*
You're right brainiac, they're crustaceans, as are lobster and prawns but they're still from the sea, thus sea-food.
Anyway, I've heard you've got a problem with seafood…
READER: *What do you mean?*
Well you see food and you eat it. Ha!! Ha!! Gone fishing!! Hook, line and sinker baby!!

Yes, it might be one of the oldest jokes in the world but it had to be done, you know, just for the halibut.
I thought salmon like you might appreciate that joke, you know, to put you in your plaice….
READER: *Alright, alright, enough with the fish puns already!!*
Soz!!

Fish and seafood in general, is low in fat, low in calories and rich in protein, vitamins and minerals.

However, some fish are better than others and the fatty, oily types of fish like salmon, trout, sardines, pilchards, tuna and mackerel, are considered the healthiest because they are a loaded with vitamins A, D and E, as well as high in Omega-3, which as we know is an essential nutrient for the body and brain.

bones

A healthy balanced diet should include at least **two** portions of fish a week, including one of oily fish and if you do, you'll benefit from a whole range of health benefits:

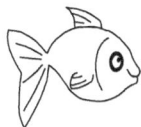

- Significantly reduce your risk of heart disease
- It can help to reduce blood pressure
- Help to lower cholesterol
- Improve your circulation
- Reduce the risk of arthritis
- Help prevent macular degeneration
- Reduce the risk of inflammatory bowel disease
- Aid lung functionality
- Help to combat the symptoms of skin conditions, such as eczema and psoriasis
- Reduce the risk of Dementia and cognitive decline
- Help to alleviate depression
- And help you to lose weight.

READER: *Wow!! Very impressive but what's that about helping to reduce weight?*
It's all to do with leptin and how the consumption of fish helps to enhance production.

'Leptin' is a hormonal message produced by the body's fat cells, which is vital in the regulation of appetite, food intake and body weight. Studies have shown that an absence of leptin in the body, or leptin resistance, can lead to uncontrolled feeding and weight gain. As you pile on the timber, the leptin signals to the brain are weakened thus appetite increases. And when weight loss occurs, leptin production is significantly reduced thus appetite also increases. A lose/lose situation.

However, a fish rich diet increases levels of leptin production, which helps to increase satiety levels, restricting appetite and reducing hunger cravings. Yep! You can't go wrong with fish and no, I'm not talking about fish-fingers.

Fish that is steamed, baked or grilled is a healthier choice than those deep-fried in fatty-batter, unless of course, you're at the seaside then I'm afraid it's the law and you **must** sample some fish and chips. As long as you eat them from a tray. With a wooden fork.

If you're desperate for fish, chips and mushy peas and you'd like a healthier alternative, then how about, grilled salmon, sweet potato wedges and chilli peas instead?
READER: *What are chilli peas?*
Aah! Another Birchy delicacy. Slap a tin of mushy peas into a pan, or blend some dried peas and mush yourself. Once peas are satisfactorily mushed, add to the pan a splash of cream, knob of butter, sprinkle of salt and pepper, some diced onions, sliced mushrooms, a pinch of chilli powder (or if you'd like it hotter, cut some red chilli, leaving the seeds in) and a few squirts of vinegar. Stir on medium heat for a few minutes and then pour onto your chosen fish and healthy chips. Thank me later.   bones

Open your mind, there's an infinite amount of cooking options out there, you've just go to experiment and find what works for you.
READER: *Fish is expensive though, isn't it?*
Nah! Not really. A decent fillet or steak can cost anything between two and five quid.
Most supermarkets have a Fishmongers now, so get acquainted, ask questions, get advice on how to cook and get your fish game on. A can of tuna will set you back less than a quid and mackerel, sardines, pilchards and salmon, can all be found in the tinned aisle and you could buy a selection and have change from a fiver.

But try to avoid battered and breaded fish from the frozen aisle.
READER: *Why, it's still fish isn't it?*
Aye but the batter and bread will be full of salt, sugar, some nasty additives and preservatives, plus the fish will be tiny, and of very poor quality. I suppose it's better than nowt but you're much better off opting for some fillets from the Fishmongers. And when it comes to the marine world, don't forget to be shellfish.

Crabs and prawns are full of nutrients and very cheap. And for those concerned about their skin, crab meat contains *'Eicosapentaenoic Acid'*, which helps **strengthen** and **firm** collagen thus giving your skin that healthy glow. Which means you can save a fortune on skincare products.
Because after all, you're worth it!!
bones

If you were so inclined, you can even get your tackle out and fish for your fish.
READER: *I don't know how to fish.*
Well you know what they say?! Give a man a fish and he will eat for the day, teach him how to fish and he will bore the pants off you telling you about his trips, and his rod, and his tent, and his flies and...

Mullet over and one day, you too could be a masterbaiter!! And if you're stuck for something to use for bait, try liquorice.
READER: *What type of fish will I catch with that?*
Oh! All sorts!!

FRUIT

Do you want a portion?

Now, I'm gonna shock you by imparting some amazing knowledge about fruit. Are you sitting down for this? Ok! You ready?
READER: *Ready?*
Fruit... is really good for you. I know. Bonkers isn't it?! Who knew?! Apart from every bloody one of you!!

There are thousands of varieties of fruit out there and each one is packed full of anti-oxidants, vitamins, minerals and nutrients. But most of us just don't get enough. Or eat enough fruit.

Five a day is the arbitrary target but it's not a limit, so try to consume as much as possible of these low calorie, low fat, fibre-enriched super-foods.

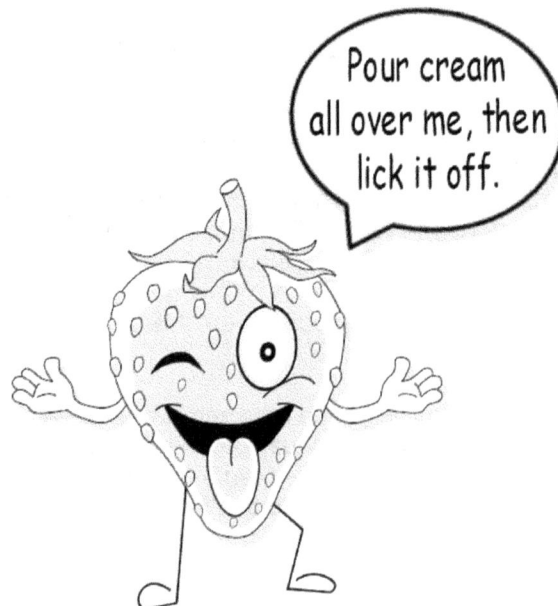

> Pour cream all over me, then lick it off.

READER: *I've heard that too much fruit is bad for me?*
Yeah, you're right. If I was you I'd just eat chocolate, biscuits, cake and packs of crisps.
READER: *Really??*

238

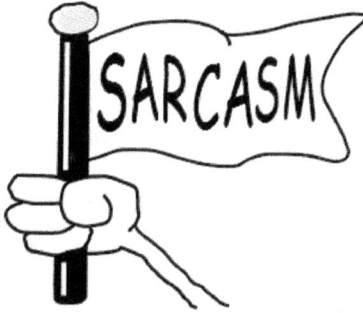

C'mon, it's like anything, the key is moderation due to fruit containing the sugar, *'fructose'* so your best bet is to eat berries because they contain less sugar than their citrus cousins.
READER: *There's not many types of berry though, is there?*
No, not at all.
Apart from Acai Berry, Bearberry, Bilberry, Blackberry, Blueberry, Cloudberry, Cowberry, Cranberry, Elderberry, Goji berry, Gooseberry, Honeyberry, Huckleberry, Josta Berry, Juniper berry, Lingon Berry, Mulberry, Raspberry, Seaberry, Strawberry and there's even Wineberries to name but twenty one.
READER: *Ok! Smartarse I was wrong, there's loads of berries.*
That's right baby!! And the best thing about 'em, is they even grow on trees.

READER: *Have you any tips to help me eat more fruit?*
I know it's a difficult choice, chocolate bar or pineapple? Biscuit or pear? Bag of crisps or a punnet of grapes? A slice of cake or a slice of banana? But if you want to get fitter, lose weight and feel healthier, then you're gonna have to opt for the fruit… sometimes, anyway.

It will help to satisfy your sweet tooth and won't increase your gut. The more you eat it, the more you'll like it.
I think one of the reasons people don't like to have fruit, is the mess. I mean, cutting up a pineapple is like performing an appendectomy, it takes surgical precision but it's worth the effort and lovely once sliced and diced. That's the pineapple, not the appendix.

And trying to unpeel an orange is very dirty work, gunge imbedded in your finger nails and juice splattered all over your face. But once peeled, everyone wants a portion. That's what they say to me anyway. Or you buy a punnet of blueberries, wash them and then inspect each individual berry like a primate scouring for ticks.
I get it. Which is why so many people opt for prepared fruit but let me tell you now, they might be more convenient but they're not as good for you. And they contain far less nutrients than fresh, unprepared produce.

As soon as they are harvested, the nutrients in fruit will begin to rapidly decrease and this will be accentuated by the preserving process which allows them to remain *'fresh'*, in their new plastic home.

Excessive freezing, pre-washed in tanks of water that contain chlorine, disinfectant, enzymes and fruit acids, this all contributes to destroying the levels of minerals and vitamins.

I mean look at an apple once it's been cut. After a few seconds it starts to brown, which is due to the polyphenols contained within the apple, reacting to oxygen exposure. In essence, once cut, the apple is beginning to rot. It's dying. And that's the same with all fruits (and vegetables).

Manufacturers try to stop this process and extend the shelf-life, initially by freezing and soaking in preservatives, and then by packing the fruit into *'Modified Atmosphere Packaging'*.
READER: *What's 'modified atmosphere packaging', never heard of it?*
This type of packaging involves altering the composition of air in plastic packs, so it contains significantly less, or no oxygen at all thus **slowing** the ageing process. That's why as soon as the plastic is perforated or removed, the fruit starts to die. Or maybe it's just desperate to breathe again.
That's why you should definitely try to avoid prepared fruit in packets, plus they're way more expensive than fresh produce.
READER: *Yes but it saves time.*

C'mon, it doesn't take that long really to slice into a fruit and cut off some pieces. If you've time to scroll through your phone looking at pathetic status updates, you've time to unpeel a mango and slice it. You've time to cut an apple into segments, or take some raspberries from a punnet and place into a bowl. It's just another crappy CBA excuse.

If you're **actively** seeking to lose weight, then you'll make the time.

If you can, try to buy your fruit from a Greengrocers, or if from the supermarket, the ones that are loose, not in that plastic, fake world packaging.

And when you want to eat the stuff, my advice is simple. Slice up a banana, chop up an apple, then chuck some blueberries, strawberries and whatever else fruit you can be fussed dissecting, into a bowl and add a few scoops of ice cream (that's scoops, not a full tub).
You'll devour that dish down in no time.

It helps get your five a day, satisfies your sweet cravings and if you've got kids, forces them to eat healthily for at least one meal a day.

Or you could whack some fruit in a smoothie-maker, complete with leaves, rind, pulp, skin, the whole shebang. Add some full-fat yoghurt ('cos that has more nutrients than sugary *'fat-free'* alternatives) and blend away.
READER: *Even the pips and seeds?*
Oh Aye!! It all adds to the flavour and it'll be a thousand times more nutritious than anything you could buy in a bottle. Although it will contain a lot of fructose therefore as I mentioned earlier, if you're making a smoothie it's best to restrict the citrus fruits.
READER: *Why, it's fruit, so by definition it's healthy?*
Common misconception. And one major reason why smoothies are not as healthy as the food industry promotes.

Keeping the fruit intact will help to retain the majority of the nutrients because most of the good stuff is contained in the outer parts of fruit anyway, but once that mechanical juicer, or smoothie-maker starts whirring, it breaks down the fruit, destroying most of the fibres and retaining the sugary fructose. This fructose gets absorbed rapidly during the digestion process and sent to the liver very quickly, just like when you drink a can of fizzy pap.

When the liver takes in more fructose than it can handle, some of it gets turned into **fatty fat fat!!**

Therefore you think you're doing yourself loads of good but you're not. It's counter-productive to your weight loss goals. However, having said that, it's far better than quaffing a can of coke, or munching on a chocolate bar or four.

READER: *What about buying fruit juice?*
No, no, no, no, no, no, no, no. **No!!**
They're just jam bloody packed with extra sugars, and preservatives, and additives, and other chemicals. They will make you fat and rot your teeth.
READER: *What, even orange juice?*
Yep, even orange juice, irrespective whether it's labelled as *'100% pure,'* or *'not from concentrate.'*

Although oranges are full of fibre, packed with vitamin C and other skin-enhancing nutrients, once blended, they are pulped and pulverised and mangled to such a degree that there's not much of the good stuff left. The flavour and taste isn't as nice as your average juicy orange, so the OJ manufacturers add **loads** of flavourings to make it more palatable (some will add sugar and artificial sweeteners too).
READER: *But they're advertised as really healthy.*
I know. It's a bloody disgrace.
An average glass of OJ can contain the equivalent of about nine teaspoons of sugar. Does that sound healthy to you?
READER: *Definitely not.*
If you make your own at home it's going to be far healthier, but your best bet will always be to eat the fruit, unfettered. You'll find that when you eat whole fruit it takes significant effort to chew and swallow, and even though they do contain fructose, these sugars are attached to the fibrous rind, and the pulp and the skin therefore they break down quite slowly during digestion. This means you don't get the sugar-rush which is common with

drinking OJ, or eating chocolate, or devouring a slab of cake. Just slice the fruit up, skin and all, chuck it in a bowl, add some cream, or ice cream, or maple syrup and spoon away.

The more you have it, the more you'll like it, I assure you.

In fact, that's another **Birchy Guarantee!!**

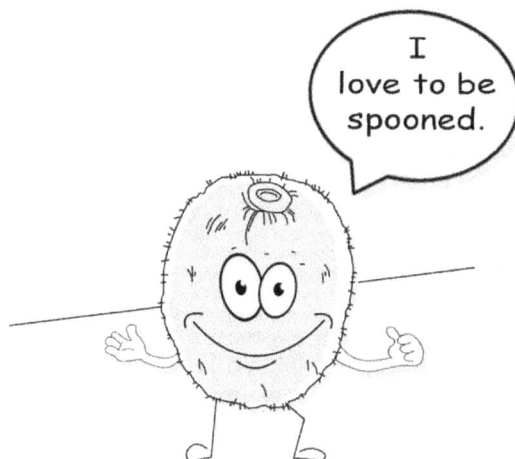

READER: *Thanks for all that but I don't really like fruit.*
Fair do's. I'm sure you've tried every fruit on the planet, so your statement is obviously true.

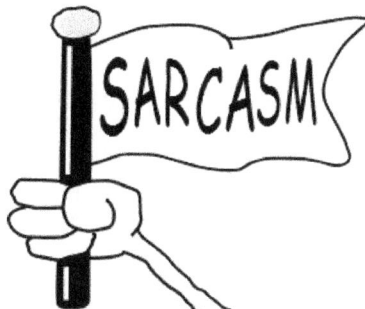

How about an Apricot?
READER: I don't think so, I'd rather not.
Blackcurrant? Tangerine?
READER: *I've heard of them, I'm not so keen.*
Mango? Melon? Physalis?
READER: *I think I'll give them, all a miss.*
Pomegranate? Lychee?
READER: *I bet they're nice but not for me.*
A Passion fruit is great when ripe,
READER: *I'm sure they are but not my type.*
Soursop? Kumquat?
READER: *Not for me and that is that!!*

Look, I'm sure there's at least **one** type of fruit that you've never tried, so the next time you're at the supermarket pop to the fruit aisle and take a gamble, play the fruit field. Who knows what you'll discover?
You might even try a Vampires favourite fruit.
READER: *What's that?*
A sanguinello.
READER: *Never heard of it.*
It's a blood orange. They're bloody gorgeous, you can count on that.

HERBS & SPICES

It's thyme for some flavour

Spice in Yorkshire used to be a ten pence bag of sweets when I were a lad but nowadays they are essential accompaniments to any meal, cooked in that there kitchen. They add what is commonly known as *'flavour'* to any dish, accentuating the taste and in addition, providing healthy nutrients on the side.

Spices can actually transform a meal by adding some serious zang, whether that's a hint of sweetness, a tart zing, or a kick of heat. I'm not talking just salt and pepper here either, there's thousands of funky herbs and spices for you to sample. Here's a selection of ten for you to sink your teeth into.

BASIL – From the mint family, there are about forty different types of Basil (or Bayzel, if you're American) each with their own unique colour and aroma. This herb is very low in calories and contains many essential nutrients and minerals including iron, potassium, and the vitamins A and K.

Depending on the variety basil can be green, white or even purple and it's highly fragrant leaves are used to season and flavour soups, poultry, red meat and vegetable dishes. It combines well with tomato and consequently appears in a wide range of Italian meals. It is also the main ingredient of the fatty sauce *'Pesto'*, which can be delicious when added to pasta but only in **small** dollops, rather than an entire jar like you normally do.
READER: *Who me?*
Yes, **you**. I've seen you. **Stop it!!**

You can buy basil in dried form but it is more nutritious when fresh, and it is best to tear basil leaves rather than chop them, as the metal from the knife can actually alter the taste.

CARDAMOM – No, not a birthday card for your Mum but a spice made from the seed pods of various plants in the ginger family. Cardamom has a strong, pungent, smoky flavour and a rich aroma, with hints of lemon and mint. Cardamom seeds are often found in Indian cuisine and are used to add a citrusy flavour to curries and basmati rice.

There are many medicinal benefits attributed to cardamom, and it is linked to healthy teeth and gums, offers relief from gastrointestinal issues, can help to lower cholesterol and aid in the improvement of blood circulation.

In the mystical world of Aromatherapy, it is thought that cardamom possesses aphrodisiac properties and is used as a cure for impotency, erectile dysfunction and premature ejaculation.
Which will be great for **you!!**
32% of MALE READERS: *Me?*
Yes, you. Apparently!! Therefore if I was **you**, I'd be adding cardamom to all my meals. Pop it in your granola for some added bite, your sarnies for extra crunch and enhance your **meat and two veg!!**

CAYENNE PEPPER – Ok! It sounds like an American pop star (I've got all her albums) but this herb from the chilli family offers a whole host of health benefits, in addition to adding hot, spiciness to any dish. Cayenne pepper is thought to increase metabolism, reduce blood pressure, lower cholesterol, ease stomach problems, clears sore throats, improve digestion and relieve muscle pains. It could probably help to solve world peace if given a chance.

And for those slaphead readers out there, Trichologists are now conducting studies using cayenne pepper to help increase hair growth. Who knows, that miracle cure maybe found in this wondrous, powdered spice.
Cayenne pepper is also used for seasoning and a sprinkle or four can add some fire to a stew, salad, soup or sauce. It even works in dishes that don't begin with an *'S'*.

Personally, I like to add cayenne pepper to my scrambled eggs but you'll find it adds some **Oomph** to baked potatoes, ice-cream, tea, lemonade, pasta, fish and rice. It's also great in chocolate cake, not that you're bothered about that type of thing.

CINNAMON – is a popular spice found in all sorts of recipes, as well as being the name of a dog that stars in a well-known USA comedy about Nerds and Geeks and Space and stuff. *'Yes Penny, I will marry you and have your children'.*

Cinnamon, with its seductively sweet aroma is often added to biscuits, cakes and puddings but this versatile spice is also used in curries, stews and rice dishes.

Back in the days of *'Cleopatra'* (no, not the band from Manchester, the Pharaoh), cinnamon was more valuable than gold. Nowadays you can buy some sticks or a jar for less than a few quid but the reason it was so treasured was down to its astonishing health benefits.

Cinnamon has a high concentration of anti-oxidants and when consumed has been found to significantly reduce blood pressure, lower cholesterol, help to prevent Dementia and improve insulin sensitivity.

Cinnamon has been used in Chinese medicine and Ayurveda for thousands of years and is revered for its medicinal qualities...
READER: *Hang on, isn't all this like that Homeopathy malarkey, its rubbish isn't it?*
Look, if I've cut my arm and someone offers to rub a plant over the wound, I'll politely tell them to go forth and multiply. With themselves. But plants, herbs and spices are **full** of anti-oxidants, minerals and vitamins, and that fact cannot be disputed. Therefore if you absorb these nutrients via your diet, it stands to reason that you'll benefit.

That's one of the main points I'm trying to communicate about food, and the importance of nutrition. Carbohydrates, fat, fibre, minerals, protein and water are all **essential** for life, and we obtain these nutrients through our consumption of food.

Having as much nutritional knowledge as possible and making smart, considered choices about the foods you eat, will help **you** achieve optimum health and is the key to helping you accomplish your weight loss goals, as well as helping you to knock depression on the head.
So, can I continue imparting this wisdom, coupled with hilarious comments?
READER: *You may.*
Gracias!!

Ok! Back to cinnamon, it's gorgeous in coffee as I mentioned earlier, give it a whirl.

CORIANDER – is one of the world's most commonly used herbs due to its fresh, strong, citrus taste.
Used as a flavouring or garnish, the leaves are rich in vitamins A, C and K, calcium, fibre, iron and protein.
Coriander is used in a lot of Indian and Thai dishes and goes well with chicken, fish and meatballs.

It won't surprise you to learn that coriander has been linked with a myriad of health benefits.
It helps to lower cholesterol and blood sugar levels, improves liver functionality, helps to prevent Dementia, aids vision, eases arthritis pain and relieves mouth ulcers.

It's also good for lady problems.
FEMALE READERS: *Careful now....*
You know what I'm on about? It's that monthly surprise that seems to inspire an unrelenting desire to roller-skate, dance, jog, laugh uncontrollably and abuse your partner.

Coriander seeds contain vital anti-inflammatory properties, which have been proven to help reduce the discomfort of menstrual pain and cramps. Apparently, take a handful of seeds, boil them in water until very little water remains, leave to stand, and then drink when cool. Hopefully it works but if not, I'm really sorry regarding that thing that I *'may'*, or *'may not'* have done. What else can I do? I could rub your tummy, make you a nice cup of tea, fetch you a hot water bottle or alternatively, yes, I can fuck off and die!!

GARLIC – The King of spice.
This super-food is awesome and an excellent source of vitamin C, calcium, iron and protein.

Not only can you ward off Emo's, deter blood-junkies and repel pretty girls in nightclubs who can't stand your pongy breath, it has countless medicinal properties. Most of the health benefits are due to a compound called, *'Allicin'*. This phenomenal element is responsible for the overpowering whiff of garlic, as well as helping to strengthen your bones, boost your immune system and metabolism, reduce skin blemishes, fortify your locks (hair, not pad), reduce cholesterol, lower blood pressure, prevent Alzheimer's and fight the sniffles. These cloves of wonder will complement most dishes and can add a distinct punch, to otherwise bland recipes. It's great in mash, goes well with a roast and should be added to all tomato-based sauces to add some bite to the flavour.

You can buy garlic as a whole bulb; get it as a paste, in powder form or even as an oil. I do recommend however, that you invest in a powerful toothbrush, complete with extremely minty toothpaste and a bacteria-destroying mouthwash, if you end up consuming this uniquely, aromatic spice on a daily basis. Like what I do.
READER: *Ah! Now we know why you're single.*

GINGER – The strawberry blonde of the spice world and one of the healthiest, loaded with nutrients and funky bioactive compounds.

Ginger is another spice with a very long history of use in alternative medicine and it's been prescribed for millennia to aid digestion, reduce nausea and fight the common cold.

Ginger can help to alleviate joint pain, lower blood sugar, reduce menstrual pain, lower cholesterol, prevent gum disease, ease stomach problems, improve cognitive function and split up The Spice Girls.
Oh aye, there's more to ginger than just beer, bread and biscuits.

Ginger can be used fresh, dried, powdered, or as an oil and adds some zing-a-ling to chicken, pork, fish, potatoes, stews, soups, stir-fries and your wee willy-winkie!!
READER: *What?*
Yeah, ginger has been prescribed for thousands of years as an afro-dizzy-yak. So if you have problems with your downstairs mixer, slap some ginger…
READER: *What, there?*
No, on your meals, yer daft **wazzock!!**

NUTMEG – You'll find nutmeg dusted on an egg custard, which are one of my favourite desserts, irrespective that they're high in calories and full of fat and sugar. I chuffin' love 'em, (typed whilst drooling).

Nutmeg is another spice famed for its *'rise to the occasion'* qualities, as well as a stack of other health enhancing benefits. A little sprinkle goes a long, long way.

This sweet aromatic spice can help to relieve joint pain, soothe indigestion, strengthen cognitive function, detoxify the body, boost skin health, alleviate gum disease, reduce insomnia, increase immune system function and improve blood circulation. Blimey Charlie, spices are bloody awesome aren't they?!

Nutmeg is known as the *'winter spice'* because of its Xmas connotations and is used to flavour festive drinks, like eggnog and mulled wine. Added to a plethora of desserts, nutmeg also works well in bread, in curry, in sauces, stews, soup, in meat dishes and it gives gravy a bit of a kick as well. It's also great in bed.
READER: *Pardon?!*
This might be an old wives tale but it seems to work on some people. If you're experiencing trouble kipping, or you're feeling a bit restless, try drinking some warm milk with a dash of nutmeg.

Nutmeg possesses mild sedative properties and this will help to make you feel drowsy.

Oh! And whilst we're on the subject, never take a sleeping pill and a laxative at the same time.

Don't ask me how I know, I just do and I won't be making that mistake again.

PAPRIKA – It may sound like a perfume, or even the name of a posh lass from the Home Counties but paprika is yet another super-spice full of health-boosting nutrients. Made by grinding sweet and hot capsicum peppers into a vibrant reddish powder, it's bursting with rich flavour. Paprika will add some pizzazz to any dish but it really adds some pep to beef, rice, chicken, fish, eggs, pasta and vegetables. Heck, if you're feeling really adventurous, it pairs well with a dark, orangey, hot chocolate. Not my cup of tea but give it a go.

Paprika is a very good source of the vitamins A, C, E and K, plus the minerals, iron and potassium.
It's yet another spice that will help to reduce macular degeneration, ease arthritis and joint pain, improve your metabolism, support healthy digestion, lower blood pressure and is also thought to slow down the signs of hair loss. Although don't shampoo with it, you have to consume it.
BALD READERS: *I'm just popping out to the shops love, I'll see you later...*

But paprika is best known for its positive impact on the skin, and this is because it contains a group of carotenoids that help to protect and boost collagen.
READER: *What are carotenoids?*
Well, they may sound like robotic veggies but *'Carotenoids'* are in fact plant pigments responsible for the red, yellow and orange hues you see in many bright fruits and vegetables. Natures very own food dye.

One of the carotenoids in paprika is *'Beta-Carotene'*, which after consumption the body converts to *'Retinol'*, which is imperative for healthy skin.
READER: *I've heard of that stuff, what is it?*
Aah! Well, *'Retinol'* is that ingredient you've probably heard about during adverts for those *'expensive'* skin creams.
Apparently, *'Retinol'* helps to smooth fine lines and lessen the appearance of wrinkles, reduce dark spots and skin imperfections, brighten the skin and make pores look smaller. In the advert, this will all be said by a gorgeous air-brushed glossy-haired woman, sporting a gleaming, pearly-white-toothed-grin. And to be fair, there is some truth in that claim.

Retinol creams can cause drying and flakiness, severe reddening and **should not** be used if you have sensitive skin, but it really does work... to a microscopically small degree. Yes, it will improve elasticity and increase collagen production but it's not gonna reverse the ageing process. **Soz abar dat!!**

Retinol is just a snazzy name for vitamin A but the kind you'll find in your fancy opaque jars is a chemically created version, whereas the stuff you'll find in paprika and other fruit, vegetable, plant and spice sources, is fundamentally better for you.
READER: *Why?*
Because it's **natural!!**

During the manufacturing process to produce your glitzy anti-wrinkle cream, any natural ingredients included will have the majority of their anti-oxidants destroyed in order to create this wonder-product. And any synthetic ingredients added, will never have the same health-boosting effects of their natural equivalents because they're fake, counterfeit, poor imitations. **UN-NATURAL!!**

Mother Earth is the best dermatologist out there and you can either spend a bloody fortune on weird skincare products, (now with *'Glycobollical Acid'* and *'Phytodynamic Therapy'* etc-scummy marketing tool-etc) or you can eat your way to great skin.

TURMERIC – Talking of spices that are good for the skin, this leads me neatly onto turmeric and the last in my top-ten countdown.

Very popular with Asian and Indian cuisine, this spice looks a bit like a ginger root and when it's ground down into a powder, it has a very distinctive yellowy-orange colour. It's one of the main ingredients of chicken tikka masala but you'll find it adds some peppery kick to scrambled eggs, lamb, stir-fries, casseroles, soups, fish dishes and of course, curries.

There are some impressive health benefits attached to the consumption of this peppery spice and it relates to a compound contained within called *'Curcumin'*. Curcumin is a remarkably powerful antioxidant which has been shown to help combat depression, alleviate menstrual problems, boost the immune system, prevent Alzheimer's, reduce the risk of heart disease, relieve the pain of arthritis, lower cholesterol and improve digestion.

READER: *Woah there!! Look, I've read all about these ten spices now and it just seems too good to be true.*

Ooh! You non-believer you. **Heretic!!**

Fair do's, I can understand your reticence but I can assure you that **thousands** of scientific studies have taken place to verify these claims. I've always said *'that if you're not cynical, then you're not paying attention'*, so **you** have to assess the evidence **for** and **against**, to establish if information promoted on TV or in books and magazines, is actually true.

In anything, whether that's news, politics or amazing herby-health-giving properties.

I implore you to check out these facts yourself and then make objective decisions but as I keep reiterating throughout this book, I'm trying to help you, so why would I lie?
READER: *I suppose but...*
The proof is in the pudding, so it's up to you to try these foods for yourself. Experiment, get out of that comfort zone and take a break from the old, boring, repetitive routine. I'm trying to be as open and transparent as possible with you, so you can help change your life for the better.

Lose that weight, get fitter and ultimately, live a moderately happy, fulfilling life.

Now we're all aware of the Big C and its devastating effect on people's health and lives, well cancer specialists throughout the world are now conducting research and studies, on the amazing health properties of some herbs and spices.

Scientists have found that certain ones, which contain *'Phytochemicals'* can stimulate the immune system, restricting and inhibiting the growth of cancerous cells. There are hundreds of published, peer-reviewed studies demonstrating the anti-cancer power of spices such as cayenne pepper, chilli pepper, oregano, garlic, ginger, paprika and turmeric.

I'm not saying these are miracle foods and they will help you become invincible but they'll help.
So, if you want to transform any dish and your health at the same time, head to the spice rack and see for yourself. I've been adding herbs and spices to my meals for years. Yep, I'm a seasoned veteran.

LEGUMES

Sorry but jelly beans don't count

You may be wondering *'what the ecky thump is a Legume?'* well, I'm gonna tell ya.
Legumes are the pod-grown, edible seeds of plants and just like blokes there are two kinds, *'Mature'* and *'Immature'*.

Mature legumes are the dried seeds found inside these pods and they are also known as, *'Pulses'*.
The most common varieties include broad beans, butter beans, chickpeas, lentils and kidney beans.

Immature legumes are those that just don't want to commit, don't want to grow up, and have an irrational fear of relationships and settling down.
READER: *Sorry?*
Oops, I hear the word *'immature'* and instantly go back to conversations I've had with ex-girlfriends.

Where was I? Ah yes, immature legumes have been harvested before they mature, such as green beans and garden peas but for the benefit of this book, I'll be lumping those type of legumes in with the veggies.
A healthy consumption of legumes has been associated with helping to prevent heart disease, lowering cholesterol levels and reducing blood pressure, according to the white-coated boffinistas. This is due to the fact that mature legumes are a great source of calcium, carbohydrates, fat, fibre, iron, protein and selenium

There are over 13,000 species of legumes and here's a few that I suggest you should try:
Alfalfa...
READER: *What is alfalfa?*
Alfalfa sprouts are highly nutritious, very crunchy and nice in salads. Plus, what a fantastic word, which in my opinion should be said as much as possible.

Darling, did you get the alfalfa?
Yes dear, I purchased the alfalfa this afternoon

Yes I am mad.
Go on say the word *'Alfalfa'*, try it for yourself.
READER: *Alfalfa. Alfalfa... ALFALFA!!*
Good on you. It's such a ridiculous word, it's ace.

So, there's Alfalfa and Asparagus bean, Baby lima bean, Black bean, Black-eyed pea (no not them), Black turtle bean, Boston bean, Boston navy bean, Broad bean, Cannellini bean, Chickpeas, Chili bean, Cranberry bean, Dwarf bean, Egyptian bean, Egyptian white broad bean, English bean, Fava bean, French green bean, Great northern bean, Kidney bean, Lentils, Lima bean, Madagascar bean, Mexican black bean, Mexican red bean, Mung bean, Mungo bean, Navy bean, Peruvian bean, Pinto bean, Red bean, Red clover, Red eye bean, Red kidney bean, Rice bean, Small red bean, Snow pea, Southern pea, Soybean, Wax bean and White kidney bean, to name but 42.

Now, I'm not saying you can purchase all of these from your local Express Supermarket, so you might have to go to those oddly smelling, Health-food Shops instead but you can definitely get tinned broad beans, cannellini, chick peas, kidney beans, lentils and pinto beans from most High Streets, so give 'em a go.

Not only are legumes highly nutritious, they are also very cheap and quick to make, which makes them an important food staple for anyone's shopping list, especially in these days of austerity.

Often used as a meat-substitute, personally I like to pair them with beef, tuna or salmon but there's no law, you can add them to what you like.

They'll help you stay fuller for longer, reducing the need to snack and they're great in stews and soups, as well as being an excellent grain replacement.
READER: *What do you mean by 'grain replacement?'*
As an alternative to rice in the main, which is starchy, low in nutritional value and extremely bland when you think about it. Legumes could also replace pasta, noodles or potatoes.

For instance, *'Spaghetti Bolognese'* could be *'Kidney Bean Bolognese'*. If you're having curry, swap the rice for lentils, or pinto beans. Basically if you're trying to lose weight, which I assume you are, you've gotta make healthier choices regarding your meals. Try different food sources and then pick the ones that work for you.
I'll discuss rice and pasta later on in this section but just because it's the norm to eat them, doesn't make it mandatory. Don't follow everyone else, or conform... lead. Who knows, you might be writing a funky cook book yourself in a few years, full of fantastic refreshingly unique, highly nutritious, low calorie meals. I for one can't wait to read it.

I'd like to finish off this section by telling you about my favourite legume, *'Lentils'*.

For most of my life I'd never eaten lentils because I was put off a bit by the stereotypical image.
When you think of lentils you instantly think of crusty, afghan-jumper-wearing, mucky-dreaded, joss stick loving hippy types, smoking that funny tobacco over a pot of lentil stew, which sub-consciously put me off. And for some reason I assumed they'd be plain, insipid and tasteless.

How wrong I was. Lentils are low in calories, high in fibre, a rich source of protein, full of minerals and vitamins, and virtually *'fat-free'*. Quick and easy to make, they can help lower your cholesterol, reduce blood pressure, aid digestion and prevent heart disease.

Open a can or packet, shove 'em in a pan, sprinkle on some paprika and cayenne pepper, chuck in some veg, and tuna or beef, stir for a few minutes and then serve. Hot, spicy and bloody delicious. Very filling too. The only drawback is a few hours after consumption you will parp like you've never parped before. And boy, they will be pungent.
READER: *Oh! That's disgusting.*
Look, everyone does it and it's entirely healthy and natural, just a by-product of your digestion system absorbing nutrients.

It's not a crime, so don't be ashamed of your bottom-burps. Just think of them as the screams of dying fat.

So join me in praise of the mighty lentil:

Let's go fuckin' LENTIL,
Let's go fuckin' LENTIL,
La, La, La, LA!!! Ooh!!!
La, La, La, LA!!! Aah!!!
Let's go fuckin' LENTIL,
Let's go fuckin' LENTIL,
La, La, La, LA!!! Eee!!!
La, La, La, LA!!! YEAH!!!

READER: *You're off yer head, you!!*
It's called having a laugh... **try it sometime.**

MARGARINE

To spread or not to spread?

READER: *I've often wondered which is better for me, margarine or butter?*
Butter is considerably better for you than margarine. **Fact!!**
One comes from a cow, the other from a test tube. Next…

READER: *Woah! Hold your horses. Is that it?*
What more do you need?
READER: *Can you explain why?*
Oh! Alright then. Blimey, you want everything on a plate you don't ya?! That's your problem…..
READER: *Sorry, what?*
Err, nothing, just horsing around… so then, butter or margarine?

There have been thousands of scientific studies performed over the last fifty years or so, trying to prove that marg is better than butter. Yes, some were financed by the Margarine Manufacturers and some were independent but would you Adam and Eve it, the majority have stated that marg contains less saturated fat than butter; ergo it's deemed to be better.
READER: *But you've just said…*
Patience my child, I haven't finished yet.

Butter is a **natural** dairy product that comes from our good mates, the cows. Essentially, it's made by churning cream or milk to separate the solid components from the liquid and once dispersed, these solids form butter. Yes there will be some preservatives added to enhance the shelf-life but all in all, butter is wholly natural.

Margarine was developed as a substitute for butter and is produced by mixing a variety of oils, additives, preservatives, colourings, emulsifiers and fancy E numbers together, to form a synthetic, hotchpotch excuse for butter. Most margarine brands are nowadays fortified with vitamins, olive oil, Omega 3 and other additives that claim to lower cholesterol.

When it comes to flavour, rich, creamy butter, trumps bland marg every single time and has the added bonus of containing the vitamins A, D, E and K, as well as being a rich source of selenium.

We've been eating one of these products for thousands of years, whereas the other, we've only been eating for the last century. One is cheaper to make than the other and I'll leave you to guess which is which.

There is no doubting that butter contains saturated fat and there is no denying that margarine contains high levels of polyunsaturated fat (Transfats) but what has been debated for years is the impact on cholesterol levels and the potential for heart disease, based on these two fats.

Now I could rattle on for ages, quoting study after study but the basic conclusion is that transfats will help to raise the bad cholesterol (LDL) whereas saturated fat will help to raise good cholesterol (HDL). Thus butter is better… but ultimately, both products are full of fat therefore must be consumed in moderation.

Personally, I would always opt for the more natural food type over its synthetic and chemically created counterpart but fundamentally it boils down to taste. And that is and always will be, subjective.

I rarely have toast these days but when I do, I slather butter on it.

You can do what you like.

MEAT

As fit as a butcher's dog

Your passion for food is unquestioned,
You just love to raid that fridge,
Well I've got a culinary treat for you,
And it's called a tongue sandwich.

Back in the day when I was a wee bairn, my Mum used to love a bit of tongue...
READER: *I bet she did!!*
Hey!! That's me bloody Mam you're talking about there, have some respect.
READER: *Sorry.*
No probs, anyway, yeah me Mum used to love a slab of meat... **Behave yourselves!!**
READER: *I never said anything.*
Good, alright then.

Mum would go to the Supermarket at the weekend and buy a selection of sliced meats, which we'd have in sandwiches for our tea but because we didn't have much brass, she'd have to buy some of the cheaper cuts, which is why she ended up taking a likening to tongue. It looked disgusting to me but I had no room to talk, 'cos I used to make butties using corned beef and I can't imagine what is mushed together to make that concoction.

But that's all we could afford, so we ate it, even though it's clear that there's a humongous thick line between quality and cheap, processed, congealed shite.

Mass-produced processed meat has become another leading contributor to the obesity crisis, due to the consumption of cheap bacon, sausages, hotdogs, pates, spreads, pepperoni, salami, tinned meats and *'alleged'* meat sauces, which have very little nutritional value and are full of salt, sugar and saturated fat.

Yes, I know that we're all watching the pennies these days but if you're trying to lose weight, then I suggest that you avoid the processed stuff. And to be fair, your local Quality Butcher will offer better cuts than you'll find at the supermarket, and at very reasonable prices. So I strongly recommend you take a visit, plus they're great at making suggestions on how to cook the meat in order to achieve the best flavour and taste.

Right, let's give processed meat a good grilling over.

Years ago, me and my mates were having a lads weekend away at the seaside and on the journey up, we stopped off at a supermarket to get some quick grub and raid the cash machines.

Whilst perusing the sandwich aisle, I saw one that simply stated *'Meat sandwich'*.
Obviously, I asked myself, *'err what type of meat? Beef? Chicken? Dog? Human?'*
I didn't know, I didn't ask and I didn't pay the quid to find out.
Surely that's against some Food Advertising Standard or something but regardless, they were selling it and I weren't buying it.

And what about the horse meat scandal a few years ago, that was a complete mare for those consumers who liked ready meals but that's the gamble buying food that contains processed meat, you haven't got a clue what it is.
READER: *Ok! Well, what is processed meat?*

The term *'processed'* applies to any food type that has been **modified** from its natural state, in order to extend its shelf life, or alter the taste. With respect to meat, once the animals have been slaughtered, they are salted, smoked, cured and then treated with additives, preservatives, sugars and various other chemicals.

The resulting carcass is then ground up, squashed, pulverised, squeezed, mangled and mushed together to form chunks, mince, lumps and compressed globules of meat. Yummy, yummy, yummy, I want them in my tummy!!

Processed meat may be tasty (debatable) but it has consistently been linked with harmful effects on our health, from high blood pressure to heart disease, to bowel and stomach cancer.

One of the main reasons processed meat is so damaging, is due to the carcinogenic compounds that are released during exposure to high heat. You then gobble these up unknowingly after consuming that fry up, or that *'I've had a bad week, so I've earnt this peperoni pizza'*, or that *'I can't be arsed cooking, so I'll have a lasagne ready meal instead'*. And one of those compounds is *'Sodium Nitrite'*, which is added to processed meats to preserve the reddish, pinky colour of the meat, enhance the flavour and prevent the growth of bacteria, to reduce potential food poisoning.

READER: *What, so I can't eat processed meat anymore?*
You can do what you like.
You've got freedom of choice. I'm just explaining to **you** that those particular types of meat are fatty, high in calories, salty, of dubious origin and could potentially cause cancer. If that still appeals to you, then carry on guzzling.

As a race, humans have eaten meat for millennia but our ancestors didn't consume **meat** that had been fed on growth-promoting hormones and anti-biotics, or mished and mashed and moshed together to form these poor excuses for meat.

No, they ate animals that had roamed free in the wilds, munched on grass and frolicked about, not born and raised in an industrial slaughterhouse, shunted into cages and fed artificial grain-based feed.

Their final anguished screams, accompanied by the shocking sound of a pneumatic captive bolt, before they are then ripped mercilessly apart and fed to the mincing machine.
Stunning!!

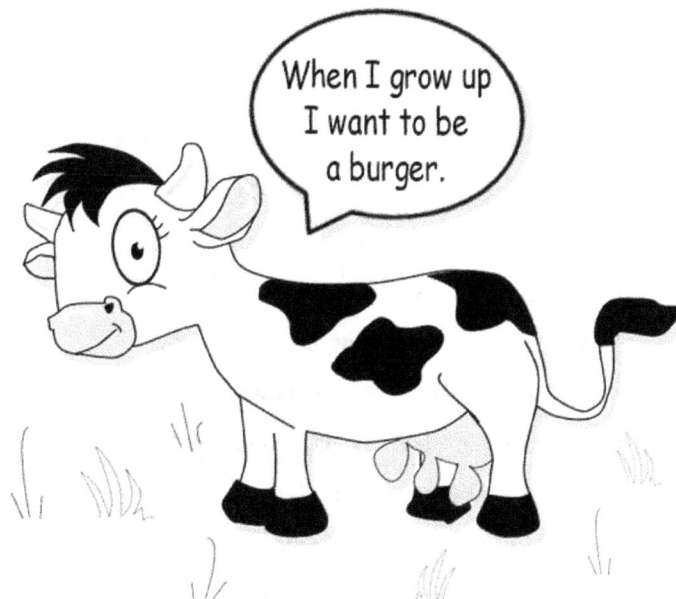

Stupid cow!!

That's why if **you must** have the meat, head to the Butchers. At least you know that the meat is locally sourced, unfettered, moderately happy, virtually additive free and actually, highly nutritious.

READER: *So now you're saying, meat is good for me?*
Definitely, meat is an excellent source of protein, B vitamins, and minerals such as iron and zinc.
Although, I'd eat red meat in moderation.
READER: *Which ones are the red meats?*
Meats that are pinky-red when raw are defined as *'Red'* meats and these include sheepies, moo-cows and piggy wigs. Meats that are white when cooked are defined as, surprise, surprise *'White'* meats, and these include chick-chick-chick-chick-chickens and other fowl, such as the one we only seem to gobble up at Xmas.

Organic meat is the kind that comes from animals that have been raised lovingly on the farm, free to bez and muck about in the safe knowledge they won't be laced with horrible additives and other chemicals.

READER: *Is beef ok?*
Hey, I love a bit of funky Friesian, especially a fillet of steak but it's very rare if I have one.
READER: *Well done…*
No, medium rare, I find that the steak is very juicy and tender when cooked this way.

Actually, beef is one of the most nutritious foods you can eat and is loaded with vitamins, minerals, antioxidants and various other nutrients which can have profound effects on your health. In fact, if you dream of being a Billy-Big-Bob, beef also contains *'Creatine'*, which is excellent for building muscle. Whether it's a casserole, spicy stir-fry, or the good ol' Sunday roast, you can't go wrong with beef.

My only beef with beef is down to the quality again, so if you're gonna chow down on cow, aim for grass-fed beef from the Butchers, not packaged, fatty, grain-fed beef from the Supermarket.

Oh! Before I forget, try to trim and remove as much of the fat as you can in order to reduce the saturated fat content. The leaner the cut of beef, the better it is for you.

Also, marinate the beef overnight in spices, red wine, lemon juice or olive oil perhaps because this will definitely enhance the flavour and tenderise the meat. If you must fry, then fry but beef (and all other types of meat) is just as nice when cooked by roasting, stewing, steaming or grilling.

Turkey mince and chicken thighs,
Braising steak and Shepherd's pies,
Hotdogs, pork chops, beefy stew,
Bangers burnt on a barbecue!!
Quarter-pounders, in a bun,
Sunday roast for everyone,
Oxtail soup with chunks of meat,
Toad-in-the-hole, bon-appetit!!
Meat balls, meat loaf, lamb for tea,
Boiled ham, mixed grill for me,
Pigging on meat for evermore,
Don't resist, you're a carnivore!!

READER: *What about offal?*
If you ask me, offal is awful.

The thought just makes me want to… **bleeuurrgghh!!**… PUKE!!

But Hey!! If you fancy a plate of internal organs or the entrails of an animal, then go for gold. The liver and kidneys especially are packed full to the gristly, spongey membrane with minerals and nutrients. So your choice mate, waste not want not but tripe, faggots and giblets, want, I do not.

I'm not gonna go through each type of animal re the meat and cuts, and so on and so forth but suffice to say, most meat is extremely nutritious and really good for you… if you buy from the Butchers. And remember, the more processed meat you consume, the more harm you will cause to your health.

Oh yeah! If someone offers you eight legs of venison for forty quid, turn it down, it's too dear!!

And if you receive an e-mail spouting that you can lose weight by just eating tinned pork, delete it immediately… it's just **SPAM!!**

MILK

Hmmm!! Calci-yum-yum-yum!!

We just can't get enough of the Udder Juice!!

Now, I'm not gonna comment on the first person who tried cow's milk and **what** they were actually doing before they ended up with a creamy moustache but it's safe to say that this visionary, has a lot to answer for. We put it in tea, pour it on our sugar-flakes, add it to porridge, we even have a mug of warm frothy milk to help us reach sleepy-la-la-land and whenever you're out, invariably you've gotta grab some on your way home.

I'm talking cow's milk here by the way, not goats, or pigs, or cats, or any other mammal that lactates in order to provide easily absorbed nourishment for its infant offspring.

For over 7,500 years we've been supping this creamy, cow secretion and there's no denying that milk is highly nutritious. It's packed with protein, chocka with calcium, mobbed with minerals and voluminous with vitamins but on the downside, it is fulla-fat. And this fat is not the **good** fat, it's the nasty, saturated, bad fat that clogs up your arteries and makes you wear elasticated trousers.

But don't worry I'm no Maggie Thatch, so I won't be taking your precious milk away from you but I do recommend you try to reduce your consumption. In fact, maybe you're lactose intolerant and don't even realise it, so it would be better for your health to cut down or even omit it from your diet completely.
READER: *What is lactose intolerance?*
'Lactose' is the sugar found in milk and dairy products, and in order for it to be absorbed into the bloodstream during digestion, it needs to be broken down by an enzyme called, *'Lactase'*. If your body doesn't produce enough lactase, the lactose becomes fermented by bacteria, resulting in stomach discomfort, bloating, cramps, diarrhoea, nausea, excessive guffing and some sufferers also experience skin complaints, such as eczema and dermatitis.

Please don't self-diagnose, if you suspect you may be lactose intolerant consult your GP for confirmation.

READER: *I have milk every day, how can I possibly cut down?*
Ok sourpuss, calm down.

Do you really need it in tea and coffee?
For example, if you normally have six cups of tea a day, make two without milk. The more you do it, the less you'll miss the blue top. Or pop a few slices of lemon in your brew, you could even try a green tea.
READER: *Eeuurrgghh!! Green tea?*
Yes green tea is disgusting, I'm with you on that but luckily many tea manufacturers have created flavoured green teas and I can defo recommend the citrus ones. I'm a big fan of the lemon variety, they're quite refreshing don't you know?!

Or you can add honey to give it some **Oomph**, or maybe a fruit tea. Just experiment and find what works for you but basically **you** need to cut down on the white stuff and this will help.

I'm not going to suggest you opt for skimmed milk because it's not milk. Period.

It's just water, flavoured with liquid paper. **Gross!!**

To replicate skimmed milk, just pour some water into a jug, add a thimble of regular pasteurised milk and shake vigorously. Never been milk but neither is skimmed. At least if you drink pasteurised milk you're getting the nutrients.

Anyway up to you, if you can stomach a liquid that is actually blue once the creamy milk has been filtered away and the resulting slop has to be dyed with milk powders and additives, in order to achieve that liquid-paper glow; then go for it, lap it up.

Alternatively, you could try coconut milk. It's full of vitamins, mineral and nutrients and I can vouch for the fact it tastes quite nice in coffee. I've never poured it in tea, so no idea if it goes well in a brew, try it.

READER: *What about coconut water?*
Aye, that's a really refreshing drink, full of nutrients and great for rehydration after a workout.
I wouldn't put in a hot beverage though but that's just me.

Oh! If you must have a big bowl of frosty-saccharin-bix, significantly reduce the amount of milk you ladle over it. Alternatively you could add coconut, or soy, or almond, or oat, or rice milk instead. Although **check** the ingredients because some of those cartons are swarming with sugar and sweeteners.

Almond milk is really nice in coffee and adds a nutty, sweet taste, which is a boon for those trying to cut sugar from their beverages.

And yes, I know that milk is full of calcium and vitamin D, which is great for your bones and teeth, so if you start to eliminate milk from your diet, there are plenty of ways to obtain your daily allowance.

Sardines, kale, almonds, leafy greens and broccoli are all **excellent** sources of calcium, and you can get your vitamin D from eggs, mushrooms, oily fish, good quality pork and if he's got his hat on, *'Sunshiii-innnne!!'*

READER: *What about yoghurt?*
Ok! How can I explain it? I know.
Natural full-fat yoghurt boosts your metabolism, whereas *'fat-free'*, sugar infused yoghurt, pumps up your spare tyre. So up to you, **sweet cheeks!!**

Oh! And never make eye contact, whilst licking the foil off a yoghurt pot.

READER: *Fair enough, what about milk-shakes?*
Oh! They're really good for you, especially if you're trying to lose weight.

READER: *Really?*

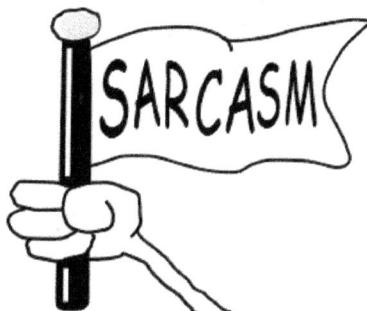

READER: *Oh!!*
Look, not only are milkshakes stuffed with saturated fat and high in calories, they're also crammed to the top with sugar and sweeteners.
READER: *But I love 'em.*
Slurp away if you're not arsed about your weight but if you are and you're committed to getting fit and losing the lard, get rid. Make your own if you must have one, at least then you'll have some control over the ingredients. You could even add fruit to replicate the sweetness.

To finish this section, I have to tell you my udderly hilarious joke about milk.

What do you get from an over-indulged, molly-coddled, pampered cow?
READER: *I don't know, what do you get from an over-indulged, molly-coddled, pampered cow?*
Spoilt milk.
READER: *Ha!... Ha! ...aah!!*

The next section may contain nuts and although every effort has been made to remove shells, some small fragments may remain.

NUTS

You need to come out of your shell

I've already mentioned AL-monds but there's other fantastic nuts out there that'll improve your health and sate your appetite, but I'm not talking about do-nuts!!

Nuts make a great alternative to chocolates, crisps or biccies when you fancy a snack but don't be fooled by the size, these tiny globules of nutrition pack a fatty punch, so beware.

If you're allergic to peanuts, then please move along, nothing to see here.
On your way... **weirdo!!**

BRAZIL NUTS
High in saturated fat, Brazil nuts should only be eaten in moderation and preferably not caked in chocolate. Three or four of these bad boys a day will help to lower cholesterol, boost metabolism, improve your skin and help to combat prostate cancer. In fact, if you really must have a choccy treat, then a few of these will satisfy your sweet craving as well as improve your health. Aye! You can't go wrong with a Brazilian.

Cashew...
READER: *Bless you!!*

Err!! Thanks but I wasn't sneezing, I was going to say **CASHEW NUTS**...

Anyway, these are an excellent source of protein, full of zinc and a handful can contain more iron than a tub of minced beef. Although high in saturated fat, the good news re cashews is that they are rich in fibre, protein and a multitude of minerals and vitamins. Linked to lowering your chances of heart disease, these sweet, crunchy wonders are awesome in curries, add some bite to a salad, or if you're a keen baker, they make a great sugar substitute in cakes, muffins and other desserts.

CHESTNUTS
Roasted chestnuts and I'm not talking about your meat and two veg, tightly packed into your boxer briefs here but a seasonal wonder-food that makes a tasty autumnal snack. Chestnuts are rich in fibre, a good source of vitamins, and low in calories and saturated fat.
They're also extremely versatile and can be used to make flour.
READER: *Flour??*
That's right. Made from dried ground chestnuts, the flour can be bought from most major supermarkets as well as specialist health-food shops and delicatessens.

'Gluten-free' and highly nutritious, chestnut flour can be used to bake bread, buns, cakes and as a thickener for soups and stews. It has a rich, chocolatey look and unsurprisingly, has a nutty flavour with a hint of honey but I warn you, it's not cheap. Mind you, what *'gluten-free'* product is these days? It's well worth it though because you can bake sweet treats that can satisfy your sugary cravings, and with the right combination of ingredients are guilt free.

Oh! Yeah!! Never eat them raw. They taste disgustingly acidic, could crack your teeth, and leave you with nasty stomach problems.

HAZELNUTS
This sweet wholesome nut is low in saturated fat, contains high levels of calcium, fibre, protein and zinc, as well as being a fantastic source of vitamin E. Consuming hazelnuts, without the chocolate and caramel casing can help boost your metabolism, lower your blood pressure, improve levels of good cholesterol and significantly reduce the risk of breast cancer, diabetes and heart disease. All in a nutshell. A brown one.
Although they can be a hard nut to crack but well worth the effort.

Commonly found in confectionery, hazelnuts do compliment well with chocolate, and whilst we're on the topic, if you must indulge in a bar, don't have more than one.

MACADAMIA NUTS
It sounds like a terrible ailment that a chap would relay to a Doctor but macadamia nuts (c'mon, it would be remiss of me not to infer a testicle/nut connotation for comedy pleasure) are a tasty delight for the nut connoisseur. These sweet, creamy, buttery flavoured nuts contain a whole range of health-promoting nutrients including vitamin A, fibre, iron and protein, which is probably why they're so damn expensive.

Although macadamia nuts are high in fat, it's the good stuff linked to reducing cholesterol levels and improving heart functionality. But they are **very** high in calories, so if you have some as a snack, don't have more than four or five at a time.

Macadamia nuts are loaded with anti-oxidants, which will help to lower the risk of breast, lung and prostate cancer, improve bone strength, alleviate dry skin, boost metabolism and even make your hair shinier.
So, do yourself a favour and get your hands on these healthy nuts.

PECAN NUTS
The rise of the Pecans. I believe it was the Romans who finally usurped the Pecans and stole their great ideas on straight roads and plumbing...
PROFESSORS of HISTORY: *I think you'll find that's poppycock!!*

Alright, alright calm yourself, but *'The Pecans'* does sound like an ancient race and if so, there would be no match for the Pecans and we'd all be speaking Pecanese… sorry, I've gone off on one again. Back to the subject in hand…

Like most nuts, the pecan is enriched with many health-benefiting nutrients, minerals and vitamins that are essential for optimum health.

The pecan has a sweet, rich and buttery flavour and…

READER: *And what?*

Well, I just keep typing the same stuff.

Bottom line, nuts are chuffin' great for you but only, **only** if eaten in moderation.

Rather than a packet of crisps, or a choc bar, or a muffin, grab a small handful of nuts instead. Packed with nutrients, sweet, crunchy and downright tasty, nuts will help you to lose weight whilst boosting your health.

So what's not to like? Oh! And walnuts contain twice as many antioxidants as other nuts. They're quite cheap and I can recommend breaking some up over your granola, yoghurt or even ice cream.

READER: *What about peanuts?*

Yeah, quite nutritious, especially the unsalted ones. Full of fibre, protein, vitamin E and numerous other minerals, you've just gotta be careful with peanut butter.

READER: *Why?*

Well you'd think that it's just ground up, pressed, whipped up peanuts, crammed and stuffed into a jar, right?

READER: *Erm! Right?!*

Wrong!! Aye that would be too difficult for most peanut butter manufacturers, 'cos they have to add salt, sugar and crappy additives to enhance the flavour.

Although to be fair, you open a jar of peanut butter and that smell is intoxicating. I have to admit; I've shoved a pinkie in and licked the contents off, on more than a few occasions. Haven't you? It's ok, don't answer that.

Peanut butter is **full** of saturated fat and **very** high in calories, with a few teaspoons serving up a whopping 200kcal and I know what you're like, **you** slap loads on your toast don't you?

READER: *Yeah!*

If it was the highly nutritious, organic type of peanut butter with nowt added at all, then slap away but when it's the salty, sugary, additivey, calorific kind, you're consuming far too many calories and as a consequence you'll increase the lard.

Watch out for **any** nutty type of spread too, 'cos they *'may'* be promoted as healthy but you'd be nutty to believe them.

So, in a nutshell that's nuts for you, they really are, the **dog's bollocks!!**   Shells

PASTA

Just like Mama used to make

I bet **you** love pasta you? As much as macaroni loves cheese.

READER: *Oh! I do. I absolutely love it.*

Yeah, I thought so.

How many times a week do you have a pasta meal?

READER: *Twice, maybe three times some weeks.*

I see. And you're trying to lose weight and find it very difficult?

READER: *Yes… oh!*

I'm sorry to say but most pasta dishes are very fattening. Creamy pasta sauces are very fattening. Grating slabs of cheese all over your piles of pasta, is very fattening. Pasta is very high in calories, which equates to more fat on your tum-tum and bum-bum.

It's gotta be one of the worst meals for anyone who is committed to losing weight.

READER: *Yeah but I can't live without pasta?*

Are you insane? You can't live without oxygen and water; you'll live an extremely healthier and longer life without pasta. But calm down, I'm not saying you've gotta get rid of it completely but you're gonna have to radically reduce the amount of pasta you gobble every week.

Think about the pasta meals you have now. Stop drooling.

No doubt you cover the entire plate with a huge mountain of pasta. Then you add a dash of Bolognese, a few chunks of melted cheese and mix together. Right?
READER: *Sort of, yeah!*
Well, that pile of pasta is just going to be transported from the plate, to your arse or belly.

Essentially it's a mound of potential energy (carbs), its fuel. And if you don't burn it off, it sticks to you as fat. That's why marathon runners, tri-athletes, swimmers and cyclists, eat **massive** heaps of the stuff before a race. This potential energy is used to fuel them throughout the event.

What do you do? Eat a gargantuan plate of pasta, wash up (if you can be arsed) and then lounge in front of the box. Can you see the problem?
READER: *I suppose.*

It may be a filling, cheap and quick meal to make but the main problem with pasta is portion control.
You should flip the amounts you currently eat.
READER: *What do you mean?*
You only need a handful of pasta. The rest of the plate should consist of meat, vegetables and preferably a home-made sauce. And if you must grate cheese all over it, then reduce the amount. **Significantly!!**

To be fair, pasta per se (that's not a new dish by the way) is not full of fat but generally the pasta we seem to consume has very little nutritional value because it is made from processed, heavily refined flour. Therefore I recommend that if you do eat pasta, always try to buy the fresh kind. At least it's made from eggs, and does contain more nutrients than the doughy, durum wheat type you buy in a packet.

Brown pasta is actually full of fibre and contains a small amount of protein but tastes like cardboard although who knows, you might like it.

READER: *So pasta isn't that bad then?*
Well, in essence, I suppose not. It's the fatty, creamy sauces, slabs of cheese and the fact that the dish itself is generally low in meat and veg, 'cos it consists of loads and loads and loads of pasta.

Up to you obviously but if you do reduce the amount you shove on a plate; you'll improve your chances of losing weight. If you continue to pile it on, you'll pile it on.

And never. Please, never ever, ever buy a ready meal pasta dish. Especially Lasagne.

Irrespective of the flashy sounding nutrients the manufacturers **pretend** the dish contains, invariably, it will be full of saturated fat, sugar, salt, sweeteners, additives, preservatives and fake cheese.
And possibly meat… of a rather questionable origin.

Ok! It might taste alright but it's heading straight for your bingo wings and rhino-legs.

Right, talking of Italian dishes that contribute to worldwide obesity levels, let's discuss pizza.
READER: *You're gonna ruin pizza for me as well, do you hate me?*
No, no, not at all. I don't hate you but if I had to urinate and you were on fire, you would burn… kidding, I'm kidding. No, I'm trying to educate you, explain the risks, then you can shove owt you want into your gob but when you keep piling on the flab, you'll know why. Unless of course, **you** take my HELP on board and start losing that lard.

PIZZA

There's always room for another slice

'Deep-pan', 'thin and crusty' or stuffed with *'garlic-sausage'*… we all love pizza don't we? You can't top 'em.
READER: *Well you can. Ham, mushrooms, cheese…*
Wooosshhh!!

Pizza is just like sex.
READER: *What do you mean?*
Well, when it's good, it's good!! But when it's bad, it's still pretty good.
READER: *Ooh! Cheesy!!*
Aye, they say a pizza joke is all about the delivery.

Enough pizza puns now, they're dough-ing my head in.

Hmmm!! Pizza. Look, you know what I'm gonna say.
READER: *Moderati…*
Nope, never eat them ever again.
READER: *AARRGGHHHH!!*

Yeah, it's all about moderation. Rather than cutting a pizza into eight slices, cut it into six.
READER: *Err! What?*
If you're trying to lose weight, then eating takeaway pizza is not going to help. But I understand that you are human, so omitting these from your diet may be nigh on impossible. Therefore it's all about cutting down. If you used to order pizza twice a week, make it once a week. If it's once a week, make it once a fortnight and so on. If you used to order a large, order a medium. If you used to order a medium…

READER: *Order small?*
Exactly. If you ate four slices of garlic bread beforehand, just eat three next time and then two, etc, etc.
I can guarantee that when you start losing the timber, you won't want to ruin your good work by scoffing a takeaway pizza that is just full of processed, fake, oily, salty, doughy shite. I'm not even gonna discuss the shocking quality of ingredients you'll find in a takeaway pizza, suffice to say they're cack!! Which is probably the appeal, we know it's bad for us so that's why we like it. You know, like that *'bastard'* you just can't seem to give up… **idioso!!**

Anyway, if you must have a pizza, make your own. At least then you can control the toppings and make it healthier.

READER: *But that will take longer.*
Bloody hell, it'll take about half an hour at the most. You know, about the same amount of time it takes for some spotty urchin on a moped to deliver your order.

Just think of it. You can overload your own pizza with quality ingredients. Actual tomatoes for the sauce. Mushrooms that aren't mouldy. Meat from the Butcher's. Freshly cut peppers. Real cheese grated on the toppings. Imagine. That's a utopian world for the pizza-lover.

No doubt you prefer one type of topping over another, so you can get rid of the stuff you're not so keen on and heap on the stuff you love. Nutritious and healthy, at a fraction of the price.

You can buy readymade dough or make your own but at least you're not limited to toppings the takeaway joint dictates you're allowed. You could even put the toppings on thick crusty bread, a ciabatta, tortilla wraps, heck, even a chicken breast if you so wish. The only limit is your imagination. Give it a go. In fact, you could get your kids involved, experiment with different toppings and sauces, who knows, you may even end up opening your very own, healthy pizza restaurant.

TIP-TOP-TASTIC!!

Paul Birch

Right, what other food group can I wreck? I know…

POTATOES

So, you like spuds?

Potatoes are the number one crop in the world and billions of these starchy buggers are consumed every single day.

I eat chips for my tea and chips for my supper,
With fish, mushy peas and a nice, hot cuppa,
I love whipped and creamy, fluffy mash,
With salt and pepper and corned beef hash,
I like to shovel beans on my jacket spud,
It's my favourite lunch, it tastes so good,
Waffles and wedges and bubble and squeak,
I skin and peel potatoes every day of the week,
Hash browns for brekkie and roasts at dinner,
I eat tatties every day and I'm not getting thinner!!

READER: *But I thought potatoes were good for me?*
It depends. Yes and no. Sometimes.
READER: *Clear as bloody mud, thanks!*

Ok! Potatoes are actually quite low in calories, an excellent source of vitamin C, and the skins contain a healthy portion of fibre and potassium. They are very starchy, which has a detrimental effect on your blood sugar levels but that's not the big issue. The problem is how they are cooked and what you have with them.

Take mash for instance.
You boil your spuds (killing most of the nutrients) and let's say you use twelve small potatoes. That's about 1500kcal. Naturally, no-one eats just plain mash you're not a philistine, so you add butter, milk, maybe even cream.
Now crank that calorie count up to over 2000kcal.
I assume that you'll be serving this mash to more than yourself, so let's presume this will be shared by three people in total.

One serving will equate to about 700kcal. And that's just the mash. If you've made a roast, you've then gotta count the meat, Yorkshire puddings, other veg, gravy, as well as six or seven roasties too. That one meal can then register over 3000kcal, which is considerably more than your recommended daily allowance.

To cut the calories and save the nutrients, reduce the amount of spuds and add other veg to the mash mix. And rather than boiling, you could cook the potatoes in a slow cooker, or steam them perhaps.
READER: *How would you steam them?*
This is how I would do it but feel free to jazz it up with your own selections.

260

Put six or seven unpeeled (washed) small potatoes in a microwave-proof dish, throw in some sliced carrots and chunks of turnip, add a dash of milk and a smidge of butter. Place a microwave-proof lid securely over the dish and zap for five minutes.

Take the bowl from the microwave and spice that baby up. Add some sliced garlic, salt and pepper, maybe some paprika, coriander. Chuck some chopped onions in too, or leeks, experiment, see what works for you.

Mix and stir, then microwave for another three or four mins. After the ping, mash the beejesus out of the soft, fluffy, spuddy, carroty, turnipy mixture and serve. Perfect mash, low in calories and full of nutrients.

The carrots and turnip bulk up the mash and enhance the flavour. They contain significantly less calories than spuds but still have a creamy, fluffy texture when mashed. **NB:** *Try adding avocado, I did it today and they were lush.*

Baked potatoes aren't too bad for you either.
A large spud contains about 300kcal, it's what you ladle all over them that is the issue.
READER: *Like what?*
Butter for one thing, a tiny knob is not so bad...
READER: *Speak for yourself!!*
Blimey, get your mind out of the gutter; I'm just trying to warn you to **ration** your butter.
Don't drown the thing in butter or marge, 'cos you're doubling the calorie count and increasing the saturated fat.
Then there's cheese. A few sprinkles, fair do's but if you're slapping half a wedge of cheese over your tattie, then **stop it!!**

Coleslaw is fundamentally a healthy dish. Finely shredded cabbage and carrot, nutrient-tastic. However, it's drenched in saturated fatty mayo. A dribble of coleslaw is fine; just don't go mad with the mayo (same principle with tuna, heavy on the tuna, light on de mayo).

Chilli-con-carne is really good for you, so put loads on for me, as long as you're aware that if you're having this for lunch you won't need loads of food for your evening meal because you'll have consumed half your R.D.A. at lunch-time.

What else have we got re spuds?
READER: *Roasts?*
Roast potatoes, drizzled in goose fat. You crunchy, fluffy, beautiful **buggers!!**

Yeah, I love roasties too but it brings me back to Marky-Mark and the Funky Moderation Bunch, again. A few is fine but they are **heavy** on the calories because they absorb the fat during cooking, so be careful. The more you consume the less weight you'll be losing each week.

Oh Yeah!! That reminds me, have you heard of *'Acrylamide'*?
READER: *No, I don't think so.*
Really? Well you should have, 'cos I mentioned it earlier in the book... why do I even bother?!!

Anyway, acrylamide is a toxic substance produced when starchy foods are roasted, fried, or grilled for too long at high temperatures. So what, I hear you ponder? Well, acrylamide has been linked with causing cancer and the more food you eat that's burnt, the more at risk you are.
READER: *Fair enough but we've all gotta die of something, right?*
Yeah, of course.

It's easy to be blasé about death when you think it'll be decades before it happens but just imagine that conversation. Spend a few moments just picturing the scene.

Initially you're sat in the Doctor's waiting room, nervous and anxious about their prognosis, then you're called in for the moment of truth...

> **DOCTOR**: *Its bad news I'm afraid. There's no easy way to say this but you've tested positive for cancer.*
> **READER**: *Oh! No! Are you sure? Is it terminal?*
> **DOCTOR**: *Unfortunately, yes. You have a very aggressive form of cancer and our tests indicate that you only have a few months to live. There's medication that could delay the inevitable but this could give you a month, maybe a few extra weeks and you will be in considerable pain throughout.*
> **READER**: *Is there no cure?*
> **DOCTOR**: *I'm sorry, but I'm afraid not.*

No doubt there'll be tears. Many, many tears. Then it's over to the seven emotional stages of grief. A rollercoaster of emotions from shock, to anger, to depression. And finally, acceptance.

You'll start to regret all those things you never got round to doing. All the events you'll miss in the future. Your family and friends growing older. The travel you wished you'd experienced. All those dreams you had.

Over. The end. No more.

Sod that, right? We're all gonna die but if we can put it off as best we can, then it's worth trying don't you think?
READER: *Definitely, yes.*

Ok then. Back to acrylamide.

In order to avoid consuming any food that contains acrylamide, firstly avoid processed potato products like waffles and oven chips because they are very likely to contain traces of this horrible substance.

If you're cooking your spuds in t'oven, whether it's a jacket, wedges, chips, or roasts, make sure you remove them once they have obtained a golden yellow colour, not a mucky brown one. And if they are burnt, either chuck 'em or cut the charred section away. It's the same principle with toast. My Great-Gran used to tell me that burnt toast put hairs on your chest, now its cancerous tumours!!

Oops, nearly forgot. Any crisp lovers out there?
97% OF READERS: *Hell yeah!!*
Well, crisps also contain traces of acrylamide, as do crackers, cereals, biscuits and sliced bread.
READER: *Is there anything I can safely eat?*
Loads of stuff.

Look, I'm just informing you of the risks, you can do what you like once you're in the comfort of your funky kitchen, with the motivational wall art and the table cloth that matches your slippers.

But if you continue buying processed food, which you no doubt will because it's difficult to escape, make sure the products have as **few** ingredients as possible. The less ingredients, the better it will be for you. Alternatively, go natural.

And on that subject, sweet potatoes are a thousand times **nicer** than the regular spud. Subjective but true.

> I like you,
> I bet you're really
> nice.

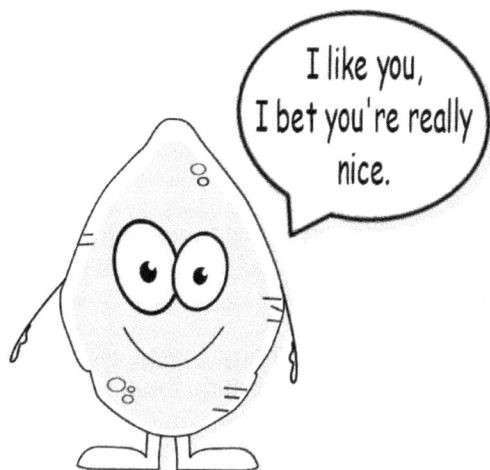

READER: *Why are they better then?*
If you'd had sweet potato wedges, seasoned with sea salt and pepper, you wouldn't quibble but fair enough I'm here to educate.

Sweet potatoes have fewer calories, less fat and less starch than their white counterparts.

They're full of vitamin A and bloody gorgeous as jackets.

Try 'em, you'll love 'em.

GUARANTEED!!

QUINOA

(pronounced keen-wah)

Are you keen on quinoa?
READER: *I'm not so quinoa.*
Have you tried quinoa?
98.36% of READERS: *No.*

'Gluten-free' and an ideal substitute for rice or pasta, the demand for quinoa has risen sharply over the last few years and it's become a bit of a darling in the world of clean-eating.

By the by, *'clean-eating'* to me is a load of pigs gonads. It's just not feasible in the long-term and you end up craving all the alleged **naughty** stuff, so you rebel, feel guilty, then quit and that's just not a good way to live your life. That's why, if you follow my advice and become active, you can still eat the naughty stuff but in moderation, which is a much better way to live, allowing you to be moderately happy for the rest of your life.

My opinion, feel free to disagree... but you're wrong.

Quinoa is low in calories, full of protein, calcium, vitamin E and fibre, and substantially more nutritious than rice, pasta or couscous. Creamy, with a nutty flavour, quinoa could replace starchy carby spaghetti in a Bolognese, starchy carby rice in a chilli, or starchy carby spuds in a stew. It also adds some **Oomph**, to a salad.

READER: *How do you make it?*
Same as you would rice, it's very simple, quick to make and extremely filling. Personally, I like to add it to stir-fries and I find it complements beef and fish the best. But hey, that's me. You can even buy it in packets to be micro-waved and they have very few added ingredients, so they pass the Birchy processed-food test.

I'm very keen on the quinoa, try it and then you might be keen on the quinoa **too!!**

RICE

It's great when you're hungry and you want 2,000 of something
(Courtesy of Mr Mitch Hedberg R.I.P.)

In the same manner as pasta, rice has become a staple of our diets but rather than just having a small handful, it seems to be the norm to pile mounds and mounds of the stuff onto our plates. Rice is another processed, refined grain and with respect to weight loss, these types of grains should be your enemy.
READER: *Why?*
Starchy foods play havoc with your blood sugar levels, and offer very limited nutrients (if any), mess with your digestive system and due to the amounts consumed, increase your timber. Significantly reduce the amounts you consume and you'll be amazed at how much weight you'll lose.

Rather than piling the rice (and pasta) on your plate, opt for alternatives such as Couscous, Quinoa, Chick peas, Lentils, Butter beans, Borlotti beans or Kidney beans. You might grimace at this suggestion but I can assure you, once they're on your plate you'll find that they have similar consistencies and tastes to rice (and pasta), plus they're substantially healthier for you.

READER: *But rice is so quick and easy to make. And it's cheap.*
So are the alternatives. Just excuses again, unwilling to even try something that is unfamiliar, out of your comfort zone. A break from the ol' routine. I've said it before and I'll say it again, *'if what you're doing now isn't working, it isn't working'*. Therefore it's time to try something different.

I'm not gonna bang on about it anymore but just like pasta, the more you pile on the rice, the more you'll pile on.

SALT

(Sodium Chloride)

I was gonna make a joke about sodium but Na, I don't think I'll bother.
READER: *I don't get it.*
Think about the periodic table and the chemical element for sodium being…
READER: *Oh!!*
No, 'Na'.

The consumption of salt will have no specific bearing on your weight loss, but it will have a massive impact on your health and well-being.

READER: *I hear it all the time but why is salt so bad for me, I thought I needed it?*
We do need it, you're right. The problem is that we're consuming far too much on a daily basis through foods we have no idea contain salt and as a consequence, putting our health at risk.

Salt is necessary to aid digestion, muscle contraction, control fluid balance and a fundamental component of the nervous system.

Our wonderful, amazing bodies (yep, even yours) regulates how much salt it contains but when sodium levels become too high or too low, imbalances can result, setting the stage for disease.

If levels are too high, we get thirsty and drink, which allows the kidneys to eliminate the salt through urination. And if levels are too low, we eat. It's very rare that you will consume too little salt in your diet but if that was the case you could end up having a heart attack. Don't worry, very unlikely.

Too much salt puts a strain on your kidneys and increases your blood pressure, leading to potential strokes, kidney stones, kidney disease and in some cases, heart attacks,

And if there are any diabetics or asthma sufferers out there, high salt intake can also exacerbate your symptoms, which may lead to more serious health risks.

The recommended daily allowance of salt for adults in the UK is 6g per day (2.4g of sodium) which is about a teaspoon, however in other countries this figure can be as little as 2g.

If you live on a diet of processed, packaged food your salt intake can be up to ten times the RDA. Therefore reducing the amount of salt you consume is essential for your health, so watch out for any food source that 'may' contain high levels of sodium.

READER: *Like what?*
Well…

There's salt in fish and salt in chips,
Salt in vinegar and hummus dips,
There's salt in cereal and pasta sauce,
In packaged food, its par for the course,
There's salt in soup and salt in cheese,
There's even salt in frozen peas,
Biscuits, ketchup, burgers too,
Check those labels, you must do,
There's salt in crisps and processed meat,
So please be careful, what you eat,
'Cos there's salt in cake and salt in bread,
Too much salt and you'll end up dead!!

Ok! A quick guide on how to decipher the food labels. As we know, salt is also called 'Sodium Chloride', so rather than quoting the figure for salt on the label, those cheeky manufacturing scamps will sometimes state the amount for sodium.

They're trying to confuse you, deceitful gits!!

To calculate how much salt you may be consuming based on the sodium figure, multiply the sodium level by 2.5. For example:

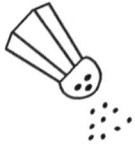

2g of sodium per 100g = 5g of salt per 100g, which is **too bloody high!!**
So, please try and avoid foods that contain this much salt

If the figure is over 1.5g salt per 100g (or 0.6g sodium) it's high, and you should be careful how much you consume. An adequate salt level would be about 0.3g salt per 100g (or 0.1g sodium).

Like everything else I've prattled on about in this book, you can take my advice with a pinch of salt or you can embrace it, use it, embrace it and be fitter, thinner and healthier than you've ever been.

If you can manage to reduce your intake, I recommend you treat yourself on the weekend with a few grains… a slice of lemon, and a shot of **tequila!!**

Bad decisions, optional.

! ! ! WARNING ! ! ! RANT IMMINENT ! ! ! WARNING ! ! ! RANT IMMINENT ! ! ! WARNING ! ! ! RANT IMMINENT ! ! !

SUGAR

The Devil's dandruff

Right, you might wanna set your phone to silent, put the kettle on and make a brew, 'cos it's another Birchy rant coming and it's gonna be a long 'un.

Here we go.
White and **deadly!!**
No, I'm not talking about US Cops policing the hood, I am talking about sugar.
Sugar is a drug.
A highly addictive, legalised drug that is omnipresent throughout the food industry. And it will make you **FAT!!**

Sugar is the leading contributor to the worldwide obesity crisis, it's horribly debilitating, it's energy sapping, it destroys neurons in the brain and it's **fuckin' gorgeous!!**

You want to lose weight and stay healthy? Eat as little sugar as possible, end of story, morning glory.

I'm not just talking cane sugar here either because it's the chemically manufactured sugars which are equally to blame. In fact, they're probably worse.
READER: *Sorry, what are you talking about?*
I'm talking about those artificial sweeteners, the Step Brother and Sisters of sugar such as Aspartame, Saccharin, Stevia and those ones that end in *'ose'.*
READER: *End in 'ose'?*
Yeah, you know the ones, Fructose, Glucose, Lactose, Maltose and Sucrose.

And that's not the end of it either because there are other sweeteners too, like:

Acesulfame-K, Cyclamate, Erythritol, Isomalt, Lacititol, Maltitol, Mannitol, Sorbitol and Xylitol.

Doesn't stop there, we're also consuming international sweeteners as well which are slowly creeping into UK produce, like:

Crystalline Fructose, D-Tagatose, Fruit Juice Concentrates, Glucose Syrup, Glycerol, High Fructose Corn Syrup, Hydrogenated Starch, Maltodextrin, Molasses and Neotame.

As consumers, the main issue regarding these synthetic sugars is we know sweet F.A. about them really, yet they're in virtually 90% of every processed, packaged product in the supermarket.

We've only been consuming these sweetened products for the last fifteen to twenty years, so it's not abundantly clear whether they cause long-term ill effects in humans, or not. However, what cannot be disputed is that **thousands** of scientific tests have taken place on mice and rats, and the majority of these artificial sweeteners have proven to be carcinogenic, cause brain tumours, incite heart problems and cause infertility.
READER: *But we're not mice.*
You're right. Or rats.

There are clearly physiological differences between human beans and rodents, but we do actually share a surprising amount of biological similarities. We're both warm-blooded mammals, we eat similar food and we live in the same environments (check under your floorboards for confirmation). We have comparable organs which are controlled by hormones, and a temperamental nervous system. In addition, we react similarly to disease, infection and injury.

<u>FOOD MANUFACTURERS of the WORLD</u>: *Aah! Yes but Aah! We categorically state that any animal's response to a certain procedure or medication, actually tells us nothing about the likely human response. Therefore we poo-poo these spurious claims.* Well, ta for the response, Food Manufacturers of the world.

So as consumers, should we just ignore it? Perhaps! Perhaps! But like our lil' furry rodent friends, you know and I do that we're addicted to sugar and synthetic nectar and it's rotting our teeth, eroding our gums, increasing the lard and causing serious health problems such as diabetes, liver damage, high blood pressure and heart disease.

The suggested daily allowance for sugar in the UK is 30g (7 teaspoons) yet the average Brit consumes about 20 teaspoons of sugar a day. A day!! **A fuckin' day!!**

And for little sprogs, the RDA should be about 24g which they surpass just by quaffing a can of coke. That's in addition to eating their wholesome sugary flakes, white bread sarnies, packs of crisps, sweetie-fruit-juice, cheese-strings, yoghurts, biccies, choc bars, waffles, pasta and any other crap they shove down their gobs before their bedtime story.

I mentioned coke earlier in the book but half of **ALL** fizzy drinks sold in the UK will contain the equivalent of about 7 teaspoons of sugar, in every can. And we let kids drink them all the time.

This is why Dentists earn so much dosh. It's like shooting suicidal fish in a barrel.

The UK Government have a cunning plan, they've got the answer to solving this problem… a sugar tax. But I'll tell you now, a sugar tax will not work.
<u>READER</u>: *Why not?*
<u>UK GOVERNMENT</u>: *Yeah, why not?*
If you add ten pence to the price of a can of ginger beer, or a chocolate bar, or some cereal, or white bread the consumer will buy them anyway. What's ten pence in the grand scheme of things?

Plus, to reduce the impact, Supermarkets will discount their prices anyway because, oh I don't know, profit margins and all that. It's all about the dosh to them; they couldn't give a shite about the wellbeing of their customers. As long as their trolleys are full of cheap, processed, packaged shite they're golden. There's no accounting for taste, well there is and Supermarket Accountants are shouting, *'Kerching!!'*

No, it's up to **you** to reduce your consumption of the sugary stuff, and to educate your children as to the true **value** and **quality** of food. No one else will and to be fair, it's no-one else's responsibility.
It's up to you.
<u>READER</u>: *How?*
Yep, I understand it's easier said than done but that's' why I'm trying to help ya.

Ok! Here goes, let's look at sugar in more detail.

WHAT IS SUGAR?
Sugar is a carbohydrate.

Now, there are different kinds of sugar, starting with simple sugars which the boffins call, *'Monosaccharides'*, like fructose, galactose and glucose. Then there are complex forms, called *'Disaccharides'*, such as lactose, maltose and sucrose.

These descriptions relate to the amount of chemical bonds joined together to form the compound and the more chains and branches, the more complex the compound.

Without getting too technical (and I failed Chemistry at school, remember, although I might take it again, yeah I will, I'll add that to my bucket list), the complex sugars take longer to be broken down by the body and thus have less of an impact on blood sugar levels. What's that mean to you? Well, in essence, simple sugars are bad 'uns, 'cos after consumption they will ramp up your blood sugar, leading to a slump, cravings, snacks and subsequent lard.

But sugar is actually a natural ingredient that has been part of our diet for thousands of years, providing essential energy for the body.

The most important sugar we consume is *'Glucose'*, which is the primary energy source for your brain, major organs and muscles. Without it, they would not be able to function properly.

Therefore sugar is essential for life.
READER: *Now we're talking.*
Don't reach for the cupcakes just yet; it's a bit more complicated than that.
READER: *It always is with you.*

Some sugars can be found naturally in juicy fruit, crunchy vegetables and creamy milk, whereas other sugars are created by the wannabe Bond villains in Food Manufacturing plants.

However, the body does not distinguish between the different types of sugar, and breaks them down through digestion in exactly the same way. Although their impact on the body will differ, depending on the **type** of sugar consumed.

Your digestive system acts like a warehouse, which ships out the natural good stuff to your muscles, skin, blood and organs etc, etc and piles the sugar and processed crap into that room at the back that no-one goes in. You know the room, it states *'Fat Store'* on the sign.

Anyway, here are the **four main sugars** we consume on a daily basis.

Sucrose

This is the crystallised, processed, heavily refined white stuff you buy in bags and store in bowls, and is also known as *'table sugar'*.
Sucrose is a hybrid sugar made from glucose and fructose, and when consumed it's broken down rapidly, elevating blood sugar levels.
It is extracted from the stems of sugar cane, the roots of sugar beet, and can be found naturally in certain fruits and plants but has absolutely diddly, nutritional value.
Sucrose is the go-to sugar that we use to sweeten drinks or for baking, and can be purchased as bags of Granulated, fine Caster, brown Demerara, or as powdered Icing sugar.

Fructose

Incredibly sweet, fructose occurs naturally in fruits, vegetables and honey.
Therefore every time you munch on an apple, chew a carrot, or stir some honey in your disgustingly bland, green tea you're consuming nature's nectar.
The lovely Food Manufacturers realised that because fructose is considerably sweeter than sucrose and cheaper to produce, it's been added to a whole raft of food sources, from ready meals to chewing gum, fizzy pop to *'fat-free'* yoghurt.

Lactose

Otherwise known as *'milk sugar'* because it's contained in...
READER: *Milk?!*
Ten points.
You probably know someone who won't stop yapping on about being *'lactose intolerant'*, well to be fair a lot of us are and don't even realise it. Although all infant mammals can tolerate lactose, only humans consume it into adulthood. Mind you, if cows could make ice cream, maybe they would too.

Children possess enzymes that help to absorb lactose, with no ill effects, whereas some adults stop producing this enzyme and after consumption of dairy products, suffer bloating and abdominal discomfort. Nowadays you can buy dairy products that are *'lactose free'* but some of these will contain artificial sweeteners to replicate the sugary taste.

Maltose

Also known as *'malt sugar'*, maltose is mostly found in germinating grain, particularly barley, and is not as sweet as its syrupy Sisters fructose, glucose, and sucrose.
You'll find maltose in malted drinks and beer.
Luckily you don't drink much alcohol, so you probably don't consume hardly **any** of this sweet stuff... ☺

Ok, so that's a basic summary of the four main sugars but **why** are they so bloody addictive, and **why** do they make you fat?

You've had a bad day at work, so you get home, change into your onesie, make yourself a brew and then slump down on the sofa to watch the box with a nice choccy bar. Those barely chewed, creamy chunks of chocolate slide down your gullet, to enter the complex, intestinal, merry-go-round that is the digestion process.

Once absorbed, those sweet lumps of salvation start to immediately impact on your blood sugar levels, which sets alarm bells ringing in your central nervous system (CNS), alerting the pancreas that something's amiss.

To combat this surge in blood sugar, the pancreas springs into action and secretes the hormone insulin, to control and regulate that excess saccharin, by allowing cells to absorb the glucose.

Now, when there's an overload of sugar in the blood the CNS interprets this significant rise as an indicator of **stress**, releasing the hormones *'Cortisol'* and *'Epinephrine'* to calm the heart and reduce blood pressure. This leads to the dreaded sugar crash, ultimately resulting in your blood sugar spiking and then dramatically dropping below normal levels. Essentially, this is your body screaming and stamping like a spoilt little child, *'I want more sugar!!'*

You start to feel sluggish, tired and irritable and you may scream at your partner, even though it's not their fault. Hey! Why change a habit of a lifetime?!

So what do you do? You could ignore this temporary feeling by having a drink of water, going for a walk, or placing your fingers in your ears shouting *'La, la, la, I can't hear you!!'* Alternatively, you could cram some cake into your gob so the process starts again. But the more you give in to these sugar crashes, the more insulin resistant you become and in the worst case scenario, this could eventually lead to Diabetes.

ADDICTION

Whilst the sugar crash/CNS/pancreas/insulin carnival is underway, there are a series of neurological processes taking place too, which help to exacerbate your cravings and yearning for sugar.

The consumption of sugary delights sends sweet, syrupy messages to the brain, activating your reward system by triggering dopamine receptors. And dopamine has a lot to answer for in your life.

Whenever you experience elation, it's down to *'Dopamine'*. When you're checking out that hottie at work and you're consumed with lust, thank your friend dopamine. Do you remember that first date and you felt anxious, excited, agitated and all in a tizzy? Yep? Down to dopamine.

When you're relaxed, it's dopamine. In the throes of passion, dopamine.

Smirking as you reveal a full-house at poker, going bonkers celebrating a 96th minute winner, or gobbling down a gateau, dopamine will have been playing havoc with your brainwaves.

READER: *What is it?*
Dopamine is merely a chemical signal between neurons, but it's the resulting feeling this creates that elicits excitement and happiness.

The first time you consumed sugar this will have triggered the release of dopamine, which led to your first *'sugar high'*.

And your brain loved it.

Whether its sex, drugs, gambling, internet shopping, alcohol or fig rolls, once the initial dopamine high was achieved, your brain wants to **relive** the sensation.

However, repetition dilutes the dopamine impact, lessening the emotive high and it can only be attained through over-consumption.

Which leads me neatly back onto sugar.

When we consume these sweet foods regularly and in large amounts, the dopamine reward is weakened and unsatisfied, we crave more… and more… and **more!!**

Like any drug, desire then leads to dependency, and then to addiction.

READER: *I thought you said sugar makes you fat, how?*
Oh aye! I forgot about that.
It's back to our good little buddy, insulin.
Insulin is a multi-functional hormone that not only assists in the regulation of blood sugar levels; it also impacts on the liver and fat storage.
READER: *But how?*
Sugar in any form (including artificial sweeteners), is a carbohydrate which is quickly absorbed into the bloodstream, in order that it can be utilised for immediate fuel. Insulin acts as a trigger for muscles, enabling them to receive this abundant source of energy and as a consequence, the body **stops** burning fat. If you live a sedentary lifestyle, your muscles will be bursting to the seams with potential energy therefore if you're not about to go for a run, or a cycle or whatever, that sugar has to be diverted and stored elsewhere.

Those excess sugars are thus converted to *'Triglycerides'* by the liver, and subsequently stored as adipose tissue.

In other words, fatty-fatty fat **FAT!!**

Therefore regular sugar consumption leads to weight gain, unless you're a fitness junkie and utilise it as energy.

MELANIE, 29 – *My God, I used to be so unhappy trying to lose weight but I know I didn't help myself. I'd come home from work hungry, so dive for a packet of crisps, sneak a few choc bars, or finish off a pack of biccies. Then I'd hide the empty packets, so my hubby wouldn't find out.*
But I was fooling no-one bar myself.
Nowadays I bake my own healthy snacks like flapjacks and granola bars, which I eat at home and take to work. In fact my colleagues start dribbling, whenever I walk into the office with a 'Tupperware' box under my arm.
I can't believe how far I've come and how much my body has changed over the last six months, for the first time in years I actually have a slim waist and shapely hips. And I'm not embarrassed to admit that I cried with joy, when I caught my reflection in the mirror after trying a bridesmaid dress for my mates' wedding. I looked great. The days of slathering bread with jam are well and truly over and it's jogging, aerobics and ballroom dancing for me now.
I can't believe it, I'm a fitty.

Look, I'd be a hypocrite to suggest that you should cut out sugar from your diet completely, so I ain't gonna do that. I for one do not want to live in a world, where I can't eat cherry bakewells. Or blueberry muffins. Or even, hot chocolate fudge cake with ice cream.

But and if it's a big butt, if **you** truly want to lose weight and are keen to get active, then you've gotta cut down.
So, it's back to choices.
READER: *But it's so difficult.*
I know, I know but I'm here to help you. It's just like walking…
READER: *What do you mean?*
It's a step by step process.

Sugar should be consumed as a **treat**, not as part of **every** meal during the day, so in no particular order, let's assess how to reduce your consumption.

HOT DRINKS

Just like the Beastie Boys, I used to like my sugar with coffee and cream but it took until I was about forty-one years old to stop. So I know how difficult it is to omit sugar from your fave beverage but it's not as tough as you think. I used to have two spoonfuls of sugar in my tea and one in coffee, and I had done since I was about twelve.
READER: *Why did you stop?*
Well, it wasn't 'cos of the lard that I stopped, although it clearly wasn't helping (love handles for me), it was because my gums were being eroded to buggery due to the plaque destroying hot, saccharin, milky pap I was drinking. So after another painful visit to the dentist, I just decided that was it, no more and I went full cold turkey.

The coffee wasn't bad because I started to add cream rather than milk, and the taste was awesome, so the transition was quite easy. However, tea without sugar tasted bloody disgusting and it took a few months to get used to the sweet-free taste.
READER: *What about now?*
I genuinely don't miss the sugar at all, I can now taste the **actual** flavours stewed from the bag, so I definitely recommend cutting it from your drinks.

Cut down gradually to give your taste buds time to adjust. Step by step.

If you currently add two teaspoons, make it one, then after a few weeks, make it a half, and then none. Add cayenne pepper or cinnamon instead, it gives both tea and coffee a bit of a zip.

Give it a go, you'll thank me.

FRUIT JUICE

<u>READER</u>: *It must be good because it's full of fruit, right?!*
Our survey says, *'No!!'*

I've mentioned OJ already but apple juice for instance, can contain about 28g of sugar in a tiny 250ml bottle. That's worse than coke. And please don't be fooled by the alleged health claims of fruit smoothies because it's complete hairy, spheroids. Whether it's cranberry, blackcurrant, grape or kiwi juice, I can assure you it will be full of sugar and artificial sweeteners. In fact, you have to be wary of most shop, restaurant and pub based drinks, from sparkling water to cider, Frappuccino's to Prosecco.
<u>READER</u>: *Prosecco, Nnnnnnnnnnnooooooooooooooooooooooo!!*
'Fraid so.
I'm gonna give you some examples of the sugary, teaspoon misery so you can decide for yourself, whether to keep scoffing.

As a guide, 5g equates **to one teaspoon of sugar** and you're allowed 7 teaspoons in total for the day.
In fact scrub that. I won't just mention how many grams, 'cos it's difficult to gauge. Therefore I'll also add **how many** teaspoons of sweet crack each product contains, then it's far easier for you to picture.

A well-known coffee house chain that originates from Seattle in the U, S of A, sells a large caramel infused Frap-a-crap-uccino which contains 64g of sugar.
I'm not even gonna do the teaspoon calculation for you because it's too chuffin' scandalous to type.

A certain fizzy drink which purports to give you the power of flight, soars in at a whopping 27.5g of sugar per 250ml can (<u>5 and a half teaspoons</u>).

A chain of coffee shops named after a Roman Emperor, offers a refreshing Iced Latte for your pleasure, which contains a generous 23.4g of sugar per serving (just under <u>5 teaspoons</u>).

A low calorie, artificially sweetened soft drink produced by a company that apparently taught the world to sing and are so up their own butt-holes, they have named a drink after *'Life'* as we know it, contains 22g of sugar per can (<u>4 and a bit teaspoons</u>).

Another fizzy drink named after an elf, or pixie and sporting a green can with white lettering, contains 22g of sugar per 330ml can (<u>4 and a bit teaspoons</u>). Must be sugary fairy dust.

A drinks company that is not guilty, sells a strawberry & banana smoothie which contains 21g of sugar per 200ml glass (just over <u>4 teaspoons</u>). Send 'em down!!

A particular Irish cider contains 20.5g of sugar in every original pint (A gnat's chuff over <u>4 teaspoons</u>). Hmm!! Refreshing.

A purple packaged, blackcurrant, vitamin C obsessed company, provides 20g of sugar in every 200ml carton (<u>4 of your silver teaspoons</u>).

Should I go on, or have I made my point?
READER: *Erm! You mentioned Prosecco?*
Yeah don't worry, it's not that bad. There's about half a teaspoon per 125ml glass, so not to worry, unless you're drinking full bottles at a time but you don't do that, do you? Do you?!
READER: *Of course not, how bloody dare you?!*
When it comes to alcohol, red wine is the best drink for you because of the anti-oxidants and polyphenols it contains. Yes it gives you a red moustache but that's a small price to pay.

Oh! And before I forget, if you order Gin & Tonic, please be aware that Tonic water can contain about 4 teaspoons per bottle... **bottoms up!!**

PROCESSED FOOD

I've mentioned it about a gazillion times but processed food contains a lot of hidden sugar, and in products you wouldn't expect. Then there's food you know is full of the sweet stuff, although you significantly underestimate the quantities, so let's take a look at some. You might want to take cover because I'm gonna unleash some hefty truth bombs here, so beware.

When you consume fruit, you think *'Yay!! Good ol' me, I'm getting one of my five a day, chalk one in the win column'*. But you still have to be careful how much you scoff because of the fructose.

Yes, you're getting the added bonus of fibre, vitamins and minerals but some of the blighters pack a sweet left hook.

Clementines can contain about 5g per orange, which isn't earth shattering but because of their size many folk are inclined to eat a few at a time, so be careful.

On the flip side, half a chocolate orange can contain over 400kcal and a whopping 5g of sugar per segment.
Per segment!!
I've been known to eat a whole one of those spherical beauties with a cup of tea. Terry has a lot to answer for and they don't even count as one of your five a day.
READER: *Sorry, how many teaspoons of sugar in a chocolate orange?*
Well, there are normally 20 segments, so that's a gi-bloody-normous, **TWENTY** teaspoons in total.
READER: *Holy flip-flops!!*
Indeed!!

It goes without saying that ice cream contains sugar but a few scoops can contain over 200 calories and over 20g of the sweet powdery stuff
(hundreds and thousands of granules = 4 teaspoons).

If you opt for a flavoured variation such as vanilla, this will contain half the sugar in two scoops. Whereas those ice creams that contain chunks of cookie dough, and sweet sauces, and biccy bits, and flakes of chocolate, you know, the good ones, well they can contain even more than 20g in just two dollops.

A tub of Jen & Berry's can contain upwards of 28 teaspoons of filthy sucre.

Therefore be careful, spooning. Who knows where it will lead...

It's no shock that choccy bars are laced with sweetness but it may surprise you as to how much.
READER: *Not anymore!*

A certain nutty bar that used to be called, *'Marathon'* (Aah! I used to love nostalgia)
contains 245kcal and 21.7g of powdered saccharin
(a heap of granules over <u>4 teaspoons</u>).

A caramel infused bar that apparently, is essential for work, rest and play contains,
wait for it… 42.6g per bar, a stratospheric <u>ten and a smidge teaspoons</u>.
In one chuffin' bar. That's well over your daily allowance, in one bar. **One bar!!**

I don't know about you but I fancy a taste of paradise?! Well, it appears that heaven on
earth contains a coco-nutty <u>8 teaspoons</u>. Hells-bells!!

An ex-girlfriend once likened me to a *'Drifter'* because I was afraid to commit. I've always assumed she meant I was like a hobo, or someone with no direction. On reflection, I'm sure she just meant I was sweet. But how sweet? About 5 teaspoons worth, it appears. **Candylicious!!**

I'm bored of chocolate bars now, so onto angelic-nutrient-enriched yoghurt. These days it seems that yoghurt is some sort of super-food. It's a treat, a breakfast alternative, it helps your gut and keeps you regular, all in one recyclable pot.

To be fair, *'full fat'* natural yogurt is brimming with dairy goodness and full of calcium, protein, vitamins and minerals. But the majority of the top selling flavoured versions contain more sugar than biscuits and cakes. The *'full-fat'* creamy yoghurt can contain just under one teaspoon in a pot, whereas some of the *'fat-free'* versions can contain well over six teaspoons. Even the yoghurt-pots designed for bairns can contain as many as 4 teaspoons in a tiny, brightly coloured pot.

Don't believe the yoghurt **hype!!**

I'm a huge lover of the cake of Jaffa, as I'm sure **you** are too. Because we're good pals now, I can freely admit that in the past I've been a bit of a Jaffa-glutton. I used to think it was fig rolls that were my *'Achilles' heel'* but it's those spongey-tangy-cakey discs of gorgeousness as well. There are twelve in a pack and I can cane them in no time. So I just don't buy them anymore. Honestly, I don't miss 'em one bit, my gums don't miss 'em and my love handles **definitely** don't miss 'em. I probably have two individual cakes a year these days, and that's only when visiting family and I'm offered one with a brew.

Jaffa Cakes are quite literally, tangerine crack and it's only whilst doing the research for this book that I now know why. Each biscuit contains 6.5g of sugar, that's over a teaspoon of sugar, **per biscuit**.
And I used to gobble up a packet, like a junkie takes a hit.
A whole packet, what about you?
READER *(after recovering from fainting)*: *OMG!! I often eat a full packet, OMG!!*
Yep, a full packet contains 78g of sugar, or for the old fashioned out there, nearly sixteen teaspoons of sugar. Sixteen… **SIX fuckin' TEEN!!**

It's a disgrace.

At least you know now, so if you carry on eating them and can't seem to lose the lard, there's a huge Jaffa shaped reason.

Next…

KETCHUP

You say *'tomato'*, I say *'salty, sugary, tomato-flavoured sauce'*. Tomatoes really are a super-food, packed full of beneficial antioxidants and a rich source of the vitamins A and C. Ketchup, although great on chips, offers zilch in the nutrient department and is a sauce **rich** in sugary sweetness. A bottle will contain about five teaspoons and is also teeming with salt. And while we're on the subject of tomatoes, be careful when you buy any flavour of tinned soup.

Tomato soup for example, can contain about five teaspoons and the creamy versions can contain about nine. That's 57 varieties of saccharin, yer buggers.

Some companies try to brag about their healthy soups, well, a certain London district-based soup company, sells a tomato infused number that contains six teaspoons of sugar **per carton!!**

Ok! Speed round.

- Those barbecue dips you get at fast food *'restaurants'*, 2 teaspoons.
- Bowl of cornflakes, 4 teaspoons.
- Lemon muffin, 6 teaspoons.
- Pain-au-chocolat, 2 teaspoons.
- 2 slices of brown bread, 1 teaspoon.
- A sprinkle of salad dressing, 1 teaspoon.
- Pasta sauce, 6 teaspoons per jar.
- Medium sized banana, nearly 3 teaspoons (I know, I was bloody shocked at that stat).
- Chicken, bacon & sweetcorn pasta salad, 2 teaspoons.
- A typical Supermarket own brand, pasta bake ready-meal, 6 teaspoons.
- Fancy Sandwich Emporium, cheese and pickle sarnie, 3 teaspoons.
- A typical Supermarket own brand, prawn curry ready-meal, 5 teaspoons.

Are you sitting down comfortably?
READER: *Oh! God here we go, yeah go ahead.*
Okay doke! 200g of toffee popcorn contains... over twenty teaspoons.

Hello, hello, are you still there?
INCREDULOUS READER: *Wha....But... N... WWWHHHAAATTTTTT??! Popcorn contains that much sugar? No, you're joking?*
Nope. Not joking, not this time. A particular brand that sounds like smooching a dairy spread, sells a 25g packet of Toffee popcorn which contains 104 calories, 14g of sugar and 2g of fat. That's a teeny, weeny bag. So when you're at home and tip a full family-sized bag into a bowl, and munch away during film night, you're just spooning sugar down your gob.

Whether its dried fruit, jam, tins of sweetcorn, packaged sarnies, ready-meals, crisps, biccies or a Victoria sponge cake, that product will be heaving with sugar. Therefore me ol' china, you're gonna have to start checking the labels. You need to become a label junkie and actually **know** what you're buying.

READER: *But they're complicated.*
They're meant to be. You wouldn't buy half the stuff, if you really knew what was in it.

If you keep in mind that 5g of sugar is the equivalent of a teaspoon, and your RDA is seven teaspoons (35g maximum) then you have a starter for ten.

Any product that has less than 10g of total sugars per 100g is ok, anything above that figure, you should try to avoid. Simple.

Example label from a natural protein, health bar:

Nutrition information	Per 100g		Per 45g bar	
Energy	2211kJ	530kcal	995kJ	238kcal
Fat		35.8g		16.1g
of which saturates		5.4g		2.4g
Carbohydrate		31.0g		14.0g
of which sugars		**13.7g**		**6.2g**
Fibre		6.7g		3.0g
Protein		18.8g		8.4g
Salt		0.005g		0.002g

As you can see, per 100g these bars contain 13.7g of sugar, and an individual bar contains 6.2g which is just a tad too high. In essence each bar would contain a teaspoon and a bit of sugar.

In my opinion it should be the law that food manufacturers display the amount of sugar (cubes perhaps) and salt (teaspoons) their food contains, **on all packaging**, so the consumer is fully aware of the risks of buying their cheaply produced crap. Sales would initially go down as a result but it would force these companies into completely changing how they manufacture their goods. The consumption of sugar by the nation would significantly reduce and obesity levels would shrink. But they won't do it because it'll cost too much dough.

Anyway back to current packaging (and I'm not talking sweet, dried, fruits here).

You've also got to pay no attention whatsoever to the packaging hyperbole, irrespective if it implies *'health'*, or states it's *'free'* of sugar or fat. For instance, *'whole grain'* sounds healthy but check the label because it may still contain just as much sugar (and salt) as it's incomplete grain sibling.

If the packet states *'Low-fat'*, or *'Diet'*, or *"fat-free"*, invariably it will be full of sugar and artificial sweeteners. **Guaranteed!!**
Check the label and if it contains any ingredient that ends in *'ose'*, or it's got *'Aspartame'*, *'Saccharin'* or any of the other chemically created sugars I've already mentioned, don't buy it. Always, always, always check the label, the more ingredients the less that product will be good for you. If you buy white bread, you're gonna end up consuming sugar whether you want to or not, so if you really do want to cut down, purchase wholemeal bread, or granary instead. But be warned, these also contain sugar, so **check the label.** If you still want to buy white rice or pasta, you're gonna end up scoffing more of the sweet stuff. You could opt for brown rice and pasta as an alternative, or you could take me up on my earlier recommendations and try bulgur wheat, quinoa, or kidney beans instead. And don't pull that sour face, I can see **you** ya know.
READER *(tentatively looks from side to side, then realises it's a book and I'm just messing)*: *You're bloody strange you!*
If you like to bake, don't go mad adding loads of powdery crack to your culinary delights.

Boost flavour by adding spices to your recipes, or honey for that sweet kick. However, you'll find that honey contains oodles of sugar too, so be careful with the amounts you add.

If you're adamant that you want to lose weight and are fully committed to reducing your sugar consumption, you'll have to start re-inventing your mindset.
READER: *How?*
If you're forever saying, *'I can't have that, it's bad for me'*, or *'I can't eat cake, it won't help me lose weight'*, you'll fail in the long run.
READER: *Why? I thought that's what you're saying?*
Far from it.
I think I've made it very clear that I don't have an issue with having the odd bun, biccy or chocolate bar. What I'm saying is that processed food is not good for you. Therefore you should try to cut it out completely from your diet. Saying *'I can't'*, doesn't clarify **WHY** you shouldn't, it just infers you're being punished. Whereas saying, *'I don't eat that type of food anymore because it's not good for me'*, implies you're fully aware of the reasoning and are dedicated to changing your identity.
You're stating to the world that you're in complete control of your diet. You're not punishing yourself, you're liberating yourself instead.

Does that make sense?

READER: *Yeah, I suppose...*

Ok! Let's look at it another way.

You're trying to lose weight, get fitter and healthier. Right?

READER: *Right.*

Unhealthy levels of sugar consumption is a barrier to that goal. Right?

READER: *Right.*

Ok! You're fully conscious of this fact and you've decided to change. Call it a *'diet'* if you will but it's not, it's a new a way of living. It's a new **mindset** because you've decided to take a different path in life. It's not that you **can't** eat a certain food; you've made the decision that you **don't** want to, anymore.

Can't implies that you want to, but you're not allowed. Whereas **don't**, suggests that you've assessed the facts, you know that it's a barrier to your weight loss goal, so you're not going to anymore.

If you say that *'you can't have crisps'*. That statement signifies that you **want** to eat the crisps but for some reason you're not allowed to. It's a temporary restriction.

If you say that *'you don't eat crisps anymore'*. That statement demonstrates that you have omitted that particular food from your diet.

No doubt you've assessed the facts and come to the conclusion that crisps contain too much fat, salt and sugar and thus are barriers to your weight loss goal. By adopting this type of mindset, you will **definitely** lose weight.

That's another Birchy Guarantee.

If you carry on saying, *'can't'* **you** will fail. **Guaranteed!!**

Do you know why you'll fail?

READER: *Why?*

Because that's what **you** did in the past, and it didn't work then and it won't work in the future.

CRAVINGS

You know the score. You start to crave something sweet; you can't stop thinking about it, salivating, desperate for that sugar rush. Then you think about the fact you're trying to lose weight and tell yourself *'no'*, you'll be good and start to scroll through your phone. Or watch the box, or pick your nose. But you can't stop thinking about the sugar. Chocolate, cheesecake, muffins, a biscuit, anything to satisfy your insatiable craving.

So you think *'sod it'* and head to the cupboard and sneak a few biccies, slice off a slab of cake, or frantically unwrap a choccy bar. You shovel 'em in your gob and then pick the crumbs from your clothes. But you feel elated, a feeling of satisfaction... for two minutes. Then what? You either eat more, or you get on with your day feeling sorry for yourself.

Rather than rushing to get your sugar fix straightaway, calm yourself. Take a few minutes to analyse **why** you want some sugar. Are you just bored? Starving? Depressed? Maybe it's all three. What you need to do initially, is have a drink. It may just be pangs of thirst you're feeling. Keep yourself busy, go for a walk. Or if you're hungry, make yourself a healthy snack. Spend a few minutes peeling, cutting, whisking and the like. This will take your mind off the sugar as you concentrate on making your meal.

Or sod that and just head for the biscuit tin. Yeah, life's bloody tough innit? So why not just relent and scoff down those snacks. Yeah you'll put on more flab, your health will deteriorate, you'll sweat more, you'll find it difficult walking up staircases, you'll have to buy bigger clothes in stretchy materials, you'll start to feel embarrassed about going out, eventually have no social life and hate yourself even more but you'll be able to eat whole blocks of cheese in your pants.

So swings and roundabouts.

But you're not bothered about all that are you? Are you?

READER: *Of course I am, you sarky git.*

Exactly. You've got to change your habits. If what you did before isn't working...

READER: *It isn't working, I know.*

That's why I keep drumming the point that if you're unhappy in your life, you'll fail miserably trying to lose the lard. If you're in the doldrums, you'll try to find solace in a bun, cake or a twelve pack of doughnuts. It won't work but you'll cheer up... for ten minutes at the most. That initial feeling of *'Ah! Sod it, a few won't make that much difference'*, will lead to guilt and remorse half n' hour later. You might start to think *'what's the point, who cares if I'm fat?'* But **you** know the answer to that question... **you** do... **you** care... a lot.

If you're busy enjoying life, walking, laughing, having fun. You won't continually seek these sugar rushes, 'cos you won't need them. And it won't matter if you do have a caramel shortbread, packet of crisps or bowl of toffee popcorn now and again. 'Cos you'll be off for a run, or a walk in the park, or doing boxercise, or joining in with the kids at the pool. Wouldn't that make **you** happier rather than scoffing a few choccy biccies and then feeling guilty about it?

Of course it would.

The less you eat crap, the less your body craves it. You stop missing it.

It's like relationships that are bad for you. Once you've finally made the decision to dump the parasitic git, it's difficult at first to get over them but once you're over that initial period, you don't miss them anymore. You move on. The issue is when you re-introduce them back into your life, the cycle begins again. Nothing has changed. If there are issues, there will still be issues. And if it's toxic, it doesn't belong in your life. Whatever it is. Respect yourself and get rid.

Therefore enjoy treats in moderation. You could even follow my example and have a *'half-seven'* every day.
READER: *What was that again?*
Basically, I don't have any sweet stuff all day but in the evening about half-seven ish I make a brew and have a slice of cake, or a flapjack, or a blueberry muffin, or a cherry bakewell (Hmmm! Cherry bakewells, just typing those words is getting me drooling. Ooh! I can't wait for 7:30pm).

I only have one (Ok! Sometimes two, or six) and that's fine for me. It works. And sometimes I don't bother at all. But if I do, it gives me something to look forward to and what's life without small pleasures? It's shite, that's what it is. As I've mentioned I'm really concerned about the state of my oral health, so that's another reason I restrict my consumption. Plus, I exercise at least 5 times a week, so any excesses I take, I know won't negatively affect my weight. So then me ol' love, packets of sweeties or Type 2 Diabetes? It's another choice. Up to you.

READER: *I get what you're saying but I couldn't live without chocolate.*
And nor should you.
But if you're gonna eat some, why have cotton when you can have organically made, luxuriously, velvety, 75% dark chocolate. In moderation. As a treat... not as your lunch.

If you're hooked on the cocoa and have a really bad habit, eating chocolate five times a day, then slowly scale it down. Have a trial separation, or only have custody during the weekend. As long as you're making positive steps, who cares if it takes you a year, even two years to finally curb your addiction. I mean c'mon, it took bloody years for you to put on the lard, it ain't coming off in a few weeks.

Sorry, there's no such thing as miracles.
GOD: *Right, that's it, you're getting a one way ticket to Hellsville, you blinkin', flippety, non-believing, heathen!!*
Please, forgive me.
GOD: *Oh! Alright then.*

Err, where was I?
READER: *Chocolate addiction.*
Aye. If you eat it five times a day, then start eating it four times a day. The week after, make it three times a day etc, etc et-cocoa-loco-cetera. If you do that, coupled with low-level exercise and enjoying life, you'll defo reduce that habit. If you want to that is?!

A sure fire way to cut your sugar and chocolate and ice-cream consumption, is via your weekly shop.
If you keep buying it, you'll keep binging and snacking and scoffing it. The less you buy, the easier it will be to stop bloody nibbling it.

Every time you purchase some processed, cheaply produced, sugary pap, you're actually confirming that you don't really care about your body and your weight. You're consciously making a decision to purchase food that is making you fat, unhealthy and depressed. Why do that to yourself? Why? Why? **WHY??!**

C'mon it's not that difficult, you've just gotta try. If you don't buy it, you don't have the temptation. Although supermarkets don't help, lowering their prices, coercing you into buying the bargains.

In fact, I need a few bits, so let's discuss those sneaky shops who are actually another leading contributor to the obesity crisis. That's right, I said it. In my humble opinion, they are GANB.
<u>READER</u>: *What's GANB?*
Bang out of order.

SUPERMARKETS

Warning – Don't go shopping when you're hungry

Back in the day, most folk would buy their grub from specialist shops. They'd get their meat from the Butchers, fruit and veg from the Greengrocers, bread and sweet treats from the Bakers, and a few bits from a supermarket. Nowadays, towns and villages rarely have these types of shop on the high street because the supermarkets have taken over. The food industry is big business and these corporations don't want you spending your dosh in friendly bespoke shops, no, they want you to increase their shareholders profits in windowless, soulless, retail-park structures.

Mini-marts and hypermarkets are the name of the game now, hence boarded up shops up and down this sorry land. Profit and greed, leading to low quality, mass produced goods, at cheap, rear-pocket-slapping prices.

When it comes to weight loss, supermarkets make the transition to healthy eating, extremely difficult for consumers. Look at the prices for *'gluten-free'* products, damn expensive.

Organic produce, **Kerching!!** Fruit, veg, high quality meat, each product is not reasonably priced. Healthy eating is a costly business.

Therefore in these times of austerity, do you plump for the decent grub or the cheap, 2 for 1, processed pap? Of course, it's no contest.

And if you're a family shopping on a budget, it's clear you'll be searching for the bargains and who could blame you. However, **you** want to lose weight, which means you're gonna have to become a smart shopper.

I get that supermarkets offer convenience in our *'alleged'* busy worlds but by making some sensible choices when you shop there, you can still eat healthily and not break the bank. Eating healthily is **not** as expensive as you may think.

Rather than buying fruit, salad or veg in pre-sliced, pre-washed packets, buy them loose. That way they'll cost significantly less, last longer and they'll still contain all of the nutrients. Plus, they'll look real, not glistening and shiny, like fake air-brushed celebs on a magazine cover.

Raw, blemished, ugly, odd-shaped produce will always be better for you than pre-packed, decontaminated, artificially preserved pap.
READER: *Yeah but I hate using those tongs and trying to manoeuvre food into a plastic bag.*
Ooh! Sorry Princess, I mean it's really difficult to open a plaggy bag and place some veg in there with your hands.

And it'll take, ooh, all of thirty seconds. Yeah I can really see the difficulty.

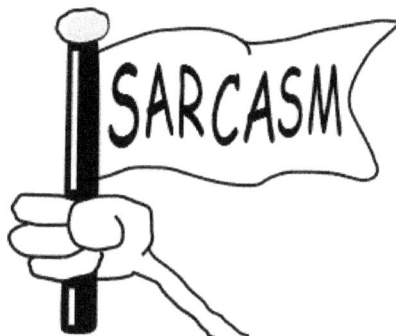

Ok! It's a minor ballache but it doesn't take **that long** and you can select the best fruit and veg, and chuck the mouldy ones back in the box. Whereas you get some right manky looking fruit and veg in some of those plastic, packaged trays. Up to you me ol' cocker!! Up to you.

Rather than buying meat or fish from the frozen aisle, head to the supermarket Butcher or Fishmonger. They're experts in their field and can actually explain how best to cook the meat in order to enhance flavour and taste. With the fish, they normally plaice the fillets in oven-proof bags, so they can easily be cooked on a baking tray with the minimum of effort.

Oh! And they're far cheaper than their frozen, breaded, neatly packed, salty mates.

If you must buy some bread, rather than opting for the sugary, processed, heavily refined, preserved, sliced, packet bread, buy the *'baked in store'* bread instead. Yes, you'll have to slice it yourself but blimey, I'm sure you can spare twelve seconds from your busy scrolling schedule. It'll be slightly healthier and you'll save some dough, which we all knead to do in these times of austerity.

Don't rush to purchase these *'buy one, get one free'* offers. Invariably the products are low quality, processed shite. You should become a snip-savvy customer instead.
READER: *Snip-savvy, what do you mean?*
Cut out coupons from magazines to get some discounts

Even better, you should try and do your big shop when the supermarket staff start to place those yellow & red *'reduced'* stickers on products that are about to reach their *'use-by-date'*. Don't be proud, you can get some right bargains. Fresh fish, fruit, meat and veg that has *'allegedly'* reached its *'about-to-be-chucked-in-the-waste-bins-round-the-back'*, date. You can actually freeze the fish and meat. The fruit and veg, you can have for your tea, although to be fair there's no rush, 'cos invariably they're still fresh enough to be consumed at a later date. It's scandalous how much food gets chucked just cos it's reached this supposed *'use-by-date'*.

To summarise, I strongly recommend that you try to buy your meat from a Butchers, Fish from a Fishmongers, fruit and veg from a Greengrocers and avoid processed, packaged food. And ready meals. And frozen food. And crisps. And pasta. And rice. And all that other bad stuff I've mentioned.

If there's a Farm shop nearby get visiting, you'll be amazed how cheap they can be, plus the quality of eggs, potatoes and the like, are substantially better than owt you'd get from a supermarket.

Oh! And if a food requires a commercial… avoid it.

Paul Birch

THERMOGENICS

The heat is on

READER: *What the hell is thermogenics? Is it another form of exercise?*
Yeah, it does sound like an aerobics class. No, you'll love this.
'Thermogenesis' is the metabolic process your body performs whilst burning calories to produce heat. Without getting too technical (because it's a scientific minefield), by consuming specific *'thermogenic'* foods, this will help increase your metabolism so you'll effectively burn more fat.
Sounds good?
READER: *Definitely. Which foods do that then? That sounds ace!! Tell me more…*
Alright, well calm down they're not miracle foods but by adding them to a healthy balanced diet, coupled with positivity, enjoying life and some moderate exercise of course…
READER: *Of course!*
…well, they will help speed up your metabolism and increase the melting of that there lard.

So the next time you're doing a big shop, your shopping list should include the following timber torching, chunk charring, blob burning, fat frazzling, flab frying foods:

DAIRY – Cottage Cheese

FREE RANGE EGGS – Eggs from caged hens contain significantly less nutrients than their roaming, playing, mucking about, happier cousins

FRUIT – Apples, Avocado, Blackberries, Pears and Raspberries (I know the plural of avocado is *'avocados'* but it looks weird hence the omission)

HERBS & SPICES – Basil, Black Pepper, Cardamom, Cayenne Pepper, Cumin Seeds, Garlic, Ginger, Mustard and Turmeric

MEAT & FISH – Chicken Breast, Lean Red Meat, Salmon, Tuna Steak, Turkey and Venison

MISC. - Aloe Vera Juice, Apple Cider Vinegar, Chocolate (85% cocoa), Coconut Oil, Flaxseed Oil, Green Tea, Kidney Beans, Lemon Juice, Lentils, Quinoa and Salsa (any opportunity to say *'salsa'* should be embraced – squirt it on your alfalfa, then we're talking!!)

NUTS - Walnuts

VEGETABLES – Asparagus, Broccoli, Butternut Squash, Cabbage, Chilli, Kale, Mushrooms, Red Onions, Red Peppers and Spinach

In theory, if your entire diet consisted of those specific thermogenic foods, you'd lose weight in no time. You'd be full of vitality, glowing with energy and your dinner would make you thinner.

Go on, give thermo a go.

What you gotta lose? Apart from melted lard **of course!!**

282

VEGETABLES

Fart your way to good health and weight loss

READER: *OMG!! I hate vegetables!! I can't stand 'em!!*
I'm sick of people saying that because I bet you don't. What you **hate**, is vegetables that have been boiled within an inch of their life.

And I agree. Boiled veg is rank. It destroys essential nutrients, impairs flavour and makes the veg all mushy and pasty, and quite frankly, unappetising.

Vegetables are **full** of nutrients, anti-oxidants, vitamins, minerals and believe it or not, flavour. But how you cook them, will determine the taste. You could go hardcore and eat them raw, you can steam them, roast 'em, stir-fry 'em but don't, please don't **ever** boil them again.

It won't surprise you to learn that I'm a veg devotee.

For the last decade, I have eaten veg for the majority of my main meals. My family think I'm nuts 'cos I rarely eat pasta or rice, but I'm healthy, I'm fit, thin and I can fart for England.

Yep, I'll admit, I'd give it twenty minutes before you follow me into the bathroom. That's the only downside from eating a diet loaded with veg, there's definitely a stench from your number two's.
But then, all shit stinks... **even yours!!**

So if you lose loads of weight by eating more veg, it's certainly a small price to pay.

Therefore I'm gonna try to persuade **you** that vegetables are freakin' awesome and you'd be a fool not to add as many as you can stomach, to every main meal. A fool, **I tells ya!!**

I want you to read this section and rather than say *'you hate veg'*, I want you to say, *'OMG! I ate vegetables!! And lost loads of weight'*.

READER: *You don't want me turn veggie do you?!*
No, no, no. Don't worry, you can still eat the meat, although it defo wouldn't do you any harm if you did become a vegetarian. I mean, you don't see many fat veggies... **just saying!!**

Anyway, how can you say you don't like vegetables, have you tried them all?
READER: *Well, no.*
Exactly!!
There are **thousands** of vegetables out there, all bursting with flavour and packed full of vitamins and minerals. I can't dig them all up to explain their virtues, so I'll just mention a few. And don't skip this bit, or else you can't have dessert later.

Oh! And if I put a plant in the veg family, or a pulse or bean, please forgive me, I'm just lumping them all together for convenience.

You don't really need me to tell you that **ALL** veg will contain specific essential nutrients, vitamins and minerals, therefore I won't labour the point re each type, I'll just mention the odd fact to help clarify their benefits. And they're all low in calories and virtually *'fat-free'*, so bulk up, to bulk down.
And, and, **AND**... nutritious **CAN** be delicious!!

BEETROOT – For some reason, old fogies used to love eating beetroot sarnies. Maybe they were forced to eat them when at school during World War Two or summat but irrespective these rich, deeply purple wonders, are nutritional super-foods. So don't ignore them. Consumption of beetroots boosts blood flow, and has been proven to reduce the risk of heart disease and lower blood pressure. Even Olympic athletes quaff beetroot juice, to aid recovery and boost stamina due to its high concentration of calcium, fibre and the vitamins A and C.

283

Pickled, fried, steamed, juiced or even raw, beetroot is great in salads, soups, or a creamy risotto.

You just can't beat **the beet!!**

BROCCOLI – Yeah, sometimes the bits might get stuck between your teeth but biscuits will stick to your butt. Yes they look like miniature trees but the fake foliage works well in salads, stir fries, curries and soups. The longer you cook them the softer and mushier they get, so I recommend stir-frying or steaming for a crunchier taste. Spice them up with cayenne or chilli-pepper.
Hot Damn!!
They are also members of the *'cruciferous family'*, which has nothing to do with Jesus before you ask. What it does mean, is these bad boys will enhance your flatulence. Can't be avoided but remember, it's just fat dying.

BUTTERNUT SQUASH – These phallic beauties are extremely high in zinc, and are great roasted in t'oven, mashed or as the main base for soup.
READER: *They look far too much hassle to chop up.*
First time I cooked with butternut squash, I went on *'You-Tube'* to find vids on how to cut 'em up. You can find anything on *'You-Tube'*.

Anyway, they're simple to chop up. Slice down the middle, spoon out the seeds, then shove in the oven for about half n-hour or so. They'll go soft, and then you can use them as an alternative to mash, or add them to your stir-fry. Not that difficult and they are bloody gorgeous, well worth the mediocre effort.

Plus, how great is it to say *'butternut squash'*? Add some salsa and alfalfa to your butternut squash and then you're really cooking.

CABBAGE – A superfood wrapped in a leafy red, white, green or purple package (calm down!).
It's full of calcium, fibre, iron, potassium, selenium and the vitamins B1, B2, C and K.

There are a myriad of health benefits linked to the consumption of cabbage that relate to your skin, hair and overall health. Add it to soup, chuck it in a stir-fry, juice it, or throw it in a salad but as a member of the cruciferous family, you may want to make sure you have plenty of air freshener around a few hours after you eat it.

What's orange and sounds like a parrot?
READER: *I don't know.*
A carrot.

CARROTS – Rabbits love 'em, so who are we to judge?
I used to like carrots, like men like shoe shopping. But it was because I'd always eaten them as part of a Sunday lunch, and invariably they were boiled, so tasted disgusting.

I changed my opinion after eating some raw carrots and realised they were really nice, especially dipped in hummus. I now add them to all my stir-fries and they are great mashed, far healthier than tatties.
You can also make *'gold soup'*…
READER: *Hold on, hold on, what the bloody 'ell is 'gold soup'?*
Oh! It's just soup made with 18 carats, sorry, I mean *'carrots'*… sorry, worst joke, **ever!!**

They're also awesome in cake. Cake. **Cake!!** Not many vegetables can say that, although I am yet to taste *'broccoli au-chocolat'*.

Carrots are rich in vitamins A, C, and K, and packed full of fibre and iron.
They also contain *'Beta-carotene'* which will help to improve skin, the immune system and your vision. And that is snow joke.

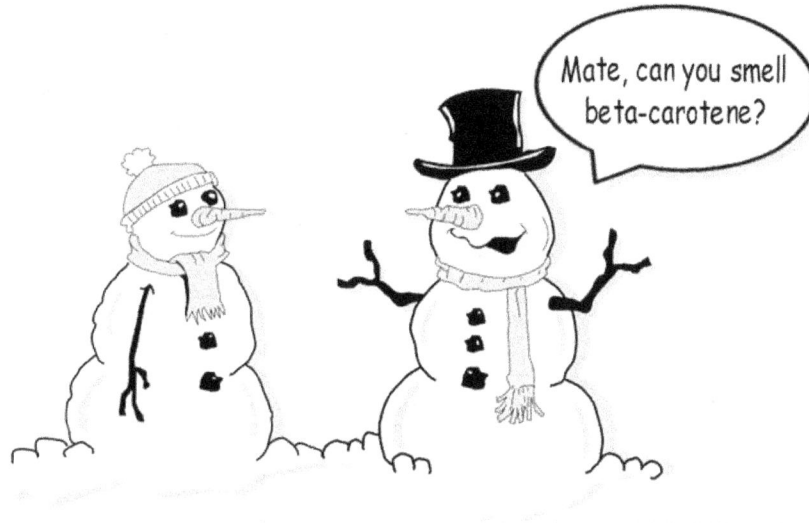

Mate, can you smell beta-carotene?

CAULIFLOWER – It might look like a brain but **you'll** be the clever-clogs if you add one of the healthiest foods on this planet to your newly, vegetable enriched diet. Absolutely chocka with nutrients and who doesn't love a bit of cauliflower cheese?
READER: *Not me.*
Damn you, you cauli-cynic.
It's quite trendy these days to use grated cauliflower as a substitute for rice, or flour for bread.
Well, I say this is one fashion you'd be wise to follow. I'm partial to cauli-rice myself, although I've not tried the bread. I'll add it to my ever changing bucket list.

Curried cauli is a treat to behold and even though I mentioned that barbecue sauce was teeming with sugar, roasted cauli dipped in bbq sauce is de-lish!! Try it and tell me I'm wrong. Go on, I dare you.

CELERY - Is 95% water and very low in calories. It's also disgusting, so avoid at all costs.

KALE – I'd never even heard of kale until about two years ago, now it's every bloody where.
Another veg full to the brim with anti-oxidants and vitamins n' that, but it's definitely an acquired taste.
I like it in stir-fries, goes really well with beef I reckon but for some reason it's ubiquitous with smoothies. I've tried a couple and they make me wanna vom!! You might love 'em though, so experiment, see what happens but don't blame me if you retch a vibrant, green, torrent of liquid, down your nice blouse or whistle n' flute.

LETTUCE – I don't have any lettuce jokes but if **you** do, lettuce know.
Anyway, lettuce is not just for salad and ruining sandwiches. It's a great accompaniment to any stir fry but add it near the end, so you only cook it for about thirty seconds. That way it doesn't destroy the many, many, many, many, many nutrients it contains and still retains some crunch.

The problem with trying to cook lettuce is it just turns to watery mush and that's not nice for anyone, so in this case, less is more with lettuce.

MANGE TOUT – Del Boy's fave veg. If you can stomach it, mange tout is full of isaflavones that help to break down stored fat. That's right, tweacle, mange tout is a fat destroyer. Load it up. Nutrients? Full of 'em. Tasty? In a stir fry, definitely. Mange tout is one of the few vegetables I can actually eat raw and they are good for dipping into hummus, and those other dips we only seem to buy for parties.

MUSHROOMS – Why did the mushroom go to the party?
READER: *Was it because, he was a fun-gi?*
No!! It's because he was invited like everyone else.
Okay, over to mushrooms.

I absolutely **love** 'em. Lightly fried in butter, button mushrooms are chuffin' lush and add some top flavour to any dish. Naturally they're full of the good stuff, especially potassium, selenium and vitamin D. Yep, shrooms are definitely magic and you can conjure up some divine dishes by adding some chopped, sliced or whole mushrooms to a meal. Mushroom soup is really nice with loads of black pepper and garlic but they're also great grilled, stir-fried, roasted, steamed or even eaten raw, although be careful if you pick your own in the wild, 'cos some of 'em are toxic.

If you buy them from the Supermarket or Greengrocers, I recommend trying Chanterelle, chestnut, enoki, morels, oyster, porcini, Portobello and shitake. There are thousands of varieties but I can't type them all here... 'cos I don't have that mushroom.

ONIONS – Tissues at the ready.
Peel the onion and you'll find layers and layers of anti-oxidants which are so good for you, it'll make you cry. Ok! They might whiff a bit but whether eaten raw, sautéed, steamed, roasted or fried, onions will add a kick to any dish. I'm not gonna go all homeopathy on ya ass, but the health benefits ascribed to consuming onions will make your eyes water. There's too many to list here, suffice to say, onions are a true super-food. And before you ask, no, onion rings are not good for you. There are loads of different varieties of onion, such as chives, leeks, garlic, green, pickled, red, spring, sweet and white, yeah there's loads but I can't think of anymore, so that's shallot.

PEAS – Give peas a chance!!
I'm not talking frozen or tinned peas here by the way, I'm talking the positively pleasant sugar-snap peas. Really high in vitamin C they add a sweet, crunchy tinge to stir-fries and actually make a nice snack.
READER: *A snack, are you kidding me?*
Hey, I tell ya, I love to pop 'em down raw. Yeah, I'm bonkers me!! Give 'em a go, then if you like them too, we can be like two peas in a pod.

Garden peas are alright too, I just find them a tad bland. Obviously I never boil them, sacrilege, so I add them to a stir-fry, caked in butter and draped in chilli-pepper. They're not bad then. Actually they do make a lovely creamy soup. With chunks of ham. And chicken. And loads of black pepper. Wang some mackerel in as well. **Yum-diddly-umptious!!**

But remember they are not **the only** vegetable out there, which if you watch any TV adverts seems to be the case. So pair them with as many other veg as you can.

PEPPERS – I'm a massive fan of red, hot, chilli peppers and I love to sing their praises. Did you know that they contain about seven times as much vitamin C as an orange?
READER: *No, I did not know that.*
Well, erm... they do.

If you want to spice things up in the kitchen, cook naked, or if that's maybe going a little too far, chuck some chilli's into any hot dish to give it some **sizzle!!**

Yep, I add them to my stir-fries but you'll find they complement any beef dish, and go really well with tomatoes.

If you're a little bit wary of some spice in your life, you can always wimp out and eat the non-fiery bell peppers, which are also bursting with nutrients.

Do you want to know an interesting fact about bell peppers?
READER: *Do I?!*
I don't know if you're being sarky or not but anyway, peppers range in colour from green, to yellow, to orange, to red and this reflects the different stages of the ripening effect.

<u>READER</u>: *That is interesting, thank you for this astounding knowledge... give me the flag...*

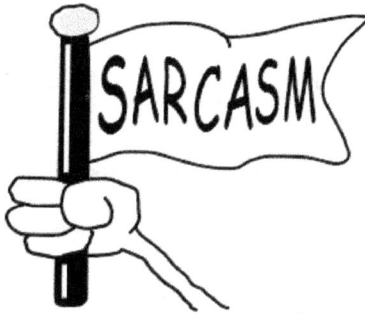

Green peppers are picked before they ripen and therefore are less sweet than their juicier cousins. They can be eaten raw but if you do cook a pepper, only grill, steam, or fry for a few minutes to retain their crunchiness; otherwise they'll go all soft and watery.

Stuffed peppers are nice too. Chuck 'em in t'oven for about an hour and they're great stuffed with a mixture of quinoa or rice, and some other veggies.

Make sure you turn the oven on though.

That's the end of this short bell pepper section. Yeah, you can't go wrong with peppers of any variety, the only one I don't like is Doctor.

RUNNER BEANS – Full of calcium and fibre, runner beans taste great steamed with a touch of sea salt. Also known as *'green beans'*, *'French beans'* or *'stringy beans'*, they're rich in fibre and vitamins and great in stews, soups and with your Sunday roast.

But whichever way you cook them, whether it's grilled, fried or roasted, only cook for a few minutes otherwise you'll ruin the bean. And you don't wanna ruin the runner bean.

SPINACH – This leafy veg is heaving with nutrients and unquestionably deserves to be known as a super-food. Spinach is a rich source of iron and zinc, as well as loaded with calcium, fibre, protein, and the vitamins A, C, E and K. For those *'Popeye'* fans, if you pop a tin of spinach down your gullet you will not suddenly develop humongous muscles, instead, you'll probably end up puking your guts out. I recommend adding spinach to a stir fry, soup, stew, mash, or mixed in with rice and unsurprisingly, spinach does go very well with olive oil.

SPROUTS – This vegetable is...
<u>READER</u>: *Sprouts?! Sprouts?! Are you insane? I hate sprouts!!*
Ok! Sprouts defo have a bad rep but they can be very nice, depending on how they are cooked.
If you boil them, yuck!! But if you cut them into quarters, and mix them in a pan with some vegetable oil and bacon and onions and chilli-pepper and mushrooms, they are awesome.

Think of cooking as like being a DJ and remix the old hits into stonking, banging, original, gastronomic, flavoursome compositions. **Get your funk on!!**

That's why cooking shouldn't be a chore but cathartic and fun. Turn the box off, get some tunes playing and get remixing those dishes. Forget techno, make it Gastro!! Gastro!! **Gastro!!**

You don't want the blues when you're in the kitchen, so think of your meals at the moment as easy listening, elevator music but with some imagination and vision it could be psychedelic, new wave, jazzy, trip-hop. So add some sophistication to your culinary palette.

And cooking is just like life, without music it would be flat.

Anyrode back to sprouts. These balls of goodness are crammed full of fibre, protein and loads of minerals and vitamins. But they're just not fashionable so they get overlooked for the trendy new veg on the chopping block. Which is a shame, 'cos for most of the year they're extremely good value and actually very tasty, so you should try to add them to your hot meals.

The only minor downside is they will make you toot. It'll be like a brass band emanating from your glute region but that's not a major reason to avoid them.

So c'mon, drop some sprout bass and shake, shake, shake, shake the room. **Boom!!**

I'm telling ya, the more veg you consume the more weight you'll lose. Replace your mounds of rice and pasta, with piles of veg instead. I mean to be fair, pasta and rice are quite plain really, so spicy vegetables will taste significantly better anyway. There are endless possibilities regarding how you cook veg, the only limit is your imagination and stubborn resistance to change.

As ever, up to you, just another suggestion but if bright colours make us happy, why do we eat bland, pale, lifeless looking food?

I know I keep mentioning stir-fries, so to give you an idea of how I cook mine here's a typical example of a Birchy dish:

Instructions

- Get a fair sized wok, add a ¼ cup of water, a few drizzles of olive oil, a generous knob of butter and glaze with sprinkles of black pepper, cayenne pepper, paprika, sea salt and a dash of Henderson's relish
- Set on low heat
- Slice two carrots, a red pepper, a wedge of red cabbage and then add to dish – shake wok and stir
- After a few minutes, throw in some sliced courgette, seven or eight whole sugar snap peas, a diced small red onion, four or five sliced mushrooms, a dozen whole green beans, a small sliced red chilli pepper and mix abaht
- Chop up two cloves of garlic and mix in with the veg
- After a few more mins, add some prepared chunks of salmon, or tuna, or beef and stir in to the melee
- Add some Puy lentils, or kidney beans, or chick peas, or quinoa
- Shake in some more black pepper, bit more butter and stir for a few more mins
- Slap onto a big plate
- Gobble that veg and meat extravaganza… slowly… remembering to chew and savour the tastes and flavours
- Wash up, relax and enjoy the rest of the evening
- An hour or so later, release a series of SBD's
- Apologise to anybody else in the room or blame the dog

I eat that type of meal probably six times a week and I have done for the last decade…
READER: *Don't you get bored of eating the same meal?*
As if… no way man!!

I've mastered the art of cooking this dish, so that I know it's gonna be lush and I always enjoy it.

The veg is crispy, juicy and spicy and I just adore them cooked in this way. I always make such a massive pile, that I'm never hungry after eating, and it sorts me out until the next day. Full of nutrients, virtually *'fat-free'*, quick to make and cheap to purchase.

The recipe for weight loss and that's another **Birchy Guarantee!!**

Have a go, play around with the spices, different types of veg, add cream, spicy lamb, curried pork, whatever, create your very own stir-fry bonanza but all in all, experiment.

Yo! Yo! Yo! It's time for some freestyle veg, so Ladies & Gentlemen, clap your hands together, wave your hands in the air like you actually care, and enjoy my wholesome, roasted, vegetable wrap…

I love vegetables, from my head to-ma-toes,
If you loved 'em too, you'd fit in your clothes,
So don't push veggies to the side of the plate,
These nutritious foods will help you lose weight,
Packed with vitamins and minerals too,
Veggies are great, they're so good for you!!!
Cucumber, courgette, butternut squash,
Before you cook 'em, just give 'em a wash,
Artichokes are ace and pumpkins are smashing,
Runner beans steamed and turnip's a-mashing,
Corn on the cob, rhubarb and custard,
Asparagus tips, smothered in mustard!!!
Roasted parsnips and cauliflower cheese,
Beetroot sarnies and popping some peas,
Stir-fried veggies and a creamy, spicy soup,
Who cares if you guff, if you fart, if you poop,
It's a small price to pay, if you're sick of being fat,
Get your VEGGIE game on, stop being a PRAT!!!

READER: *Well, thanks for that. Erm, I though a tomato was a fruit?*
Ok! Betty Botany, from a pedantic point of view a tomato is a fruit, but c'mon it's a bloody vegetable and we all know it.

And by the by, **fresh** tomato soup is extremely healthy for you. They might be squishy but tomatoes are full to the core with vitamin A. C, E and K, plus a fabulous anti-oxidant called *'Lycopene'*.
READER: *What's lycopene?*
Lycopene gives a tomato that bright, reddish hue and when consumed this compound can provide a multitude of health benefits, from lowering the risk of heart disease to reducing blood pressure.
Lycopene consumption has also been linked to improving your eyesight, which reminds me,
www.maculardegeneration.org

READER: *What's that?*
Oh! It's a site for sore eyes. **Boom!!**
Yes, I am **always** that funny, I'm **hi-bloody-larious!!**

Now, it's over to something warm, wet and filling… SOUP.
If you still can't stomach veggies, even when stir-fried or roasted or grilled, then either add them to soup, or make some soup yourself. If you're trying to lose the lard, you should really try and eat soup whatever the weather.

READER: *What, even when it's hot outside?*
Of course! So you can't have soup in summer? Who says, the government? It's not against the law, so sod 'em. We don't have seasons anymore anyway. Therefore if you fancy soup, have it. In fact buy a soup maker, I implore ya and shove your veggies in there. You see, your stomach takes a lot more time to absorb soup than solid meals, therefore you feel fuller for longer. Stopping you reaching for those damn, sugary snacks. Win/win.

Consuming vegetable based soup will help provide you with loads of nutrients, in a simple, easy to cook dish and it's always comforting eating soup. Add some curry powder to 'em, just don't mop it up with loads of salty, sugary, processed white bread.
READER: *Oh!! You take the fun out of everything you.*

Another dish to try is *'Ratatouille'.*
READER: *What's that?*
Oh! It's delightful. A veggie dish containing aubergine, courgettes, onions, tomatoes and peppers, lightly fried in garlic and vinegar, then stewed in t'oven for a bit. Feel free to chuck some beef or chicken in with it too, and even extra veg if you so feel the desire. Any excuse to say *'ratatouille'* should be grasped at every opportunity. Especially if you try and say it in a Welsh accent.
Go on give it a go, after me... RAT-A-TOU-ILLE!!
READER *(in faux Welsh accent)*: *RAT-A-TOU-ILLE!! You're a tosspot.*
Yes I am, thanks for noticing. There are thousands of ratatouille recipes on t'internet so have a gander and get cooking.

HARRY, 31 - *Since I've started eating more fresh fruit and veg, it's had a really positive knock-on effect with the kids. Instead of having cupboards bursting with biscuits, crisps, popcorn and chocolates, our kitchen table now has a tower of apples, bananas, carrots, grapes and sugar snap peas that the bairns can help themselves to whenever they're feeling peckish.*
I feel like it's setting them up for a healthier future and I don't want to see my kids getting obese.
And Birchy, I know you used to say, 'monkey see, monkey do!!' well, in our family you're right!!
Obviously the cycling has helped with me losing weight but 'cos of the positive results, I'm on such a health kick now that I'm even growing my own veg in the garden. Carrots, peas, courgettes, the bloody lot and I have to say, they taste so much better than store-bought veg. My Dad has an allotment so I'm getting him to add more variety to his patch, and family and friends now pop round hoping to cadge some free veg off us. I never would have thought about doing anything like this if I hadn't spoken to you mate.
Cheers Birchy!!

Look, don't worry, I'm not recommending you become a vegetarian or heaven forbid, a vegan but by eating more veg and making it a major part of your dinner, you'll lose weight and that's what it's all about, isn't it?! Isn't it?! **ISN'T IT?!** The body needs **forty specific nutrients** on a daily basis in order to function properly, and no single food will provide all of these. But if you eat a diet rich in vegetables, you'll get most of 'em.

Alrighty then, here's a joke to finish this section.

How do you know when someone is vegan?
READER: *I don't know?*
Don't worry, they'll tell ya.

So now you know what to eat, let's get to the kitchen and see what's cooking.
Hmm!! It smells delicious...

THE KITCHEN

If you're trying to lose weight… know your place

If you're trying to lose weight, then evidently your current diet is not conducive to this goal. Therefore you have got to try and **BAKE THE FIT UP** in order to **WAKE THE FIT UP!!**

Already, I can your inner voice saying *'I haven't the time to prepare, or cook food on an evening'*. Really? **Really?!** Are you being true to yourself there? Or is it, 'cos you can't be arsed?!

If you can spend hours in front of the box watching soaps and reality pap, then you've got more than enough time to cook a decent healthy meal of an evening.
READER: *Yes but I do like to relax on an evening after a hard day at work.*
I getcha!! Well, don't ever moan about your weight again.
READER: *What do you mean?*
Look, if you truly want lose weight, I mean, you're actually **desperate** to, then you'll decide enough is enough re your previous lifestyle, take a timeout, re-evaluate and make some significant changes for the better in order to succeed.

But if you're just **pretending** that you want to lose weight, then fine, that's your decision but that negates your ability to bang on about your weight 'cos you're not really arsed about it.

Harsh but oh so true.

READER: *You make it sound so easy.*
That's 'cos it is.
Back in my pre-healthy-nutrition days, when I used to make my evening meal, I'd bang a few bits on a baking tray and shove 'em in t'oven. Wait half n' hour and then serve with beans or packet pasta.
READER: *What type of things?*
Breaded fish, breaded chicken, pies, jacket spuds and meals for one. I used to love spending time in the kitchen. I didn't cook, I just loved sitting in there.

But over the years and especially in the last decade, I've completely changed my diet.

I'm no chef by any stretch of the imagination; all I generally do is slap loads of veg in a wok and make my own funky creations. I like fish, so I'll either buy packet salmon flakes, or tins of mackerel and tuna, then add them to my veggie-stir fry.

Or I'll purchase a fillet of salmon or tuna steak, sprinkle some herbs and spices over it and chuck that on a baking tray, shove in t'oven for half n' hour. Serve on plate, with veggie medley.
READER: *Is that all you ever eat?*
For my main meals, yes. Some form of fish or meat, and a heap of veg.
Nutrients aplenty and keeps me full. Cheap too, 'cos I don't buy loads of packet stuff and frozen crap.

And I make regular trips to the Greengrocers to get my veg.
READER: *Why not the supermarket?*
Well, I like to support my local Greengrocers and c'mon, those guys know their onions. And carrots. And broccoli. And cabbage…

But I admit that it's easy peasy for me, 'cos I'm a single chap and just shop for one. I appreciate it's far harder to shop for a family but you can still adopt the same principles, you've just gotta make some changes.

Ok! Here's some food for thought.

As I've mentioned **you** should limit the amount of processed, packaged food you buy, but if you do have to get it **always** check the labels. If you don't know what the ingredients are, then you don't want to know. Step away from the aisle and buy something else.

If you do purchase some frozen tat, you can funk them up by adding fresh vegetables and quality meat to add bulk to the dish, as well as adding some, what we call, flavour, taste, anti-oxidants etc, etc. Avoid monotony in your diet, experiment because ad nauseam will make you sick.

If you're about to cook a frozen pizza, do me a favour and before you chuck it in t'oven, slice it into four.
READER: *Why, will that make it cook more evenly?*
No. But once you've cut it into four, it's far easier for you to get each piece and throw them in the bin.
Don't buy them ever again, make your own or grab something that has **actual** nutrients instead. As I keep rattling on, food should offer **VALUE**.

> **KATIE, 38** - *I was sick and tired of eating the same things and feeling the same way. Fat, tired and morose. My plate was always covered with mounds of starchy carbs, followed by a huge dessert. Ready meals were my salvation because I didn't know how to cook but I felt terrible!*
> *I needed to change.*
> *I wanted to make healthy, delicious meals because I knew it would help me feel better. I'm so glad we met up and discussed food as well as fitness.*
> *I took on board your advice, started to read cook-books, in fact I even started sharing recipes with my colleagues at work. It became fun trying out new dishes. Yeah, some of them didn't always taste so appetising but I got quite good at cooking. I still had pasta and rice now and again but I did like you said and cut down the portion sizes, bulking the meal up with meat and veg. Coupled with the walking, I've lost loads and I can tell you now, I'm not wasting all that effort by ruining my good work.*
> *Meals for one, they can do one!!*

Learn **HOW** to cook. Spend time reading recipe books and try some of them out. Baking, steaming, roasting and whatever else, are not difficult to master, they just take practice. Pressing a few buttons on a microwave, is not cooking. You have a kitchen, no doubt full of expensive machinery and fancy cutlery and utensils and whatnot... **use 'em!!**

Got a chopping board? Use it.
A spice rack? Use the spices, it shouldn't just be for decoration.
A soup maker? Definitely use that. You know, after you've wiped the dust off it.

And if you haven't got one, buy a wok. They are ace and you can create your very own, stir-fry mishmash. Yep, you should definitely wok up and smell the possibilities.

Taste is subjective and just because the fancy chefs on the telly might scoff at your orange juice pork roast, or beetroot flapjacks, if you like it then who cares.
So try your hand at making your own pies, stews, curries, sauces...
READER: *Sauces?!*
Aye why not? That way you can control what goes in them and add ingredients that **you'd** like to see in a particular sauce, that perhaps you can't buy in a processed jar from the supermarket.
Fancy some vinegar in a tomato sauce? Add it. Entirely up to you.

Here's one for you. Get your foil game on.
READER: *What foil game?*
I've done this trick several times to cut corners and save me a bit of time, plus it reduces the amount of washing up that needs doing after, which is always a bonus. Think about that, CBA gang.

For example, make a pouch with some foil, similar in shape to an envelope. Slap a fillet of salmon in there. Cut some veg up, then chuck that in the foil pouch too. Add some herbs and spices, a splash of Hendersons, close pouch and delicately place in t'oven for half n' hour.

Go about your business, take pouch from oven. Open slightly to pour some of the watery juice away and then serve on plate (or save the juice and use it the next day to marinade meat, or as a sauce).

I'm telling you, it works wonders and tastes great.

On a weekend, try and spend a bit of time cooking and preparing dishes which you can eat in the week. After all, you've got loads of *'Tupperware'* and *'Clingfilm'* in that cupboard gathering dust, why not actually use it?!!

If you start to prepare your food for the week, it'll save you time after a busy day at work.

Once defrosted, bang it in the oven or even the microwave whilst you get on with all those other jobs you need to do. You could set aside one day a week for meal prepping. It'll take a few hours, tops. You know what they say, fail to prepare, prepare to fail.

Put your mobile away for an hour, switch the box off, put on some toons and get your kitchen freak on. Boogie-baking, it's the future. Get the kids involved too, they can help slice and dice and chop. **And** they can wash up afterwards. It's a nice bonding experience and they might even learn that cooking, doesn't just involve the whirr/ping of a microwave.

READER: *Ok! I'll give it a try. Any tips for eating at work?*
Yeah, don't put mackerel in the microwave. Your colleagues will hate you and it's a pain in the posterior to get rid of the fishy stench.
READER: *I meant…*
Yeah, yeah I know.

I would always recommend that you bring in a packed lunch. That way you can control what ingredients you scoff, and you're less inclined to make a rash, unhealthy decision on your lunch hour. Plus, it will stop you buying crappy meal deals from the sandwich shop. You know the ones, a sarnie on white sugary bread with low quality meat, coupled with a packet of salty, sugary crisps, followed by a can of fizzy, saccharin infused pop. *'No deal, Noel'.*

You could even stop bringing money to work, which will prevent you from heading to the tuck shop or snack machine. Ideally you want to eat a meal at lunch that will **stop** you from snacking until you eat again in the evening. Oats, eggs, quinoa, soup, lentils, kidney beans, meat and veggies, will all help you accomplish that by keeping you fuller for longer.

It's not the law that you have to eat a sandwich at lunch you know, so change your dietary habits.

If you work shifts, don't change how you would normally eat just because the mealtimes are different. If you're working nights, you want to eat a really big meal before work and have an early breakfast. That way, it will prevent you from snacking just for the sake of it.

And here's a little warning to conclude this section. It's very difficult to out-exercise a bad diet.
Now, talking of exercise…

Pre and post workout food
So you're happy with yourself and proud that you've completed a decent workout.
After your gym session you're likely to get a bit peckish. So, do you opt for a low calorie recovery snack, or do you reward yourself with a bun, bacon butty and a saccharin infused milkshake?

Most people opt for the latter, and can eat in upwards of a 1000kcals after they've conducted a workout.

But even though you might've spent an hour at the gym or jogged for forty-five minutes, you may only have burned about 500kcals.
READER: *Is that all?*
Yep!! Although the harder you train, the more calories will be burned. That's up to you of course.

Therefore if you're gobbling up 1000kcals after a bit of exercise, you don't make any positive gain and instead you'll have a 500kcal deficit. Let's say this continues over the weeks, you'll probably decide to quit the gym because even though you're putting in all that effort, you're gaining weight rather than losing it.

READER: *I've done that you know. Well, what can I do to change it?*
It's simple. After your workout, sup some water and have a low-energy snack such as porridge, scrambled eggs, soup, salad, granola, fruit or even nothing at all.
READER: *Nothing?!*
Yeah, there's no law that says you have to eat after a workout. Why not have a 500kcal gain and just eat normally for the rest of the day?!

If you continue to fall into the trap of rewarding yourself with treats after a gym session or a run, this is completely counter-productive and negates the time and energy expended.
You're trying to lose weight here, not put it on.

So stop wasting your time.

You don't have to eat anything **before** an exercise session either, if you don't want to.

Be aware that if you do, that food will be utilised immediately as energy during your workout thus stored fat will not be touched. If you do require some pre-exercise fuel, try eating bananas, or a small bowl of porridge, or some scrambled eggs about an hour before conducting any activity. This will provide ample enough energy for the workout.

Water is especially important whenever you conduct exercise. Therefore please make sure you have a few glasses before and after, plus a few sips during your session.

As a consequence of physical exertion, you will end up sweating therefore water is **the best way** to replenish the lost fluid in your system.
'Isotonic drinks' are quite good but don't waste your dosh on expensive, very high in sugar, sports drinks.
READER: *Is sweat, your fat crying, like people say?*
No it bloody well isn't.
That's just a complete myth to sell expensive sportswear.

We sweat in order to cool our bodies down during exercise, or heightened episodes of stress, such as wolfing down a hot vindaloo.

Your brain sends a signal to over three million glands in your body, for them to let the floodgates open and release sweat. And sweat is a funky smelling, clear fluid, made of water, salts and electrolytes, which when evaporated, helps to **lower** the bodies temperature.
It does not contain any element, of adipose tissue.
READER: *So how does fat, die?*
Fat doesn't really melt or burn, instead it is broken down into tiny molecules, and combines with oxygen to be utilised as energy.
But only, yes only, after the body has run out of its preferred energy source, *'Glucose'* (sugar). Which means Ladies and Gentlepeeps, the less sugar you consume in your diet, the more **fat** will be broken down to be utilised as an energy source. Ergo, the more energy you need, the more fat cells are used and the more weight you will lose.

See? It's making sense now, innit?!!

Let me bust another **myth** for you.

You may have noticed that after an energetic workout your top is drenched in sweat, so you head over to the weighing scales to check on your progress. Hallelujah!! The number on the scale has gone down. **Yippee!!** You've lost some timber.

Not exactly, I'm afraid.

Nope, you haven't dropped a few pounds of fat, what you've lost is a fair amount of fluids, which is **why** you need to replace that lost weight with some refreshing water to avoid dehydration.

Now, I'm often asked why a client will initially lose over a stone quite quickly during a diet, or new exercise regime, yet this tapers off to just about a pound/two pounds a week. This is down to water. Adipose flavoured water.

Whenever you start to lose the lard, water is the first thing to go. All fat stores contain water and there's a distinct difference between *'water-weight'* and *'fat-weight'*. Those first few weeks of exciting weight loss, consist of a teeny amount of fat and a few litres of water.
That's normal.

A pound of fat equates to 3500 calories and looks like a large, bulbous, dumpy, disfigured orange.
Okay, imagine that blobby citrus fruit attached to your stomach, or arse, or thighs.

If you've lost a pound of fat in a week, be proud of yourself because underneath your fleshy coat, you have lost some fat... equivalent to the size of a swollen, rotund, flabby orange.

It's not to be sniffed at... 'cos it would be disgusting.

In fact, a healthy weight loss **should** be about half a pound to two pounds a week. So be thankful the dial is going in the right direction. And keep going.

Just think, that's half a pound or two pounds of fat **you** shouldn't need to lose again.

Weighing scales can be misleading because the dial doesn't take into account the undigested food, the alcohol in your system, the stresses in your life, your hormones, water retention, sugar synthesis etc, etc.

So don't just focus and obsess about the numbers on that scale, and let it dictate your mood for the rest of the day. Instead, equate your weight loss by how you look, how you feel, your energy levels, how your clothes fit. Or how happy you are.

But let me also warn you, that your body doesn't want you to lose weight...
READER: *I'm sorry, what the fu...?*
Yep, you heard me right.

Buckle up for some more truth bullets.

When you start to lose weight, your CNS kicks in and burns fat at a lesser degree because the *'survival mechanism'* kicks in due to this new **stress** placed on the system.

And gaining weight is a predictable consequence of rapid weight-loss because your hormones will **increase** your appetite to counter-act this depletion in calories.

Therefore calorie restriction isn't the answer... HELP is the answer.

And as I keep prattling on about, you shouldn't just focus on one element of HELP over another. Because they **do not** work in isolation.

Healthy eating needs to be mirrored with enjoying life, acting positively and conducting moderate exercise.
That's why *'diets'* and *'diet clubs'* don't always work, 'cos they omit those fundamentally important factors.

Which leads me nicely onto the wonderful world of weekly subscription, slimming clubs...

Paul Birch

SLIMMING CLUBS

The diet starts… on Monday

I've briefly mentioned slimming clubs already in the book, but I just wanted to reiterate a few points because we're nearly at the end of our journey and I'm trying to give you as much helpful info as I can, before I depart… for a jog.

Slimming clubs per se are a great idea.

Similar folk all trying to reach a common goal, supporting and encouraging each other, sharing tips, socialising with like-minded individuals. **Awesome!!**

I've attended some *'slimming club'* classes as part of my research and they are run by enthusiastic, caring, empathetic people who work extremely hard to promote their ethos but they only work for the slimmer, if they put in the hard yards too. Otherwise, it's just a waste of dosh, time and effort.

I've read the promotional magazines of these slimming clubs and they are brilliant.

They make sensible recommendations for meals, offer real-life examples of slimmers who've successfully lost the timber, and make numerous lateral suggestions to aid long-term weight loss.

But how many of their slimmers do **you** personally know who are happy, who are fit and above all, slim?
READER: *Erm…*
Yep!!
So what's the problem?

The problem is effort, the problem is nutritional knowledge, the problem is positivity, the problem is lack of fitness, the problem, is these slimmers still have fundamental issues with their personal lives and that's why they've failed.

Maybe you're one of those people that say *'well I've lost weight in the past using slimming club diets'*. If that's the case, that means you will **never** lose weight in the **long-term** because you've only found a temporary solution. Which is not a lifestyle.

You didn't like it because you stopped. No doubt it was punishing, you constantly craved food and as soon as you quit, you went back to the same ol' routine as you had **before** the slimming club diet.
Am I right?
READER: *Erm… well, maybe…*
I'm right.

So what's the point joining again?

Look, if you do decide to sign up with one of these *'slimming clubs'* (again or for the first time), I wish you the best of luck. If you adhere to the strict principles of their *'diets'*, you *'may'* even manage to achieve your weight-loss goals but will you be happy? Evidence has shown that the successful slimmers from these *'clubs'* are **always**, without fail, people that have **also** embraced fitness as part of their weight loss regime. Therefore, you could cut out the expensive middle man and take on board my HELP instead.

Won't cost you an extra penny, you've already bought the book. You know what to do now and there's no weekly subscription fee.

Unless you want to set up a *'Standing Order'*?
No?!!

Your choice… alternatively, rather than strict calorie restriction how about regulated calorie reduction? You could try slim fast, or you could trying fasting to be slim.

FASTING

The hunger game

I don't advocate fasting to ridiculously unhealthy levels but controlled, intermittent fasting, can work wonders if you're trying to lose weight.

It has become quite trendy these days to go on the *'5:2 diet'* and based on the success stories, I can certainly see the appeal.
READER: *What is it?*
The idea is based around calorie reduction. On five days of the week you eat your recommended calorie allowance, 2500kcal for blokes and 2000kcal for the ladies. On the other two days, you only eat about a third (or less) of your *'recommended'* calorie intake.

Many folk that have undergone this quite drastic lifestyle change, have noticed significant weight loss, increases in energy levels, heighted awareness, and improvements in overall health and wellbeing.
READER: *Sounds brilliant.*
Yeah, it works, for **some** people but you should be careful regarding any form of calorie restriction, and be warned that weight loss can **plateau** as a result.

Your body is an astonishing, complicated piece of machinery and not eating enough calories can cause a series of metabolic changes, both positive and negative.

Once you've consumed a hearty meal, or un-nutritious one for that matter, your digestive system goes into overdrive and spends a few hours stripping down and processing that food. Immediately, there is a readily available source of energy swimming throughout your bloodstream therefore the body will choose to use this fuel, rather than break down the fat you have stored.

However, during periods of calorie restriction, your body cannot access a recently consumed meal to use as energy, so it will break down the fat stored in your body to burn as energy.

Whenever you're in a fasted state, without a ready supply of glucose your body is **forced** to adapt and pull from the only source of energy available to it, **the fat** stored in your cells. Thus by default, weight loss starts to occur.

But like I said earlier, your body is an amazing piece of machinery and once it **senses** there is prolonged energy restriction, the central nervous system readjusts to accommodate these new set of circumstances. This leads to what is commonly known as *'starvation mode'* and your metabolism slows down to a sustainable level, in order to deal and cope with the reduction in calories. Whether it's down to fasting or a calorie restrictive diet, your body will always react in this specific way and as a consequence, weight loss grinds to a glacial pace.

This process explains why yo-yo dieters tend to put on weight quite rapidly once they quit their diets.
READER: *What do you mean?*
Ok! During diets and fasting, once the intake of calories drops below a certain level, the body clearly has to adapt and thus will start to digest your muscle cells, as well as body fat, in order to produce energy. As we know, muscles require more energy to sustain than fat therefore if you're repeatedly losing muscle mass, you're inevitably going to slow down your metabolism, which over time, results in it becoming harder and harder to lose weight. Put simply. A slower metabolism, means fat is burned at a slower rate, a faster metabolism, leads to fat being burned at a faster rate.

Yo-yo dieting means your metabolism and hormones are all over the place, as they react and reset to meet calorie restrictions, then calorie overloads, then back to restrictions etc, etc. Weight loss can be rapid but on the flip-side, weight gain occurs just as quickly.

That's why *'diets'* don't work. C'mon you know the answer... HELP yourself, that's' the answer.

READER: *But you said fasting leads to long-term weight loss didn't you?*
I did, I did yeah.

READER: *How?*
If for instance, the 5:2 becomes your norm and you **consistently** consume food in this manner for a few months and more, the body and as a consequence your metabolic rate, gets used to functioning at a lower energy level, and can adequately deal with these protracted periods of **voluntary** starvation. And if you're consuming less than your weekly calorie allowance, by default, you will lose weight. **Guaranteed!!**

But *'diets'* will **always** be difficult to follow if they involve a form of calorie restriction, which forces **you** to disrupt your lifestyle in a way that is just not sustainable. And as soon as you quit the diet, the weight will inevitably creep right back on. This is why I'm so against these temporary measures to attain weight loss. They don't address the major issues in your life, they **punish** and **abuse** your psyche and as a result, you fail.

This cycle of rebounding leads to your perception of *'healthy weight loss'*, as a futile exercise.

It becomes so daunting that you feel it's just not worth the hassle, knowing you've failed so many times before, so you eventually stop. You develop an unhealthy relationship with food, and it becomes far easier to live a life binging and munching on crap, than adopt another pointless diet.

And I agree.

I can completely empathise with this viewpoint but it's similar to you attempting to use a trampoline, by just lying on it. You're doing it wrong. If you wake up and HELP yourself, then that is the equivalent of jumping and bouncing and messing about on the trampoline. It's actually fun.

EATING DISORDERS

They're no joke

Mentioning fasting and calorie restriction has made me realise, there's a considerable risk that it could lead to some form of eating disorder, and I would hate for that to happen to **you**. Or anyone else for that matter.

The goal of sustainable weight-loss is not purely down to being thin, people who suffer from anorexia and bulimia are thin but they're certainly not healthy, either in body, or in mind. Moderate happiness and positivity are what it should be about.

With respect to food and wellbeing, it shouldn't be *'health why?'*

But *'healthy'*.

Therefore if **you** ever start to have an obsessive fear of weight gain, or you are in a state of denial regarding the seriousness of excessive weight loss, please see your GP as soon as possible.

Restricting food is not healthy for you.
Inducing vomiting to rid your body of food is not healthy for you.
Using laxatives as a form of weight control is not healthy for you.
Low self-esteem is not healthy for you.
Depression and anxiety is not healthy for you.
Looking emaciated is **definitely** not healthy for you.

Society relentlessly pushes the ideal that being skinny is the epitome of body perfection. But that is complete and utter **bollocks!!**

As I've mentioned numerous times already, there is no such thing as perfection. I will say that again, there is no such thing as perfection. Stop attempting to attain it, because, look away now if you don't want to know the score... you'll fail to achieve it.

Boniness is **not** sexy.

Curves, laughter and light bondage are... so get some meat on your bones.

Which leads me neatly onto the final section of the food chapter. Save the best for last and all that.

If you want a so-called *'diet'* that will 100% guarantee weight loss, is sustainable for the rest of your life and will **never** leave you feeling hungry again.

Then it's time to go, Paleo.

THE PALEO DIET

It's prehistoric, man!!

Paleo and walking, another **Birchy guarantee** for long-term weight loss.

I could write a book about the primal diet, or *'Paleo'* as it's also known but I won't because others have written fantastic tomes dedicated to this movement. And it has become a movement.

Check out the number of sites on t'internet if you don't believe me, there were 70 million results the last time I checked.
READER: *What is it?*

Ok! Here are the main tenets of PALEO:

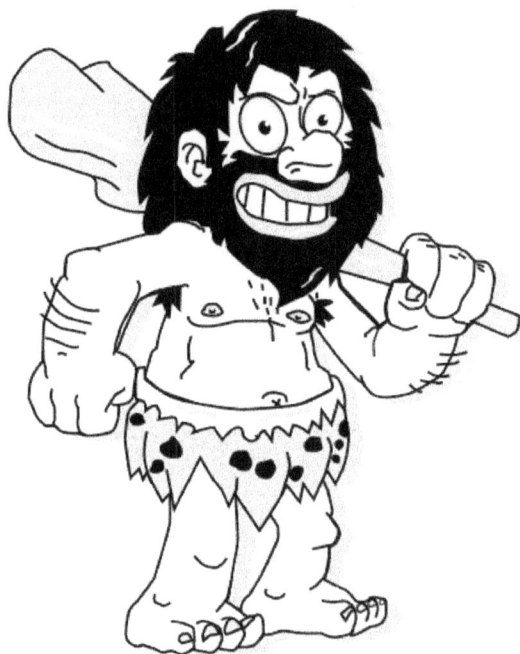

Only eat meat, fish, plants, nuts, seeds, fruit and vegetables

Drink lots of water

Walk, a lot

Muck about and try and have as much fun as possible

Sprint once a week

Lift heavy things, occasionally

Get loads of shut-eye

Try to get at least an hour of fresh air and sunlight a day

Use your noggin, by partaking in puzzles and brain teasers.

Basically it's based around *'Neanderthals'* and how your primal ancestors *'Ug'* and *'Gug'*, operated on a daily basis. I'm talking thousands of years ago here, before the advent of farming, money, flags, borders and reward points.

These brutes of nature climbed trees, lifted heavy rocks, foraged for food, they hunted, they jogged, ran, jumped, squatted, sprinted away from wildy-beasts, slept… a lot and were quite literally, to use a parlance of our times, *'fit as fuck!!'*

Not in a hubba bubba type way but supreme, physical specimens.

Yeah they probably died from infections caused by cuts, or a mild case of Ug-flu but if you could replicate their basic principles of living into today's culture, you're **golden!!**

<u>READER</u>: *But how do we know what they ate?*
We don't. But lots of bearded, dedicated Anthropologists and Archaeologists, have spent their lives assessing fossils, evaluating cave paintings and watching *'The Flintstones'* to put forward ground breaking, peer-reviewed papers, indicating and surmising what they believe they ate, and how they lived.

I think it's indisputable that they didn't eat processed food and they didn't calorie count, they fasted and binged but never, never, ever, ate tubs of ice-cream in their leopard skin pants, whilst slumped on a couch watching celebrity ice-dancing.

Paleo is just another fancy diet really, which omits manufactured and processed food.

I actually don't recommend you follow it 100%, although you could, none of my business. No, I would suggest, like me, you adopt the diet for about 80-85% of the time.

<u>READER</u>: *And the rest of the time?*
Well, I think I've made it abundantly clear throughout this book that treats are fine, in moderation.

So if you adopted the paleo diet for 85% of your life, then you can knock yourself out for the remaining 15% and eat whatever you want. I mean you don't have to, it's merely a suggestion.

For guaranteed long-term weight loss, that is. You know, **guaranteed!!**

Obviously the fitness recommendations are just that, recommendations. But walking is THE best form of exercise for **you**, by a picturesque, country path mile.

But by all means play around with the principles, add a few extra bits, take some away but ultimately stick to the main tenets, and you're cooking.

If you'd like to give it a go, then try to ease your way into the paleo lifestyle. Like any major change to your diet, don't go all in and try and alter your **entire** dietary habits in one go.

Perhaps just start with one meal a day. Or alternate days. Or just during the week, leaving the weekend to have a few treats. I don't know, whatever works for you. Just try. Attempt to make some changes in your life, or else you'll never change.

What I do recommend, is making **one** permanent change and omission **every** week.

For example:-

- Stop eating white bread, for good.
- Stop eating processed meat, for good.
- Stop eating *'fat-free'* yoghurt, stop eating crisps, stop eating pasta, just stop eating crap. You can adopt a primal diet, without acting like a primate.

Do it for good. For your **good!!**

PERSONAL TRAINING

Trust me… I'm a qualified know-it-all

Many people have asked me over the years, *'why?'* I wanted to become a personal trainer (PT). And the answer is this - I wanted to help people who have difficulty helping themselves.

Ever since I was a football playing obsessed teenager, I've been interested in fitness and nutrition but the main reason I wanted to qualify as a PT, was simply to enhance my flawed knowledge.

Therefore I have spent the last decade researching the subject by attaining qualifications, speaking to experienced personal trainers, reading books, attending seminars, listening to podcasts, conducting exercise classes and visiting gyms. But most importantly, speaking to individuals who are **desperate** to lose weight and get fit… and they failed because they didn't know how to.

This research has confirmed my contention that gyms are **not** the best answer for long-term weight loss.
READER: *Why would you say that?*
Ok! Gyms basically treat their members as *'consumers'*, trying to fob them off with exorbitantly priced annual memberships, exercise classes that have no bearing on specific fitness goals, branded sportswear to promote the club, and expensively priced energy drinks.

Gyms are not there to help **you** successfully lose weight. If they were, every gym would have a kitchen, with nutritionists explaining the virtues of healthy eating, and chefs to demonstrate cooking methods, explaining how to enrich flavour and taste.

Psychologists would conduct one-to-one counselling sessions to identify the fundamental issues that result in unhappiness, and why there appears to be an unrelenting desire to find comfort in food.

Friends and family would be invited to attend group sessions, to address levels of support and how their help and encouragement can positively or negatively, affect the fitness and weight loss goals of the member.

Doctor's would present weekly sessions discussing potential health risks and how simple changes in diet and lifestyle, can lead to prevention.

But they don't.

'Cos that would cost 'em a chuffin' fortune and they've got shareholders to think about and profit margins, and fluffy towels to sell.

- A PT can advise on the best form of cardio to suit your shape, size and fitness ability but they can't stop you grabbing those cakes that Tracey from Accounts baked and brought into work.
- A PT can assess your lifting form, or kettlebell swing but can't stop you crying when you're about to go up town and can't fit into that dress you love.
- A PT can encourage you to hold the plank position for more than thirty seconds, but they can't stop you from filling your shopping trolley with packets and tins and jars of chemically processed, sugary shite.
- Nor should they because every decision **you** make, is all down to you. **You** are the only person who can make the necessary changes. No one can do it for **you!!**

The reason I wrote this book was because I know **exactly** what is required for **you** to lose weight and get fitter but I couldn't achieve that by working as a PT. A few sessions a week on the treadmill and chatting whilst you complete a few dead-lifts, isn't going to help you change your lifestyle in order to finally banish depression… for good.

And that's what you need to do, you **need** to change your lifestyle, your mindset, your whole ethos for living. In fact, you need to kill yourself.

READER: *I'm sorry?!*

Oops!! Poor choice of words, I'll rephrase it. You need to get rid of your old mindset. Make radical changes to your diet. You have to kill your old self, to become the **new** and improved you.

You **2.0.** if you will.

Get positive, start having fun and enjoying life. Then, and only then will you start to lose weight and keep it off. Everything else will all fall into place, guaranteed. But only if you HELP yourself.

During my countless conversations with clients and potential clients, I began to compile sure-fire tips that will, in addition to the intrinsic elements of HELP, definitely improve your chances of long-term weight loss success.

Some of those clients took my advice, listened, made vital amendments to their lifestyle and lost weight, and got fitter, and became happier... others didn't and didn't.

So, like anything else, it's a choice. It's up to you. But remember, healthy nutrition and wellbeing is for life, not just the first few weeks after Xmas.

I never tried to make any dosh when I conducted my personal training, instead I asked clients to donate some money to a certain charity, that way we could both feel good about ourselves.

Practice what you preach and all that. But folk don't half waste a lot of moolah trying to lose weight and get fit, when the solutions are so simple.

Therefore I'd always begin our chats by stating the following:

> *If you want to save a fortune on gym memberships, diet pills, slimming club subscriptions, juicers, protein drinks, celebrity DVD's, meal replacement shakes, vitamin supplements, expensive trainers, branded sportswear, Apps, books, exercise classes, magazines, fat-monitors and other worthless gizmo's... eat less and walk more.*

They'd look at me with a face that could curdle *'fat-free'* yoghurt, you know, the one that you're pulling now but the point stands.

I'd then try to establish **why** they wanted to lose weight and the answers ranged from feeling miserable, their partner wanted them to, hating how they looked, sick of the teasing, or they needed to fit into a dress for a wedding.

In essence, all legitimate reasons but if one thing is missing, they would fail. And some did.

READER: *What's that then?*

Self-motivation.

READER: *How do you mean?*

Ok! You have to **want** to lose weight, otherwise you'll fail.

Now this might seem obvious, I mean you probably **want** to lose weight but you've failed in the past and could feasibly fail again in the future. But if your desire is weak, you'll **always** fail.

Too many people **pretend** that they want to lose weight. That's why they go in all half-arsed and quit after a few weeks. Determination is the **key** to success but it can be developed and strengthened like a muscle, the more you activate it, the more stubborn and resolute you'll become.

It comes down to the CBA gang again. If you can't be arsed, then you can't be arsed and you'll never ever succeed. You've got to **want** it so much that you accept that it'll take a long time but you'll persevere regardless, because the reward is so great.

If you are being coerced into losing weight by a partner or friend, and you're not wholly committed, you'll fail because you don't really **want** to change but are being forced into it.

But if you are doing it for your self-worth and happiness, then you'll start to accept it's a full-time commitment and failing isn't an option. Your desire supersedes your fears.

If you want to lose weight due to vanity, you will probably fail in the long-term. It's a losing battle.

That is **not** a legitimate reason to lose the timber and you will never be happy. There'll always be something wrong, some minor imperfection you want to change. You'll never be satisfied.

If you're looking to lose the lard because you're miserable, again, you will fail in the long-term. The **weight** is not the reason you're unhappy, it's a by-product of your overall state of sanity. It's probably down to your job, friends, family, partner, kids, money issues or some other concern. Until you quash those specific problems, everything else in your life will pale into insignificance.

If for example, you're depressed because your relationship just isn't working, will that stop you eating chocolate cereal for brekkie? **No!!**

Therefore until you address that particular issue, you'll **never** lose weight and keep it off for good.

If you're really happy living that way for the rest of your life, keep carrying on but if you truly respect yourself, you won't be, so do something about it.

If your major reason for losing the flab is down to your health, then you'll probably succeed. It'll still be difficult but you've identified the perfect catalyst for change. You've identified that being overweight is detrimental to your overall health and wellbeing therefore by losing the fat, by default your health (and sanity) will undoubtedly improve. As a consequence you *'may'* feel that you look more attractive, sexier even but that's a bonus, feeling better about yourself is the ultimate reward for your hard work. And a perfect example to set to your children, after all you don't want them to be obese do you? Do you?

The following tips related to clients that failed and those that succeeded. I'll leave you to decide which ones took the advice and which ones ignored it.

FOOD - GENERIC

Learn from the mistakes of others

Whenever you consume a meal, always eat your food **slowly**, savouring each spoon or forkful and actually do some chewing, rather than just shovelling it down your throat. Slow, controlled eating, fools your brain into thinking you are getting fuller quicker, in turn reducing your appetite.

1 Sometimes, I bet you've been two-thirds through a meal and not even realised. I mean you spent your valuable time over the cooking (or pressed the start button on the microwave), so you might as well enjoy the taste and flavour.

And if you can, try to eat at the table, rather than from a tray across your lap whilst you watch some crappy telly. If you focus on the meal rather than the TV, you're less inclined to eat more. Otherwise you end up like a robot, sub-consciously funnelling food into your mush, without even realising it.

If you're not hungry, don't eat.

2 Just because it's normal to eat at certain parts of the day, there's no law saying you must indulge and throw some grub down your gob. Don't worry you'll get your appetite back at some stage, you can't ruin them, there'll be another one round the corner.

3 When you're dishing out a nutritious and healthy, well-balanced meal, serve onto an extra plate and then freeze it. That way, some other time in the week when you're strapped for time you can defrost and voila, a quick and easy dish, with hardly any washing up. Bonus!!

Perhaps, like me, you were taught by your folks to finish everything on your plate, whether you're full or not. Yep, awesome principle in these days of austerity and global hunger but you're trying to lose the lard. Therefore if you're full, you're full. Halt. Stop. Quit spooning scran into your melon, you're full. Instead, scrape the remains into a *'Tupperware'* dish or summat and put it aside for someone else to warm up later, or add it to your meal the day after. Or have it for your brekkie. Remember, you have a recommended daily

4 allowance for a reason and excess calories, means more timber.

These days, plates are about the size of dustbin lids but instead of serving small human-size portions, we fill these plates like we're feeding a mountain lion. If you dish out the grub onto smaller plates, take some time devouring the contents, have a few sips of water and then wait ten minutes after you've finished; this will reduce your desire to opt for seconds, and thirds and *'oh go on then, I'll have some more cheesecake'*.

5 Throughout the food chapter, I mentioned that you should experiment, try different foods, deviate from your current diet and investigate new sources of food (and food sauces). Don't just shrug, puff out your cheeks and dismiss something you've never tried before. If you don't like it once you've tried it, don't eat it again but if you don't try, you won't know if you'd like it or not.

Taste is subjective and we're all different, what works for one doesn't work for the other. But I would definitely recommend that you think about the person you want to be, and eat as they would.

6 If you want to be some thin, curvy, athletic woman then imagine and picture their lifestyle and diet. If you want to be a rugged, Billy-Big-Bob-Beefcake, act, exercise and consume food as they would. Do some research and become the **YOU**, you want to be.

7 I'm not a massive fan of calorie-counting but it does work for some people, and they find it easier to assess their consumption, and evaluate weaknesses as well as identifying areas for improvement. Therefore you could start a food diary to monitor your daily consumption.

They only work however, if you're honest. If you start lying and omitting the odd biscuit, packet of crisps and those chips you nicked from your partner's plate, they won't work.

If you do opt to go down this route, try making daily changes by eating a few portions of veg a day, reducing cappuccino consumption and limiting treats. Marking these down in your diary, you can tally weekly success and perhaps reward yourself at the end of the week; by eating something naughty or heading to a lingerie boutique and **buying** something naughty. Even the lasses should give that a try.

8 Most people have a treat cupboard, or garage in some cases. But to help you in your weight loss goal, you can either stop buying them, or if you carry on, you know *'for the kids n' that'*, you could move them somewhere else in the house. As in a place that's a ballache to reach. This way, out of sight out of mind. The significant effort involved in trying to access these treats, exacerbates guilt, which *'may'* stop you from consuming. Worth a shot.

The major problem with having treats in the house (and I'm guilty of this), is if they're in the cupboard or fridge, **you know** and you can't not know what you know. Which results in you obsessing about eating them, so what do you do?
READER: *Eat them!*
Ten points to the pretty lady at the back.

Alternatively, you could place a mirror on the treat cupboard or fridge, and that way you have to face **yourself**, and your guilty mug before a raid. Guilt is actually a powerful motivational tool but don't abuse it, 'cos you'll end up hating yourself.

9

Sometimes we **think** we are hungry, when actually we are just thirsty. Our central nervous system starts turning on loads of hormonal alarms, until we stop ignoring them and either eat or drink. If your aim is to try and drop a few stone, then having a brew, sup of duck wine, or glass of moo-juice can serve as an appetite suppressant, which by default helps with the ol' weight loss.

If you do join a gym, running club or decide that you are on a health kick and *'by jiminy, you're gonna lose some timber',* then tell **everyone**.

Folk will relish reprimanding you when you err. And you will. You're only human... except **you**, you're a bit of a weirdo.

10

Your family, mates and work colleagues just can't wait to embarrass, or shame you into not eating. It's actually a reflection of their weaknesses and reluctance to change, so take it as a compliment. You're doing something about your health and weight, and they're not.

'Cos they **can't be arsed!!**

And just picture the look on their chops when you reach your weight loss goals.

Bow-chicka-fuck-you!!

Paul Birch

YOU

Yes, you!!

Place a picture of yourself that you **absolutely detest** on the fridge, cupboard at home, treat cupboard at work, or whatever in order to scare you from gorging and snacking.

Remember, everything you've tried before didn't work so invest in new ideas, embrace creativity, anything out of the ordinary in order for **you** to reach your goals.

Some people hate seeing their reflections, so don't have mirrors in the home. My advice, buy a massive mirror and face your problem head on, don't avoid it. Use it as motivation. Just looking at yourself, especially half naked, is a powerful message. It communicates better than any other medium **what** the current state of your health is.

Study the contours of your face and look at how it moulds into your chin(s). Gaze at your arms and touch the flabby, drooping skin.

Grab a chunk of your blobby midriff and rub the fat between your fingers. That's **you**. And it ain't changing until **you** do something about it. You... No-one else.

YOU!!

Once you begin your weight loss journey, put a fiver aside for each pound you lose. That way you have an added incentive to lose more lard. When you reach your first target, buy yourself an item of clothing that will only fit once you attain your ultimate goal.

No one likes to waste money, which is yet another reason to help motivate you to keep going.

Just imagine how awesome you'll look once you reach that target. **Hot Diggidy!!**

For those meditative types out there, you could try *'Aversion Therapy'*.
READER: *What's that?*
Well, you associate negative connotations and thoughts to a particular food, that way, the next time you try to eat said food your mind will conjure up lots of disgusting images, which *'may'* put you off consuming.

For example, if you want to stop eating cheese, sit yourself down in that comfy chair by the fireplace, close your eyes, relax and then start to imagine all the worst facets of cheese.

Picture a slab of stinky, putrid, mouldy cheese, with maggots and worms sliding and crawling, in and out of the rancid, oozing, moist, seeping holes... etc, etc. Do that for five minutes every day, for a week or so and the next time you leer at some Leerdammer, or gawk at some gorgonzola, you may want to reach for a sick bucket.

I can see you pulling faces, scrunching up your nose and squirming at these words but it works, for some people. Might work for you, try it and if it doesn't work, well at least you tried.

Now, after me, *'Ohmmmmmmmmmmmmmmmmmmmmmmmmmmmm!!'*

It can be a good idea to take a picture of yourself, on the day that you decide you're gonna make some changes. I'm not a big fan of the *'before and after'* pictures that you see on the t'internet because you have no idea about the history of the individuals.

They could quite easily be fitness fanatics, who got into some bad habits for whatever reason but found it very simple to start running again, or joining a gym.

When you see these visual transformations, you **assume** they were couch potatoes beforehand but that *'may'* not be the case therefore how can you trust them?
Fair do's if the person led a sedentary lifestyle before jumping onto the fitness bandwagon but you have no idea.

But you know **you**. So if you take a *'before'* pic, you can gauge how far you've come along and that photo cannot lie.

Don't worry I'm not asking you to make it your FB profile picture, or security pass for work, you don't have to share it with anyone, it's solely for you. Put it somewhere safe and take a peek whenever you're feeling down, or you've hit a few snags along the way.

It will remind you of how you looked, how you felt **before** you began your long journey to losing the timber, and **why** you're doing it.
It will motivate, inspire and reinvigorate you to continue whenever you're feeling negative.
So after 3... 1, 2, 3... **Cheese!!**
READER: *Eeuurrgghh!! Don't mention cheese, I feel sick after what you wrote earlier...*
Oops, my bad.

If you want to weigh yourself along the way to gauge progress, then I strongly recommend that you weigh yourself every week at the **same time** because this way, you have a consistent indicator of your weight.

Don't waste money on some expensive branded number either, pick a regular set, make sure that the dial is set to zero before you weigh, and you're sorted.

Don't fear the scale, it doesn't lie but it can mask the truth, so don't place too much emphasis on the results.
I've mentioned it before but let me assure you that your weight will fluctuate daily, depending on your hormones, sleep patterns, water retention, exercise, muscle mass, food intake and your central nervous system playing havoc, with your mind and body.
READER: *Water retention?*
Yep. The scale will not only reflect your current weight but it is also influenced by the amount of water you are retaining, along with any food that has not yet been digested.

As I've alluded to throughout the book, your mood, levels of positivity, health, energy, clothes and your friends and family, will tell you all you need to know about your progress.

Therefore I implore you, **do not** weigh yourself every day. It's counter-productive and a waste of energy and time.

And don't be fussed about your body fat percentage either. Yes, check it when you've reached your goal but who gives a shit when you start.

It does my head in that gyms still get the ol' callipers out to check a newbie, by gripping some fat and then informing the person of their fat percentage.

They know they're overweight, **dickweed!!**
They don't need an embarrassing procedure like that, to tell them summat they **already know!! Derrrr!! That's why they've joined the gym!!**

Obviously you have a certain goal regarding weight loss and fitness but rather than it being generic, such as *'I want to lose some weight'*, it should be **specific** and time orientated (SMART).

For instance, *'I want to lose 3 stone, by Xmas of this year, so I can fit into that green dress for the Office party'*.

This way, you have a specific target to aim for and a motivational deadline.

Otherwise you're just dreaming and the big difference between a dream and a goal, is a deadline.

The aim and date could be placed in locations around the house and at work, to constantly remind you of your goal.

But don't put too much unrealistic pressure upon yourself, be pragmatic.

Paul Birch

It's extremely unlikely that you are going to lose three stone in a month. It could take six, ten, eighteen months depending on your level of dedication, willpower and enthusiasm to adapt and change.

Just like the under-resourced and underpaid Doctors and Nurses, you've gotta have patience.

PATIENCE

Don't lose it, lose fat instead

Now, are you ready, 'cos I'm gonna release a few more truth missiles here? **Boom!! Boom!!**

It's gonna take you a **long** time to lose this weight you're trying to get rid of. A long time.
Therefore you must accept this point.
READER: *I do yeah, thanks!!*
I'm not sure that you truly do. Therefore I feel it's my duty to really emphasize, how bloody long it could feasibly take. So, I will.

Let's say that you want to lose two stone. That's a fair wedge of timber but highly achievable. There are fourteen pounds to a stone therefore that equates to twenty-eight pounds.

In simplistic terms because the body is a complicated piece of machinery, this means that **you** will have to burn 3500kcal, in order to lose one pound of fat.

I'm quite a fit bloke and to give you an indication of how hard it is to burn 3500kcal, I usually burn 1000kcal or so, after conducting one hour of sweat-induced-calf-straining-lung-bursting exercise on a X-Trainer.

That's really giving it some mind, although that figure can fluctuate depending on the incline settings, resistance and intensity. And who's to say the machine is calibrated right, so that figure of 1000kcal could be inaccurate however to simplify the following calculations, let's say it's correct.

But it won't be.

Therefore, it would take me three and a half hours of X-Trainer exertion, really pushing myself at piston-pushing-pace to burn those 3500kcal, or one pound of fat.

That's in addition, to making sure **I didn't** consume any more grub than the 2500kcal I'm permitted to gobble for each of the days I conducted a fitness session.

So, if I wanted to lose twenty-eight pounds of weight/fat from my svelte and hairy body, it would take **ninety-eight hours** of strenuous activity on the X-Trainer.

- If I attended the gym four times a week, it would take me about twenty-five weeks (six months).
- If I popped to the gym three times a week, it would take about thirty-three weeks.
- If I only used the X-Trainer twice a week, it would take about forty-nine weeks (virtually a whole year).
- And if I only went to the gym once a week, it would take a whopping **ninety-eight weeks**, which is getting on for nearly two years.

Taking those calculations in mind, on top of that, I would **never** be able to consume more than 2500kcal for any day I attended the gym **OR** those days I didn't go.

Are you getting what I'm saying here?
READER: *Err...*
It's gonna take you **chuffin' ages**, and probably far longer than you even imagined it would.
Please don't think you can undo overnight what it took **years** of cakey, chocolatey pleasure to create.

Just take a moment to think about how many times over the years you've eaten slices of pizza, scoffed burgers, devoured cheesecakes, crunched crisps, dunked biscuits and munched on muffins. And the times you've chowed down on plates of pasta, mounds of rice, buttery toast, buckets of popcorn, takeaway curries, bacon butties, scoops of ice-cream and all that other processed shite.

Then there's the beer, the vino, champers, Prosecco, cocktails and all those shots. Blimey. **All them shots!!** And what about the cream in your coffee, milk on your sugary cereal, tubs of *'fat-free'* artificially sweetened yoghurts and packaged, salty, fatty, meat sarnies at lunch.

Not forgetting your hatred of exercise and love of the sedentary life. Slouched on that comfy sofa, gawping at the idiot box, playing activity-themed video games and having afternoon naps. Then there's driving, sitting on your arse at that job you hate, taking the escalator and lift rather than the stairs, and catching the bus home from work on beautiful sunny days, instead of taking a nice gentle stroll.

All the above and more, much, much, much, much, much, much, much, much, more has contributed to your current physique. The size and shape of you. Your weight. Your jiggly bits. Your fat. **You!!**

Your weight has cost you a fortune to attain but don't let it cost **you** your health or your life.

You're not Amanda. You're you. And you can change.

In addition to patience, you're definitely gonna need the help and support of your friends and family, and you'll need to be good humoured and negativity impaired throughout. Positivity and patience are the **key** drivers to success, and will help you get through the tough times.

But don't focus on how long it will take, focus on progress instead. No matter how slow the journey, if you want it, you'll get there. And always keep in mind that every pound you lose, is another pound of unwanted fat you should **never** have to deal with again.

We all know someone who's a lil' bit chunky but they're not bothered about it, always jolly, poking fun at their size, *'watch out, big lad coming past'* or *'are you having that? If not, I'll have it'* or *'I'm starving me, I've only had 3 lunches'* etc, etc.

In fact, they might even have a nickname such as *'Jellyball-Jim'* or *'Big-Blobby-Becky'* but they don't mind they enjoy the harmless rib-tickling, don't they? Don't they?!

Maybe I'm referring to someone like **you**, someone who uses self-deprecation to **avoid** admitting the truth. Well, I've spoken to numerous blokes and lasses over the years who have similar tales and guess what, they bloody hate all them names but because they find it so difficult to lose the lard, they not only embrace them, they allow them to formulate their personality.

But it's not really them. They are **desperate** to drop the pounds, as well as the insults but don't know how. My advice to these types of people is to start respecting yourself and rather than self-deprecation, try self-confidence and self-enhancement instead.
READER: *How?*
HELP yourself.
Rather than, *'look at the size of my gut'* it should be *'check out the size of these blisters, from running'*.

I'm gonna tell you something here, extremely important info that most folk seem afraid to admit and you definitely won't hear this on the news, or read it in your celebrity-obsessed, gossip mags.

You and everyone else on this planet are **not** designed to be obese because our skellingtons, are not built to withstand the extra mass.

Hundreds of thousands of years of evolution, has led to **you** and **I** becoming *'Homo Sapiens'*. And Homo Sapiens are bipeds, not quadrupeds.

That's why obese individuals find it difficult to walk, struggling for breath as they trudge down the street, putting immense strain on their spine, hips, knee joints and leg muscles.

It's not natural.

This should not be the next step of evolution:

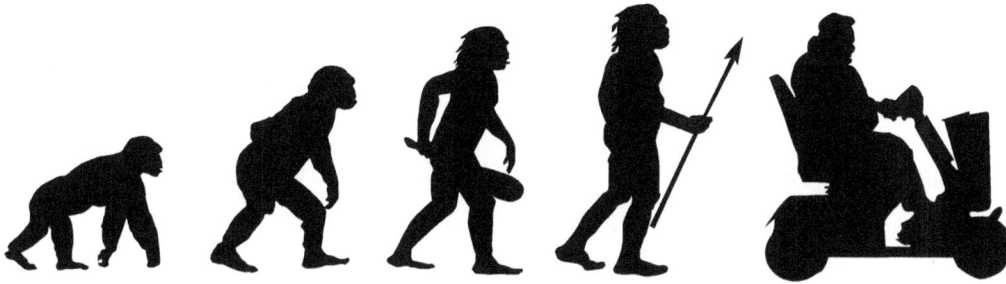

<u>READER</u>: *You're a fat shamer you.*
Well I'm **ashamed** that so many people are obese. Ok! Maybe I am a *'fat shamer'* to an extent but that phrase really pisses me off.

'Fat shaming' implies that if anyone makes a comment regarding someone's weight, by definition, they are discriminating against that person and trying to make them feel *'ashamed'* regarding their size.

My whole remit and the motivation behind this book, is to help people who **want** to drop the pounds but find it extremely difficult, not those who are more than comfortable with their weight.

If someone is *'obese'* but they are content and proud, not concerned in the slightest with their health or happiness, then fair play to them. Keep on keeping on but I would **never** abuse, or demean them in any way. It's none of my business.

It's the same principle if someone wants to smoke, or gamble or vote Tory. I wouldn't do it because it's not part of my mindset, my way of living but it's that person's choice, and they currently share the freedom to continue making those choices. Fair play to them.

In my humble opinion, *'fat shaming'* relates to this idealistic and unattainable version of perfection, and if anyone veers from this ideal, such as love handles, jowly chin, bit of a gut etc, etc morons, and they are **morons**, start to chuck insults at them.

I didn't get that memo and I'm not on board with that.

Being slightly overweight or a tad podgy is **nothing** to be worried about for anyone but if you're starting to get obese and it's negatively affecting your health, then I firmly believe **you** should try to do something about it. That's my personal outlook on life and I'm not forcing it upon you, or anyone else for that matter.

But I think it's a shame, that being *'fat'* and extremely *'overweight'* is deemed to be the modern way of living. That's a crying shame. To me, that is.

So, if **you** want my help, then I'm here and pleased to assist. Bring it on, which is why I wrote this bloody book. In fact, if you want to get in touch with me to discuss your specific issues, please do.
My e-mail address is <u>birchygoober@hotmail.com</u>.

Just don't abuse it; I'm not interested in those *'hot singles in my area'*, PPI claims, or ingenious ways to enhance my manhood.

If you don't want to talk to me, fair enough, there's plenty of other folk willing to help.

Get yourself logged on and try the web. Have a look at some internet forums that include **real life** examples of people who have **successfully** lost the lard. Read their stories. Talk to them and learn what to realistically expect. Just don't give up. Keep trying; it's worth it in the end.

Paul Birch

It's obvious that *'fat shaming'* actually demotivates a lot of people, making them feel terrible about their size and thus seek comfort in eating more food, and as a consequence they get bigger. But those individuals are no doubt depressed and unhappy with their lives anyway, and therefore **need** to make fundamental changes to their behaviour and mindset.

They need to embrace the four elements of HELP because **then** and only then, will they start to lead a contented and moderately happy life.

Which leads me neatly back to the intrinsic principles of HELP, in order to conclude this book.

Yep, sorry, it's nearly over. The lecture is about to finish.

Although no one leaves, until I say you can leave, wait for the bell.

314

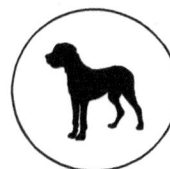

CONCLUSION

I'm sure you can appreciate now, that losing weight is not just about fitness and calorie restriction. It's about that tiny little noggin of yours, how happy you **allow** yourself to be and how willing you are to actually let yourself go and live life to the full.
It's all about HELP:

H	E	L	P
is for	is for	is for	is for
HEALTHY EATING	**EXERCISE**	**LIVING & ENJOYING LIFE**	**POSITIVE MINDSET**

To lose weight and keep the flabby, jiggly-wiggly bits off for good, it's vital that you adopt and follow each aspect of HELP.

Your mind and body works in harmony and when one element breaks down, the whole system collapses. Life is far too complicated and challenging for you to put 100% into each element but if you want to be moderately happy for the rest of your life, the more you put into each principle, the more you'll get out of life.
No-one can do it for you though. It's all down to **you!!**

It's all about choices.

Fat or thin? Happy or miserable? Negativity or positivity? Moderation or gluttony? Fitter or bitter? Couch potato or sweet potato?

It's all about how much **you** want it?

Do you **pretend** to want to lose weight or do you really, really, really, really, **really** want to lose weight?
Success or failure is all in your mind. And the more limitations you place in front of you, the more likely you will fail.

But remember, you only fail if you quit.

Over to **you**... **Good luck!!**

Actually, let me see, before I go have I forgotten anything?
Losing weight takes tenacity, patience and above all...
<u>READER</u>: *Positivity?!*
Damn right treacle!! And if you have positivity in abundance, you'll succeed, **guaranteed!!**

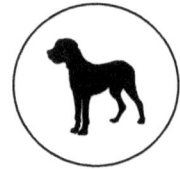

Paul Birch

LAST
WORDS

By 'eck, it's been emotional this. Who'd have thought that losing weight and fighting depression would be so challenging? Well, I did. And of course, so did **you** because if it wasn't you'd have done it already and you wouldn't be reading this.

I want to finish by comparing the act of writing a book, to someone attempting to try and lose weight and banish the blues. They're both bloody difficult to accomplish but the feeling of relief, satisfaction and pride in completion, can be measured equally.

On and off, it's taken me over twenty years to finally achieve my dream of writing a book.

That is some serious procrastination. Call Norris McWhirter (for our older viewers).

And from hearing about Amanda's suicide, to typing, doodling, editing and finishing the first complete draft of this book, it has taken me about nine months.

I might not have any bairns but I've created this bad boy and I'm as proud as punch, and there was no messy or awkward sexual encounter involved in the process. Actually… no, there wasn't.

Nine months is a **very long** time, about 274 days and for most of them I've had the pleasure of staring at my laptop screen and keyboard wondering *'what the fuck am I doing??'*

For **every** one of those 274 days, I questioned my sanity.

I'm not a writer.

I'm an opinionated, judgemental, sarcastic, worthless, deluded dreamer, drifting through life **hoping** for some magic beans to help drag me from the monotony of normality.

Every day my inner voice would scream at me *'What are you doing Birchy trying to write a book, dickhead, you're not a writer?'*

Perhaps, I should've just quit and lead a much simpler life, avoiding any attempt to actually achieve one of my lifelong goals.

If I spoke to family or friends, I'd mention what I was doing and they'd just raise their eyebrows, knowingly smirk and think *'Silly Paul, wasting his time yet again, when will he grow up?'*

Obviously I could sense this, so I'd get depressed, bathed in self-pity, agreeing with that sentiment. On some of those days, I'd feel quite low and there'd be no tip-tapping on the keyboard, instead I'd immerse myself in the comforting world of the tellybox, watching some comedies to cheer me up.

But most of the days, I'd think *'No, I can do this, I am doing this, I will do this, I am a writer. It's gonna work, this is the best thing I've ever done with my life and I'm going to succeed'.*

This was my dream, my goal, my passion and that is why **you** and the other five people who bought this book are reading these words, and will be inspired to change your life and finally live a moderately happy life.

I won't lie to you, it's been bloody tough but I've done it and if I can do it, you can do it too.

It just takes patience, a hell of a lot of positivity, passion, willingness to adapt and good humour.

There'll be days when you'll wanna quit 'cos you're having a bad day (or week) but focus on the end goal, not the temporary meaningless blips.

Don't quit, no matter how long it takes because it's worth the heartache, it's worth the effort and it's worth the pain.

And there will be pain but the more you fight it, the easier it gets.

Hey!! You've noticed my punctuation isn't great and the book is a bit contradictory sometimes, it might not flow as well as it could do, I've missed bits out and forgotten stuff but that's just like life.

That's just like trying to lose weight. It doesn't run smoothly.

'Cos it's tough, it's difficult and those things that we want and desire the most are the hardest to achieve.
If it was simple, everyone would be doing it.

Cast your mind back to the last time you went to the fair, or an amusement park.

Did you want to ride the rollercoaster or the gentle merry-go-round?

One ride looks exciting, dangerous, enthralling, fun. Whilst the other is safe, slow, comfortable, sedate. **Boring!!**

Life is just like a rollercoaster.

There are plenty of ups and copious downs.

There's loads of queueing, it's never as good as you imagine it'll be, it sometimes makes you sick, it can be scary, it's full of idiots, it's over far too quickly and it costs too much.

But it can be so much fun whilst it lasts.

Open your eyes, embrace the thrills, buckle up and **enjoy the ride!!**

All the best and luk afta thissen!!

Ding!! Ding!!

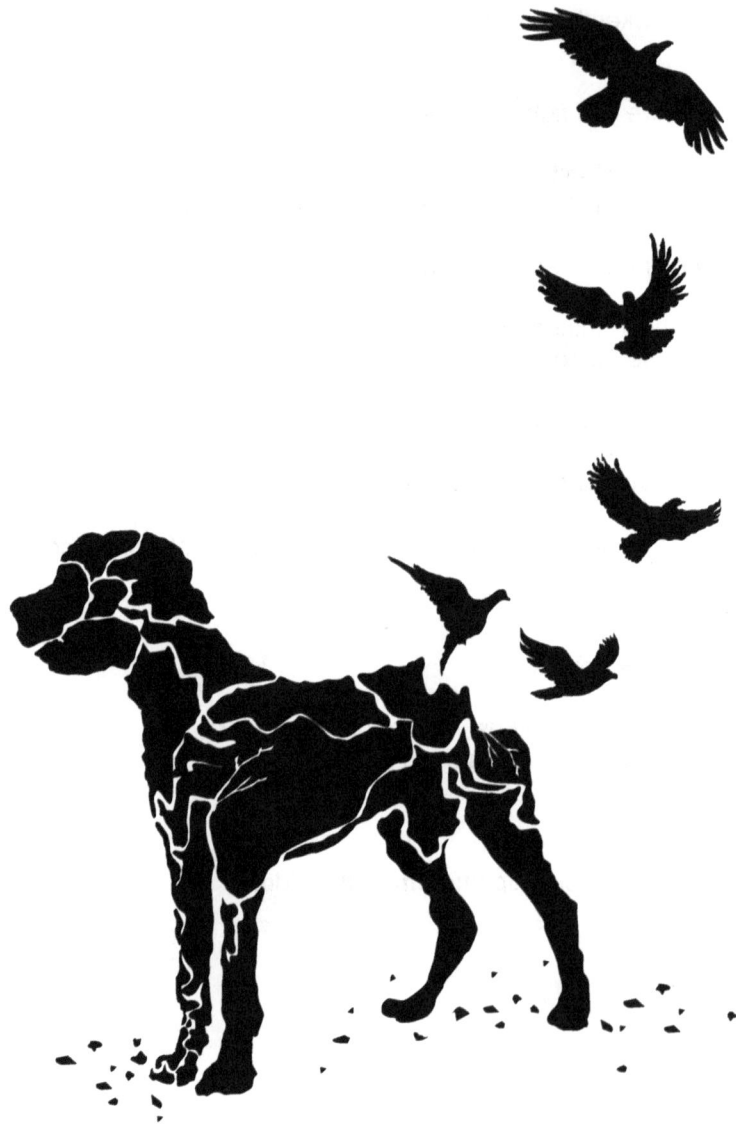

www.ingramcontent.com/pod-product-compliance
Lightning Source LLC
Chambersburg PA
CBHW080618030426
42336CB00018B/3009